Vascular-targeted Therapies in Oncology

Vascular-targeted Therapies in Oncology

Editor

Dietmar W. Siemann

Shands Cancer Center, University of Florida
Gainsville, Florida, USA

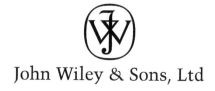

John Wiley & Sons, Ltd

Contents

Preface

Cancer has been described in the history of medicine ever since records were kept. Today it remains a major health problem worldwide. Indeed its global burden continues to increase.

Over the past few decades great strides have been made in our fundamental understanding of the causes of cancer as well as the molecular underpinnings of this disease. Research and innovative technology developments have greatly aided our ability to detect cancer at its earliest stages when it is most manageable. Insights into cellular signaling pathways have led to the pursuit of novel anticancer drugs that hold the potential of greater tumor specificity with reduced treatment side effects.

For the patient facing this disease in the year 2006, surgery, radiation therapy and chemotherapy remain the principal options. However, unlike in the past, the treatment of many advanced cancer patients nowadays involves the integration of these modes of therapy into definitive treatment strategies. This evolution in cancer therapy is largely a reflection of the clinical trial process. Indeed multi-modality therapy delivered in cancer centers by experts in these specialties is rapidly becoming the norm in cancer management.

Still, too often the cancer treatment is not curative. Additional treatment strategies are clearly needed. A variety of approaches to enhance tumor responses are under active investigation. One of these is the focus of this book – the pursuit of targeting the tumor blood vessel network. The tumor vasculature offers an attractive target for cancer therapy as it is a critical participant in cancer development, tumor growth and metastasis. Given its pivotal role, the vasculature may prove to be a tumor's most exploitable Achilles heel.

This book encompasses the past, present, and future of vascular targeting therapies. It is about what we have learned and what the future may hold. Most of all it is about endeavors to seek better treatments for cancer patients.

I feel privileged to have collaborated on this text with such an outstanding group of co-authors. To them I owe a debt of gratitude. Without their efforts and dedication this book would not have materialized. It has been a pleasure working with these colleagues. I thank them for their willingness to participate in this project, timely contributions, integrity and, most of all, their friendship. The quality of the book reflects their efforts and is to their credit.

I also would like to thank the staff at Wiley & Sons, especially Joan Marsh and Andrea Baier, who have worked diligently at bringing this book to fruition. Their assistance in matters ranging from the mundane to the complex has been untiring, invaluable and much appreciated.

Finally I would like to dedicate this book to my parents who, though no longer with us, are not forgotten.

It's the journey – not the goal.

Dietmar W. Siemann
Gainesville

List of Contributors

G-One Ahn Division of Radiation and Cancer Biology, Department of Radiation Oncology, Stanford University School of Medicine, CCSR – South, Room 1255, 269 Campus Drive, Stanford, CA 94305-5152, USA

Bruce C. Baguley Department of Molecular Medicine and Pathology and Auckland Cancer Society Research Centre, The University of Auckland, Private Bag 92019, Auckland, New Zealand

Adam W. Beck 5323 Harry Hines Boulevard, MC 8593, Dallas, TX 75390, USA

Orest W. Blaschuk Urology Research Laboratories, Room H6.15, Royal Victoria Hospital, 687 Pine Avenue West, Montreal, Quebec H3A 1A1, Canada

Rolf A. Brekken Departments of Surgery and Pharmacology, Hamon Center for Thearpeutic Oncology Research UT, Southwestern Medical Center, NB8.218a, 6000 Harry Hines Boulevard, Dallas, TX 75390-8593, USA

J. Martin Brown Division of Radiation and Cancer Biology, Department of Radiation Oncology, Stanford University School of Medicine, CCSR – South, Room 1255, 269 Campus Drive, Standford, CA 94305-5152, USA

David J. Chaplin Research and Development, Oxigene Inc., 230 3rd Avenue, Waltham, MA 02451, USA

Peter D. Davis Angiogene Pharmaceuticals Ltd., The Magdalen Centre, The Oxford Science Park, Oxfordshire OX9 5SX, UK

Graeme J. Dougherty Department of Radiation Oncology, Arizona Cancer Center, 1501 North Campbell Avenue, P.O. Box 245081, Tucson, AZ 85724-5081, USA

Shona T. Dougherty Department of Radiation Oncology, Arizona Cancer Center, 1501 North Campbell Avenue, P.O. Box 245081, Tucson, AZ 85724-5081, USA

Lee M. Ellis   Department of Surgical Oncology, The University of Texas, MD Anderson Cancer Center, 1400 Holcombe Boulevard, FC12.3056, P.O. Box 301402, Houston, TX 77230-1402, USA

Susan M. Galbraith   Bristol-Myers Squibb, Clinical Discovery – Oncology, Pharmaceutical Research Institute, P.O. Box 4000, Princeton, NJ 08543-4000, USA

Andrew M. Gaya   Department of Medical Oncology, The Clocktower, Mount Vernon Cancer Centre, Rickmansworth Road, Northwood, Middlesex HA6 2RN, UK

Sally A. Hill   Gray Cancer Institute, Mount Vernon Hospital, Northwood, Middlesex HA6 2JR, UK

Michael R. Horsman   Department of Experimental Clinical Oncology, Aarhus University Hospital, Noerrebrogade 44, Building 5, 8000 Aarhus C, Denmark

Claire E. Lewis   Section of Oncology and Pathology, Division of Genomic Medicine, University of Sheffield Medical School, Beech Hill Road, Sheffield S10 2RX, UK

Uwe Michaelis   MediGene AG, Lochhammer Strasse 11, D-82152 Planegg/Martinsried, Germany

Rumi Murata   Department of Biophysics, Institute for Cancer Research, The Norwegian Radium Hospital Montebello, 0310 Olso, Norway

Kevin G. Pinney   Department of Chemistry and Biochemistry, The Center for Drug Discovery, Baylor University, One Bear Place #97348, Waco, TX 76798-7348, USA

Joseph C. Randall   Preclinical Research, OXiGENE, Inc., 230 3rd Avenue, Waltham, MA 02451, USA

Amyn M. Rojiani   Department of Oncology and Pathology, H. Lee Moffit Cancer Center and Research Institute, University of South Florida, 12901 Bruce B. Downs Boulevard, MDC 11, Tampa, FL 33612, USA

Mumtaz V. Rojiani   Department of Pathology, University of South Florida, 12901 Bruce B. Downs Boulevard, Tampa, FL 33612, USA

Tracey M. Rowlands   Adherex Technologies Inc., Research Triangle Park, Durham, NC 27713, USA

Gordon Rustin   Department of Medical Oncology, The Clocktower, Mount Vernon Cancer Centre, Richmansworth Road, Northwood, Middlesex HA6 2RN, UK

Wenyin Shi   Department of Radiation Oncology, University of Florida, Shands Cancer Center, Gainsville, FL 32610, USA

Dietmar W. Siemann Research Department of Radiation Oncology, University of Florida, 2000 RW Archer Road, Gainsville, FL 32610, USA

Bronwyn G. Siim Department of Molecular Medicine and Pathology and Auckland Cancer Society Research Centre, The University of Auckland, Private Bag 92019, 85 Park Road, Grafton, Auckland, New Zealand

Carolyn A. Staton Academic Unit of Surgical Oncology, Division of Clinical Sciences (South), K Floor, Royal Hallamshire Hospital, Glossop Road, Sheffield S10 2JF, UK

Oliver Stoeltzing Departments of Surgery and Experimental Surgery, University of Regensburg, Franz-Josef Strauss Allee 11, 93053 Regensburg, Germany

Michael Teifel Zentaris GmbH, Drug Discovery – Pharmacology and Toxicology, Weismüllerstrasse 45, D-60314 Frankfurt/Main, Germany

Philip E. Thorpe Department of Pharmacology, University of Texas, Southwestern Medical Center, 2201 Inwood Road, NC7.304, Dallas, TX 75390-8594, USA

Peter Vaupel Institute of Physiology and Pathophysiology, University of Mainz, Düsbergweg 6, 55099 Mainz, Germany

Scott L. Young Clinical Affairs, OXiGENE, Inc., 230 3rd Avenue, Waltham, MA 02451, USA

1

Tumor Vasculature: a Target for Anticancer Therapies

Dietmar W. Siemann

1.1 Introduction

Historically, approaches to improve cancer therapy have focused primarily on achieving increased tumor cell kill. Recently however another treatment approach has garnered considerable attention. Rather than targeting the neoplastic cell population directly, this strategy endeavors to impair the tumor's nutritional support system by target the tumor blood vessel network. Vascular targeting approaches are based on the recognition that a continuously expanding vasculature is an essential requirement for tumor initiation, progression and metastasis. Indeed it is generally well accepted that most tumors remain dormant and fail to develop beyond a few millimeters in size in the absence of angiogenic growth. The therapeutic potential of targeting the tumor vasculature is therefore abundantly clear. As a consequence the field of vascular targeting has expanded rapidly and led to a large number of investigational drugs, many of which have now begun to undergo clinical evaluation. These agents are quite distinct from conventional anticancer treatments such as radiation therapy and cytotoxic drugs. Indeed the application of vascular targeting strategies as adjuvants to standard therapeutic modalities may offers unique opportunities to develop even more effective cancer therapies.

1.2 Tumor vasculature

Solid tumors require a functioning vasculature for the delivery of nutrients and the removal of toxic waste products associated with cellular metabolism. Such a vascular network can be acquired by the tumor at least in part, by the incor-

---

Vascular-targeted Therapies in Oncology Edited by Dietmar W. Siemann
© 2006 John Wiley & Sons, Ltd.

poration of existing host blood vessels. Yet ultimately tumor expansion requires the formation of new blood vessels. Thus tumor growth and survival are critically linked to a parallel proliferation of endothelial cells comprising the tumor blood vessel network. The process involved, neovascularization, is relatively uncommon in most normal tissues, but now recognized to be an important feature of solid tumors (Ausprunk and Folkman, 1977; Folkman, 1986; Hahnfeldt *et al.*, 1999). However, neovascularization invariably lags behind the aggressively expanding tumor mass (Tannock, 1970), resulting in a tumor vasculature that is morphologically and functionally abnormal and differs greatly from that found in most normal adult tissues (Schweigerer, 1995; Konerding, Miodonski and Lametschwandtner, 1995; Konerding *et al.*, 2002). It is primitive in nature, highly abnormal and chaotic. Common features of vessels comprising the tumor microcirculation are dilated and elongated shapes, blind ends, bulges and leaky sprouts, abrupt changes in diameter, extensive tortuosity and evidence of vascular compression. It is this abnormal nature of the tumor vasculature that not only gives rise to the physiologic characteristics associated with treatment failures but also offers the opportunity for novel therapeutic targeting approaches.

1.3   Impact of tumor microenvironments on cancer management

Tumor vasculature is typically characterized by dilated vessels, large intercapillary distances and accompanying decreases in vessel density. Because the vessel network that is formed in tumors is typically unable to keep pace with the rapidly growing tumor cell mass, it inevitably fails to meet the nutritional needs of the tumor cells. Indeed, the blood flow associated with this heterogeneous vasculature is often irregular, sluggish and intermittent (Vaupel, Kallinowski and Okunieff, 1989). The resultant areas of hypoxia and acidosis are common features of solid neoplasia that have been well documented (Vaupel, Thews and Hoeckel, 1996). Cells that exist in such adverse micro-environmental conditions can appreciably alter the tumor response to cytotoxic anticancer treatments. Indeed, it is now established that the presence of oxygen-deficient or hypoxic cells can not only lead to therapeutic resistance in preclinical tumor models but also have a detrimental effect on the ability to control human malignancies treated with curative intent (Hoeckel *et al.*, 1993; Nordsmark, Overgaard and Overgaard 1996; Brizel *et al.*, 1999, Brown and Giaccia, 1998; Horsman and Overgaard, 2002). Importantly, physiological pressures exerted by the tumor microenvironments also contribute to processes that favor malignant progression (Young, Marshall and Hill, 1988; Hill, 1990; Giaccia, 1996), oncogenesis (Giaccia, 1996; Graeber *et al.*, 1996) and potential for metastatic spread (Young, Marshall and Hill, 1988; Hill, 1990; De Jaeger, Kavanagh and Hill, 2001; Brizel *et al.*, 1996).

1.4 Vascular-targeting therapies

Tumor endothelium represents a key target for cancer therapy. Given its pivotal role in tumor survival, progression and spread, factors known to contribute significantly to treatment failures, agents capable of targeting tumor blood vessels have been actively pursued (Folkman and Shing, 1992; Arap, Pasqualini and Ruoslahti, 1998; Ruoslahti, 2002; Ellis *et al.*, 2001; Kerbel, 2000). Indeed it is now well recognized that strategies directed against the tumor blood vessel network may offer not only unique therapeutic opportunities in their own right but also novel means of enhancing the efficacies of conventional anticancer treatments.

Vascular-targeting therapies that endeavor to take advantage of unique features of the microvessel networks in tumors fall into two general categories based on whether they interfere with new blood vessel development or damage the established tumor vasculature (Thorpe, 2004; Ellis *et al.*, 2001; Bloemendal, Logtenberg and Voest, 1999; Siemann, Chaplin and Horsman, 2004). The first aims to inhibit the tumor-initiated angiogenic process itself. *Angiogenesis inhibitors (AIs)* seek to interrupt essential aspects of angiogenesis, most notably signaling between tumor, endothelial and stromal cells, as well as endothelial cell function in order to prevent new blood vessel formation. Strategies that have been tested include the use of drugs that interfere with the delivery or export of angiogenic stimuli, antibodies to inhibit or inactivate angiogenic factors after their release, drugs that inhibit receptor action, inhibitors of invasion and agents that inhibit endothelial cell proliferation (Scott and Harris, 1994; O'Reilly *et al.*, 1997; Schweigerer, 1995; Kerbel, 2000; Twardowski and Gradishar, 1997; Strohmeyer, 1999). Many of these agents are currently undergoing clinical evaluation. An alternative approach involves the application of therapeutics seeking the preferential destruction of the established tumor vessel network. These *vascular-disrupting agents (VDAs)* aim to cause a rapid and selective vascular shutdown in tumors, which produces secondary tumor cell death due to ischemia (Chaplin, Pettit and Hill, 1999; Chaplin and Dougherty, 1999; Blakey *et al.*, 2002; Baguley and Ching, 2002; Thorpe, 2004; Siemann, Chaplin and Horsman, 2004). VDAs can be divided into two main classes: (i) the biologics that utilize antibodies and peptides to deliver toxins and effector molecules to tumor endothelial cells and (ii) the small molecules that exploit the differences between tumor and normal tissue endothelium to induce selective vascular dysfunction (Thorpe, 2004; Siemann, Chaplin and Horsman, 2004).

Although both AIs and VDAs target the tumor vasculature, it is important to recognize that key differences between agents that affect angiogenesis and those that lead to selective vascular destruction exist (Siemann *et al.*, 2005). These differences apply not only in their mode of action but also in their likely therapeutic application (Figure 1.1). Briefly, the objective of antiangiogenic therapies is to interfere with new vessel formation, thereby preventing tumor growth and limiting metastatic potential. Consequently, antiangiogenic therapies are

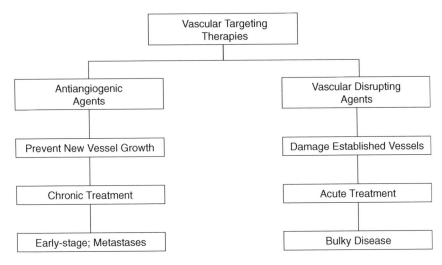

Figure 1.1 Taxonomy of vascular targeting therapies. Redrawn from Siemann *et al.* (2005) with permission

typically administered chronically over months and years. VDAs compromise established tumor vasculature and have the potential to destroy tumor masses as well as preventing progression. Such agents are designed to be used in an intermittent fashion rather than by means of long-term exposures. Given these differences, it should be clear from a therapeutic perspective that targeting the tumor vasculature with AIs and VDAs is complimentary and not redundant.

1.5   Combinations with conventional anticancer therapies

Lead agents in both categories of vascular targeting agents have now advanced into clinical trials. Yet it is in their combination, either with each other or with conventional anticancer therapies, that they will likely find their greatest utility. There are two primary reasons for this. The first is that combining vascular targeting strategies with conventional anticancer therapies may improve treatment outcomes by capitalizing on principles of enhanced antitumor efficacy, non-overlapping toxicities or spatial cooperation (Steel and Peckham, 1979). While there exists a multitude of factors associated with the clinical failures of radiation therapy and chemotherapy, abnormal tumor microenvironments, tumor progression and metastatic spread of neoplastic cells are believed to be major contributors (DeVita, Hellman and Rosenberg, 1997). Since all of these resistance factors may be affected by angiosuppressive or vascular damaging treatments, the combinations of such approaches with radiotherapy or chemotherapy are likely to improve treatment outcomes. The second reason that such combined modality approaches may have merit is that the full clinical potential of AI- and VDA-based therapies may not be realized unless they are combined with other treatments. This is because achieving tumor cures in patients with either AIs or VDAs alone is likely to be extremely difficult. In the case of the former, the complexity of pathways available for neovascularization implies that disrupting only a single aspect of angiogenesis probably will not suffice (Ellis *et al.*, 2000; Fidler and Ellis, 1994). Indeed, the greatest benefit from AIs may lie in their ability to control tumor growth. VDAs also may be best utilized as adjuvants to conventional anticancer therapies since by the very nature of their highly selective mechanism of damaging tumor blood vessels they are not able to eliminate those pockets of tumor cells whose nutritional supply is derived from blood vessels in the surrounding normal tissue agents (Siemann, Chaplin and Horsman, 2004). In light of these considerations, and given the frequent use of radiation therapy and chemotherapy in the clinical management of cancer, the continued examination of strategies combining such conventional treatment modalities with strategies directed against the tumor vessel network are certainly warranted.

1.6 Combinations of antiangiogenic and vascular-disrupting agents

Given their disparate modes of action, the combined application of AIs and VDAs is likely to lead to complementary antitumor effects. Since both the initiation of new vessel formation and the integrity of the existing blood vessel network are critical to a tumor's growth and survival, such a double assault on the tumor vasculature would appear to be a very logical approach. This possibility has been examined experimentally in studies combining a selective inhibitor of VEGFR2 associated tyrosine kinase with a microtubulin disrupting VDA (Wedge *et al.*, 2002; Siemann and Shi, 2004). The results showed that such a combination therapy could significantly enhance the tumor response beyond that achieved with either vascular targeting therapy alone. A likely explanation for these observations is that while the VDA significantly reduced the viable tumor mass, the AI impaired subsequent tumor regrowth by interfering with the re-establishment of tumor vasculature. In light of the apparent success of this treatment strategy, combinations of other agents seeking to exploit the approach of dual targeting of the tumor vasculature are currently under active investigation.

1.7 Conclusions

The concept that attacking a tumor's supportive blood vessel network could offer a means of improving cancer cure rates has received a great deal of attention in recent years. A variety of potential targets have been identified and

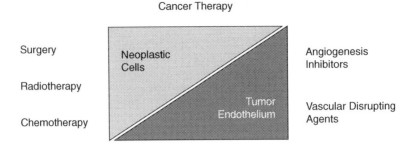

Figure 1.2 Schematic diagram of possible future anticancer therapies incorporating vascular targeting strategies into the current principal modes of neoplastic cell treatments

preclinical studies have shown that compromising the tumor vasculature can indeed lead to favorable tumor responses at low toxicity. Importantly, combining VTAs with radiation and chemotherapy has demonstrated that treatment outcomes of conventional anticancer therapies can be improved by the inclusion of such agents. Whether or not these data can be extrapolated to cancer patients remains to be established in clinical trials. Still, the experimental studies themselves have raised many additional fascinating questions concerning possible future applications of vascular targeting treatment strategies. Given their possible future clinical impact, the continued pursuit of agents exhibiting the ability to affect the growth and survival of tumors by targeting their endothelium is clearly warranted. Perhaps it is not too much to imagine that future definitive treatment for advanced cancer patients (Figure 1.2) might not only involve the integration of surgery, radiation therapy and chemotherapy, but encompass vascular targeting approaches as well.

Acknowledgments

Work from the author's laboratory referred to in this article was supported in part by Grants RO1 CA84408 and RO1 CA89655 from the National Institutes of Health.

References

Arap, W., Pasqualini, R. and Ruoslahti, E. (1998). Cancer treatment by targeted drug delivery to tumor vasculature in a mouse model. *Science* **279**, 377–380.

Ausprunk, D. and Folkman, J. (1977). Migration and proliferation of endothelial cells in preformed and newly formed blood vessels during tumor angiogenesis. *Microvasc Res* **14**, 53–65.

Baguley, B.C. and Ching, L.M. (2002). DMXAA: an antivascular agent with multiple host responses. *Int J Radiat Oncol Biol Phys* **54**, 1503–1511.

Blakey, D.C., Westwood, F.R., Walker, M., Hughes, G.D., Davis, P.D., Ashton, S.E. and Ryan, A.J. (2002). Antitumor activity of the novel vascular targeting agent ZD6126 in a panel of tumor models. *Clin Cancer Res* **8**, 1974–1983.

Bloemendal, H.J., Logtenberg, T. and Voest, E.E. (1999). New strategies in anti-vascular cancer therapy. *Eur J Clin Invest* **29**, 802–809.

Brizel, D.M., Dodge, R.K., Clough, R.W. and Dewhirst, M.W. (1999). Oxygenation of head and neck cancer: changes during radiotherapy and impact on treatment outcome. *Radiother Oncol* **53**, 113–117.

Brizel, D.M., Scully, S.P., Harrelson, J.M., Layfield, L.J., Bean, J.M., Prosnitz, L.R. and Dewhirst, M.W. (1996). Tumor oxygenation predicts for the likelihood of distant metastases in human soft tissue sarcoma. *Cancer Res* **56**, 941–943.

Brown, J.M. and Giaccia, A.J. (1998). The unique physiology of solid tumors: opportunities (and problems) for cancer therapy. *Cancer Res* **58**, 1408–1416.

Chaplin, D.J. and Dougherty, G.J. (1999). Tumour vasculature as a target for cancer therapy. *Br J Cancer* **80**, 57–64.

Chaplin, D.J., Pettit, G.R. and Hill, S.A. (1999). Anti-vascular approaches to solid tumour therapy: evaluation of combretastatin A4 phosphate. *Anticancer Res* **19**, 189–195.

De Jaeger, K., Kavanagh, M.C. and Hill, R.P. (2001). Relationship of hypoxia to metastatic ability in rodent tumours. *Br J Cancer* **84**, 1280–1285.

DeVita, V.T., Hellman, S. and Rosenberg, S. (1997). *Cancer: Principles and Practice of Oncology.* Lippincott-Raven, Philadelphia, PA.

Ellis, L.M., Liu, W., Ahmad, S.A., Fan, F., Jung, Y.D., Shaheen, R.M. and Reinmuth, N. (2001). Overview of angiogenesis: biologic implications for antiangiogenic therapy. *Semin Oncol* **28**, 94–104.

Ellis, L.M., Takahashi, Y., Liu, W. and Shaheen, R.M. (2000). Vascular endothelial growth factor in human colon cancer: biology and therapeutic implications. *Oncologist* **5** (Suppl. 1), 11–15.

Fidler, I.J. and Ellis, L.M. (1994). The implications of angiogenesis for the biology and therapy of cancer metastasis. *Cell* **79**, 185–188.

Folkman, J. (1986). How is blood vessel growth regulated in normal and neoplastic tissue? *Cancer Res* **46**, 467–473.

Folkman, J. and Shing, Y. (1992). Angiogenesis. *J Biol Chem* **267**, 10931–10934.

Giaccia, A.J. (1996). Hypoxic stress proteins: survival of the fittest. *Semin Radiat Oncol* **6**, 46–58.

Graeber, T., Osmanian, C., Jacks, T., Housman, D., Koch, C.J., Lowe, S. and Giaccia, A.J. (1996). Hypoxia-mediated selection of cells with diminished apoptotic potential in solid tumors. *Nature* **379**, 88–91.

Hahnfeldt, P., Panigrahy, D., Folkman, J. and Hlatky, L. (1999). Tumor development under angiogenic signaling: a dynamical theory of tumor growth, treatment response, and post-vascular dormancy. *Cancer Res* **59**, 4770–4775.

Hill, R.P. (1990). Tumor progression: potential role of unstable genomic changes. *Cancer and Metastasis Reviews* **9**, 137–147.

Hoeckel, M., Knoop, C., Schlenger, K., Vorndran, B., Baussman, E., Mitze, M., Knapstein, P.G. and Vaupel, P. (1993). Intratumoral pO_2 predicts survival in advanced cancer of the uterine cervix. *Radiother Oncol* **26**, 45–50.

Horsman, M.R. and Overgaard, J. (2002). The oxygen effect and the tumour microenvironment. In *Basic Clinical Radiobiology for Radiation Oncologists*, G.G. Steel (ed.). Arnold, London, pp. 158–168.

Kerbel, R.S. (2000). Tumor angiogenesis: past, present and the near future. *Carcinogenesis* **21**, 505–515.

Konerding, M.A., Miodonski, A.J. and Lametschwandtner, A. (1995). Microvascular corrosion casting in the study of tumor vascularity: a review. *Scanning Microsc* **9**, 1233–1244.

Konerding, M.A., van Ackern, C., Fait, E., Steinberg, F. and Streffer, C. (2002). Morphological aspects of tumor angiogenesis and microcirculation. In *Blood Perfusion and Microenvironment of Human Tumors*, M. Molls and P. Vaupel (eds). Springer, Berlin, pp. 5–17.

Nordsmark, M., Overgaard, M. and Overgaard, J. (1996). Pretreatment oxygenation predicts radiation response in advanced squamous cell carcinioma of the head and neck. *Radiother Oncol* **41**, 31–39.

O'Reilly, M.S., Boehm, T., Shing, Y., Fukai, N., Vasios, G., Lane, W.S., Flynn, E., Birkhead, J.R., Olsen, B.R. and Folkman, J. (1997). Endostatin: an endogenous inhibitor of angiogenesis and tumor growth. *Cell* **88**, 277–285.

Ruoslahti, E. (2002). Specialization of tumour vasculature. *Nat Rev Cancer* **2**, 83–90.

Schweigerer, L. (1995). Antiangiogenesis as a novel therapeutic concept in pediatric oncology. *J Mol Med* **73**, 497–508.

Scott, P. and Harris, A.L. (1994). Current approaches to targeting cancer using antiangiogenesis therapies. *Cancer Treat Rev* **20**, 393–412.

Siemann, D.W., Bibby, M.C., Dark, G.G., Dicker, A.P., Eskens, F.A.L.M., Horsman, M.R., Marme, D. and LoRusso, P.M. (2005). Differentiation and definition of vascular-targeted therapies. *Clin Cancer Res* **11**, 416–420.

Siemann, D.W., Chaplin, D.J. and Horsman, M.R. (2004). Vascular-targeting therapies for treatment of malignant disease. *Cancer* **100**, 2491–2499.

Siemann, D.W. and Shi, W. (2004). Efficacy of combined antiangiogenic and vascular disrupting agents in treatment of solid tumors. *Int J Radiat Oncol Biol Phys* **60**, 1233–1240.

Steel, G.G. and Peckham, M.J. (1979). Exploitable mechanisms in combined radiotherapy–chemotherapy: the concept of additivity. *Int J Radiat Oncol Biol Phys* **5**, 85–91.

Strohmeyer, D. (1999). Pathophysiology of tumor angiogenesis and its relevance in renal cell cancer. *Anticancer Res* **19**, 1557–1561.

Tannock, I.F. (1970). Population kinetics of carcinoma cells, capillary endothelial cells, and fibroblasts in a transplanted mouse mammary tumor. *Cancer Res* **30**, 2470–2477.

Thorpe, P.E. (2004). Vascular targeting agents as cancer therapeutics. *Clin Cancer Res* **10**, 415–427.

Twardowski, P. and Gradishar, W.J. (1997). Clinical trials of antiangiogenic agents. *Curr Opin Oncol* **9**, 584–589.

Vaupel, P., Kallinowski, F. and Okunieff, P. (1989). Blood flow, oxygen and nutrient supply, and metabolic microenvironment of human tumors: a review. *Cancer Res* **49**, 6449–6465.

Vaupel, P., Thews, O. and Hoeckel, M. (1996). Tumor oxygenation: characterization and clinical implications. In *rhErythropoietin in Cancer Supportive Treatment*, J.F. Smyth, M.A. Boogaerts and B.R. Ehmer (eds). Dekker, pp. 205–239.

Wedge, S.R., Kendrew, J., Ogilvie, D.J., Hennequin, L.F., Brave, A.J., Ryan, A.J., Ashton, S.E., Calvete, J.A. and Blakey, D.C. (2002). Combination of the VEGF receptor tyrosine kinase inhibitor ZD6474 and vascular-targeting agent ZD6126 produces an enhanced anti-tumor response. *Proc Am Assoc Cancer Res.* **43**, 1081 [abstract].

Young, S.D., Marshall, R.S. and Hill, R.P. (1988). Hypoxia induces DNA overreplication and enhances metastatic potential of murine tumor cells. *Proc Natl Acad Sci* **85**, 9533–9537.

2

Abnormal Microvasculature and Defective Microcirculatory Function in Solid Tumors

Peter Vaupel

Abstract

Newly formed microvessels in most solid tumors do not conform to the normal morphology and function of the host tissue vascularity. Blood vessel formation and tumor vasculature can thus be described as a pathophysiologic system that is maximally stimulated, yet only minimally fulfilling the metabolic needs of the rapidly growing tumor mass. This leads to (i) a spatial and temporal heterogeneity in tumor blood flow, and (ii) a metabolic micromilieu uniquely different to that of normal tissues. It is characterized by O_2 depletion (hypoxia and anoxia), extracellular acidosis, hypercapnia, bicarbonate deprivation, excessive lactate levels, glucose depletion, energy impoverishment, expansion of the interstitial space, interstitial hypertension and interstitial fluid flow. These "hostile" parameters which are heterogeneously distributed within the tumor mass – both spatially and temporally – may be (directly or indirectly) responsible for selection of aggressive cells, tumor progression and acquired treatment resistance.

Keywords

Angiogenesis, tumor microvasculature, tumor microcirculation, tumor blood flow, microenvironment, hypoxia, acidosis, lactate accumulation

2.1 Introduction

Most, if not all, solid tumors begin as avascular aggregates of malignant cells. 'Microscopic tumors' exchange nutrients and catabolites with their surroundings by simple diffusion (Brem *et al.*, 1976; Vaupel, Kallinowski and

Vascular-targeted Therapies in Oncology   Edited by Dietmar W. Siemann
© 2006 John Wiley & Sons, Ltd.

Okunieff, 1989; Vaupel, 1994). The growth of an avascular three-dimensional aggregate of tumor cells is therefore self-limiting (up to 1–2 mm in diameter). Rapid tumor growth, tumor progression, invasion, local spread and distant metastasis to other organs or tissues following the avascular growth period are possible only if convective transport (nutrient supply and waste removal) is initiated through nutritive blood flow, i.e. flow through tumor microvessels that guarantees adequate exchange processes between the microcirculatory bed and the cancer cells. This notion has led to the dogmatic assumption that both tumor growth and tumor spread are dependent on rigorous angiogenesis (for a review see Sivridis, Giatromanolaki and Koukourakis, 2003). This implicates that vascularization is a prerequisite for tumor growth. However, at the same time, tumor vasculature can also be an 'Achilles heel', a condition that is discussed in this chapter.

2.2 Basic principles of blood vessel formation in tumors

When considering the continuous and indiscriminate formation of a vascular network in rapidly growing tumors, five different mechanisms have to be considered (Carmeliet and Jain, 2000; Ribatti, Vacca and Dammacco, 2003; Vaupel, 2004):

- angiogenesis by endothelial sprouting from pre-existing venules,

- vascular co-option,

- vasculogenesis,

- intussusception and

- vascular mimicry.

Angiogenesis

The avascular (= prevascular) growth phase characteristic of a 'dormant' tumor and the vascular phase, in which 'explosive' growth ensues, in many solid tumors are separated by the 'angiogenic switch'. This switch is 'off' when the effect of pro-angiogenic molecules is balanced by that of anti-angiogenic molecular players. It is 'on' when the net balance is tipped in favor of angiogenesis (Hanahan and Weinberg, 2000). Pro- and anti-angiogenic molecules can be released from cancer cells, endothelial cells (ECs), stromal and inflammatory cells or can be mobilized from the extracelular matrix (Carmeliet and Jain, 2000; Ribatti, Vacca and Dammacco, 2003). The 'angiogenic switch', a pivotal and early event in tumor progression, greatly depends on one or more positive regulators such as growth factors, permeability regulating factors, migration stimulators, proteolytic enzymes (balanced with their inhibitors), extracellular matrix molecules and adhesion molecules (see Table 2.1). *Vascular-specific growth factors* include vascular endothelial growth factors (VEGFs) and their receptors, the angiopoietin family (Ang) and Tie receptors and the ephrins. *Non-specific factors* comprise platelet-derived growth factor (PDGF), fibroblast growth factors (FGFs), transforming growth factor-β (TGF-β), tumor necrosis factor-α (TNF-α), epidermal growth factor (EGF) and several others.

A central inducer of growth of new blood vessels is VEGF (originally identified as vascular permeability factor, VPF). Expression of VEGF is regulated by hypoxia (Semenza, 2000; Pugh and Ratcliffe, 2003), hypoglycemia (Shweiki *et al.*, 1995), acidosis (Carmeliet and Jain, 2000), activation of oncogenes or deletion of tumor-suppressor genes that control production of angiogenesis regulators (Kerbel, 2000), cytokines and hormones (M. Neeman, personal communication).

The process of angiogenesis is extremely complex and requires balanced interactions with biologic redundancy. Major steps in the 'angiogenic cascade' include (besides the 'angiogenic switch' and upregulation of pro-angiogenic molecules, binding of the latter to specific endothelial cell receptors and ligand–receptor interaction):

Table 2.1 Angiogenic proteins regulating tumor angiogenesis and major actions of these growth factors (selection)*

Factors	Major actions
A. Specific factors	
VEGF	increases vascular permeability, promotes proliferation and EC migration, upregulates proteases for matrix degeneration, inhibits EC apoptosis, stabilizes vessels
Ang-1	stabilizes endothelium, suppresses EC apoptosis, promotes vessel maturation and vascular hierarchy, stimulates sprout and lumen formation, inhibits hyperpermeability
Ang-2	antagonizes Ang-1 signaling, destabilizes endothelium, promotes endothelial sprouting
Ephrins	guide vessel branching, determine EC specialization
B. Non-specific factors	
PDGF	promotes EC proliferation and migration, stimulates pericyte and smooth muscle cell recruitment, stimulates DNA synthesis in ECs
FGFs	stimulate proliferation and migration of ECs, promote EC tube formation, induce and synergize VEGF
TGF-β	regulates proliferation and migration of ECs, regulates vessel maturation, stimulates production of extravascular matrix
TNF-α	stimulates angiogenesis and tube formation
EGF	stimulates EC proliferation

* Adapted from Yancopoulos *et al.*, 2000; Papetti & Herman, 2002.

- dilation of existing vessels,

- EC activation,

- hyperpermeability of postcapillary venules and vessel destabilization,

- localized degradation of basement membrane,

- matrix remodelling (degradation of extracellular matrix in response to activation of matrix metalloproteinases, formation of a new provisional extravascular matrix by leaked plasma proteins),

- migration of ECs,

- cell–cell contacts, sprout formation,

- extension of sprouts by EC proliferation,

- tube formation, fusion to form vascular loops,

- (non-mandatory) recruitment of pericytes and smooth muscle cells and

- (improper) vessel maturation.

These different steps are partly concurrent, partly in series and sequential. They occurr in different parts of primary tumors and in metastases at the same time.

Vascular co-option

Tumor cells often appear to co-opt vessels; i.e., they can incorporate pre-existing vessels within a vascularized host tissue to initiate vessel-dependent tumor growth as opposed to classic angiogenesis (Ribatti, Vacca and Dammacco, 2003). Later in the co-opted vessels ECs release angiopoietin-2 (probably by autocrine action), which leads to vascular destabilization and vascular collapse. The resultant hypoxia and nutrient deprivation then yield an upregulation of VEGF and 'secondary' angiogenesis (Ellis *et al.*, 2001).

Vasculogenesis

For vasculogenesis, *de novo* vessel formation through incorporation of circulating endothelial precursor cells (angioblasts) from bone marrow or peripheral blood is mandatory.

Intussusception

In intussusception, interstitial tissue columns insert into the lumen of pre-existing vessels and lead to partition of the initial vessel lumen (Patan, Munn and Jain, 1996).

Vascular mimicry

In central areas of melanomas *de novo* generation of blood channels without the participation of endothelial cells has been described. A contribution of cancer cells to the wall of tumor vessels has also been reported for tumor entities other then melanomas (Ruoslahti, 2002; Ribatti, Vacca and Dammacco, 2003). The concept of vascular mimicry is still however being discussed as controversial (McDonald, Munn and Jain, 2000).

2.3 Tumor lymphangiogenesis

Although the metastatic spread of tumor cells to regional lymph nodes is a common feature of many human cancers, it is not clear whether shedding tumor cells utilize existing lymphatic vessels or whether tumor dissemination requires *de novo* formation of lymphatics (Ribatti, Vacca and Dammacco, 2003). The notion that tumor microcirculation may be supported by a newly formed, tumor-induced lymphatic network has so far not been convincingly confirmed. VEGF-C, VEGF-D and their corresponding receptors have been identified as specific lymphangiogenic factors in several tumors (Jussila and Alitalo, 2002; Ribatti, Vacca and Dammacco, 2003). It has been proposed that functional lymphatics in the tumor margin are sufficient for lymphatic metastasis, because the tumor center was found to contain no functional lymphatics (Padera *et al.*, 2002). The intratumoral lymphatic vessels are usually collapsed (compressed) due to the high interstitial pressure caused by the growing tumor mass in a confined space. In the tumor periphery VEGF-C causes lymphatics to enlarge, collecting interstitial fluid and metastatic cancer cells (Carmeliet and Jain, 2000).

2.4 Tumor vascularity and blood flow

As already mentioned, the key players in tumor angiogenesis are VEGF, the angiopoietins, the ephrins and their corresponding receptors. However, their excessive production causes the formation of structurally and functionally abnormal blood vessels (Figure 2.1). The tumor vasculature can be described as a system that is maximally stimulated, yet only minimally fulfilling the metabolic demands of the growing tumor that it supplies (Hirst and Flitney, 1997).

Microvessels in solid tumors are often dilated, tortuous, elongated and saccular. There is significant arterio-venous shunt perfusion accompanied by chaotic vascular organization, which lacks any regulation matched to the metabolic demands or functional status of the tissue. Excessive branching is a common finding, often coinciding with blind vascular endings. Incomplete or even missing endothelial lining and interrupted basement membranes result in an increased vascular permeability with extravasation of blood plasma and of red blood cells expanding

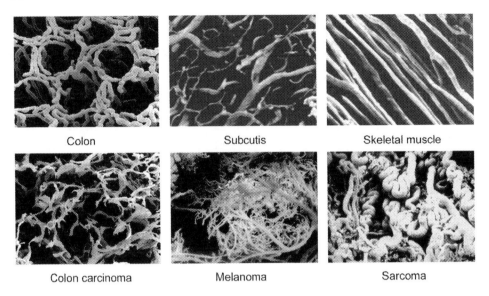

Figure 2.1 Differences in vasculature between normal tissues (upper panels) and malignant tumors (lower panels; courtesy of Professor M.A. Konerding, Dept. of Anatomy and Cell Biology, University of Mainz)

the interstitial fluid space and drastically increasing the hydrostatic pressure in the tumor interstitium (Table 2.2). In solid tumors there is a *rise in viscous resistance to flow*, due mainly to hemoconcentration (Figure 2.2). Aberrant vascular morphology and a decrease in vessel density* are responsible for an *increase in geometric resistance to flow*, which can lead to an inadequate perfusion (Figure 2.2). Substantial spatial heterogeneity in the distribution of tumor vessels and significant temporal heterogeneity in the microcirculation within a tumor (Gillies *et al.*, 1999) may result in a considerably anisotropic distribution of tumor tissue oxygenation and of a number of other factors, which are usually closely linked and which define the so-called metabolic microenvironment. Variations in these relevant parameters between tumors are often more pronounced than differences occurring between different locations or microareas within a tumor (Vaupel and Höckel, 2000; Vaupel, Thews and Höckel, 2001; Vaupel *et al.*, 2003b).

Blood flow can vary considerably, ranging from 0.01 to 2.0 ml g^{-1} min^{-1} (Figure 2.3). Tumors can thus have flow rates similar to those measured in tissues with a high metabolic rate, or can exhibit perfusion rates comparable to those of tissues with low metabolic turnover. Flow data from multiple sites of measurement show marked heterogeneity within individual tumors. However, tumor-to-tumor variability seems to be more pronounced than intra-tumor heterogeneity (Vaupel and Höckel, 2000).

---

*Blood vessel density provides little information on vascular function!

Table 2.2 Major structural and functional irregularities of tumor microvessels (updated from Vaupel, Thews and Hoeckel, 2001)

1. **Blood vessels**
   Missing differentiation
   Loss of vessel hierarchy (disorganized vascular network)
   Increased intervessel distances
   Existence of avascular areas
   Large-diameter (sinusoidal) microvessels
   Elongated, tortuous (convoluted) vessels
   Contour irregularities
   Saccular microvessels, blind endings
   Aberrant branching*
   Haphazard pattern of vessel interconnection
   Incomplete endothelial lining, fenestrations
   Interrupted or absent basement membranes
   Presence of lumen-less endothelial cell cords
   Existence of vessel-like cavities not connected to the blood stream
   Existence of tumor-cell-lined vascular channels ('vascular mimicry')
   Arterio-venous anastomoses (shunts)
   Vessels originating from the venous side
   Missing innervation
   Lack of physiological/pharmacological receptors
   Lack of smooth muscle cells
   Poor or absent coverage by pericytes
   Absence of vasomotion
   Absence of flow regulation
   Increased vascular permeability, plasma leakage
   Increased geometric resistance to flow
   Increased viscous resistance to flow
   Unstable flow velocities (about 85% of all microvessels**)
   Unstable direction of flow
   Intermittent flow, regurgitation (about 5% of all microvessels**)
   Flow stasis (about 1% of all microvessels**)
   Plasma flow only (about 8% of all microvessels**)
   Formation of platelet/leukocyte clusters***
   Thrombus formations
   Formation of RBC aggregates
   Reduced Fahraeus–Lindqvist effect
   Acidosis-induced rigidity of RBCs

2. **Lymphatic vessels**
   Commonly infiltrated by tumor cells (periphery)
   Flattened vessels without lumen (center)
   VEGF-C- and VEGF-D-induced growth at tumor margin
   Inadequate lymphatic drainage in the tumor center
   Interstitial fluid flow
   Interstitial hypertension

* Konerding, Fait and Gaumann, 2001.
** Kimura et al., 1996.
*** Baronzio, Freitas and Kwaan, 2003.

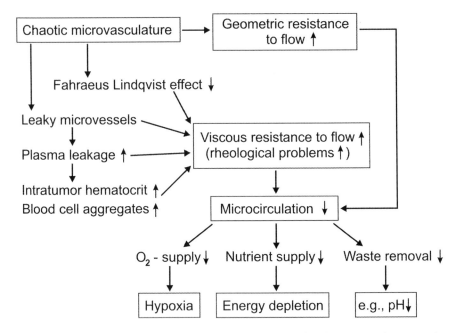

Figure 2.2 Flow-chart describing the mechanisms responsible for the increase in geometric and viscous resistance to flow caused by structural and functional abnormalities of the tumor microvasculature, which lead to a hostile tumor microenvironment

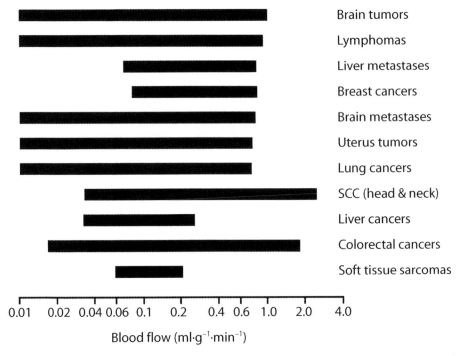

Blood flow (ml·g⁻¹·min⁻¹)

Figure 2.3 Variability of blood flow rates in solid tumors (SCC = squamous cell carcinomas, modified from Vaupel and Höckel, 2000)

2.5   Volume and composition of the tumor interstitial space

The interstitial compartment of solid tumors is significantly different from that of most normal tissues. In general, the tumor interstitial space is characterized by

- an expansion of its volume, which is three to five times larger than in most normal tissues (Figure 2.4),

- high interstitial hydraulic conductivity and diffusivity,

- a relatively large quantity of mobile, i.e. freely moving fluid in contrast to normal tissues where almost all of the fluid is in the gel phase, and

- a quick spread of water soluble agents (e.g. contrast agents) due to significant extravascular convection.

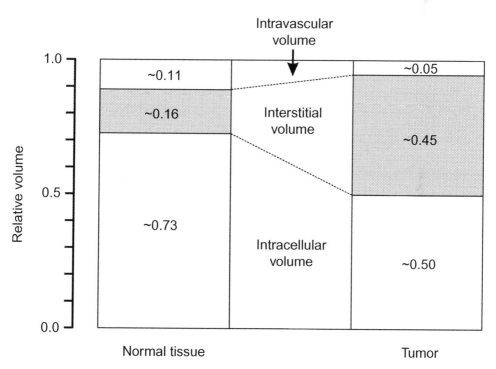

Figure 2.4   Mean relative volumes of the intracellular fluid, the vascular compartment and the interstitial fluid space in malignant tumors (right panel) and in normal tissue (left panel; adapted from Vaupel, 1994)

2.6 Fluid pressure and convective currents in the interstitial space of tumors

The growing tumor produces new, often abnormally leaky microvessels but is unable to form its own functioning lymphatic system. As a result of this and due to a large hydraulic conductivity, there is a significant bulk flow of free fluid in the interstitial space. Whereas in normal tissue convective currents in the interstitial compartment are estimated to be about 0.5–1 per cent of plasma flow, in human cancers interstitial water flux can reach 15 per cent of the respective plasma flow (Vaupel, 1994; see Figure 2.5).

After seeping copiously out of the highly permeable tumor microvessels, fluid accumulates in the tumor matrix and a high interstitial pressure builds up in solid tumors. Whereas in normal tissue the interstitial fluid pressure is slightly subatmospheric or just above atmospheric values, an interstitial hypertension with mean values of 15 mmHg and above develops in cancers (Jain, 1994; Milosevic *et al.*, 2004). Due to these increased interstitial fluid pressures, fluid is squeezed out of the high- to the low-pressure regions at the tumor/normal tissue interface.

2.7 Evidence, characterization and pathogenesis of tumor hypoxia

Clinical investigations carried out over the last 15 years have clearly demonstrated that the prevalence of hypoxic tissue areas (i.e. areas with O_2 tensions (pO_2 values) ≤ 2.5 mmHg) is a characteristic pathophysiological property of locally advanced solid tumors and that such areas have been found in a wide range of human malignancies: cancers of the breast, uterine cervix, vulva, head and neck, prostate, rectum, pancreas, brain tumors, soft tissue sarcomas and malignant melanomas (for reviews see Vaupel and Kelleher, 1999; Vaupel, Thews and Höckel, 2001; Vaupel, Briest and Höckel, 2002a; Vaupel, Mayer and Höckel, 2004; Vaupel and Höckel, 2002).

Evidence has accumulated showing that up to 50–60 per cent of locally advanced solid tumors may exhibit hypoxic and/or anoxic tissue areas that are heterogeneously distributed within the tumor mass. The pretherapeutic oxygenation status assessed in cancers of the breast, uterine cervix and head and neck is poorer than that in the respective normal tissues and is independent of clinical size, stage, histology, grade, nodal status and a series of other tumor characteristics or patient demographics (Figure 2.6). Data do not suggest a topological distribution of pO_2 values within a tumor. Tumor-to-tumor variability in oxygenation is greater than intra-tumor variability. Local recurrences have a higher hypoxic fraction than the respective primary tumors, although there is no clear-cut difference between primary and metastatic malignancies (Vaupel and Kelleher, 1999; Vaupel, Thews and Höckel, 2001; Vaupel, Briest

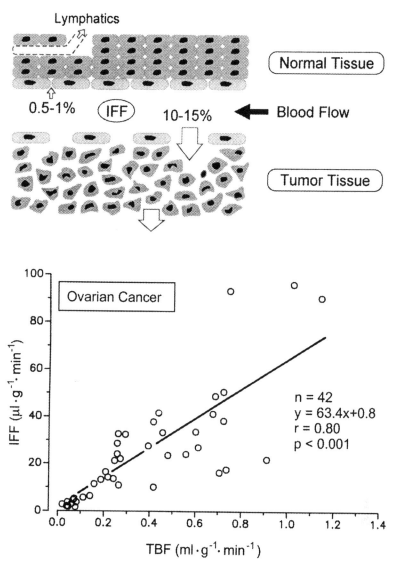

Figure 2.5   Interstitial fluid flow (IFF) as a function of blood flow (TBF) in xenografted human ovarian cancers (lower part). Schematic representation of convective fluid currents in normal and tumor tissues (upper part; adapted from Vaupel, 2004)

and Höckel, 2002a; Vaupel, Mayer and Höckel, 2004; Vaupel and Höckel, 2002).

Hypoxic (or anoxic) areas arise as a result of an imbalance between the supply and consumption of oxygen. Whereas in normal tissues or organs the O_2 supply matches the metabolic requirements, in locally advanced solid tumors the O_2

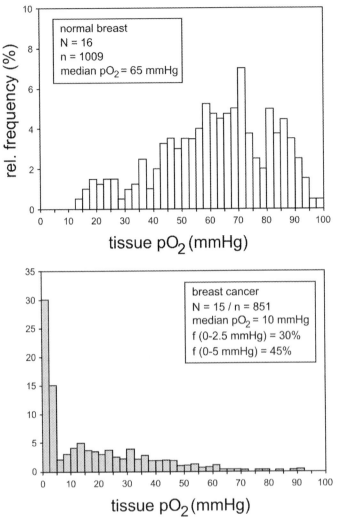

Figure 2.6 Frequency distributions (histograms) of oxygen partial pressures (pO_2 values) measured in normal breast (left panel) and in locally advanced breast cancers (T1b–T4). N = number of patients, n = number of pO_2 values measured, $f(0$–$2.5\,mm\,Hg)$ = fraction of pO_2 values between 0 and 2.5 mm Hg, $f(0$–$5\,mm\,Hg)$ = fraction of pO_2 values between 0 and 5 mm Hg

consumption rate of neoplastic (as well as stromal) cells may outweigh an insufficient oxygen supply and result in the development of tissue areas with very low O_2 levels.

Major pathogenetic mechanisms involved in the emergence of hypoxia in solid tumors are

- severe structural and functional abnormalities of the tumor microvessels (*perfusion-limited* O_2 *delivery*),

- a deterioration of the diffusion geometry (*diffusion-limited* O_2 *delivery*) and

- tumor-associated and/or therapy-induced anemia, leading to a reduced O_2 transport capacity of the blood (*anemic hypoxia*).

There is abundant evidence for the existence of substantial heterogeneity in the tissue oxygenation status, predominantly due to the former two mechanisms (see Table 2.3).

Perfusion-limited O_2 *delivery* leads to *ischemic hypoxia*, which is often transient. For this reason, this type of hypoxia is also called 'acute' hypoxia, a term that does not, however, take into account the mechanisms underlying this condition. Hypoxia in tumors can also be caused by an increase in diffusion distances, so that cells far away (>70 μm) from a nutritive blood vessel receive less oxygen (and nutrients) than needed. In Figure 2.7, profiles are calculated based on *in vivo* data (Vaupel, Kallinowski and Okunieff, 1989; Vaupel, 1994). pO_2 = oxygen partial pressure (outer left ordinate); tissue glucose (Gluc), ATP (outer left ordinate), and lactate (Lac$^-$) concentrations (inner left ordinate) are given in $mg\,dl^{-1}$. pH_e = extracellular pH value (right ordinate). The hypoxic region

Table 2.3   Causative factors of tumor hypoxia (modified from Vaupel, Thews and Hoeckel, 2001)

1. Perfusion-limited hypoxia[a]
    - Abnormal structure and function of microvessels
    - Transient flow stasis (ischemia)

2. Anemic hypoxia
    - Tumor-associated anemia
    - Therapy-induced anemia

3. Diffusion-limited hypoxia
    - Enlarged diffusion distances
    - Adverse diffusion geometry

4. Hypoxemic hypoxia
    - Plasma flow only
    - Microvessels arising from venous side
    - Liver tumors supplied by portal vein

5. Toxic hypoxia
    - HbCO formation (in heavy smokers)

[a] The question of whether 'acute' hypoxia in tumors is a far more serious problem than 'chronic' hypoxia cannot be answered at this time and is still a matter of controversial discussion. Furthermore, the relative contribution of each hypoxia type in a tumor at any given time has not yet been conclusively investigated.

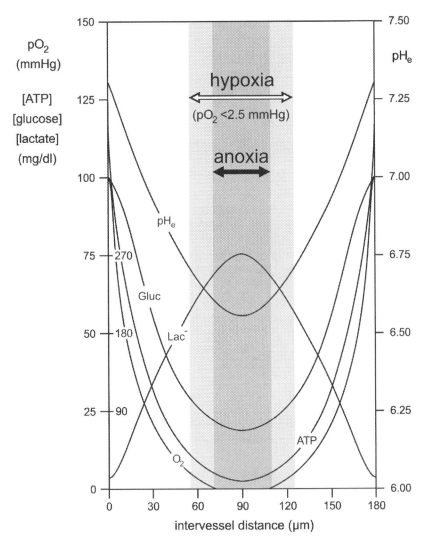

Figure 2.7 Schematic representation of 2D profiles of relevant micro-environmental parameters within the intervessel space of tumors (adapted from Vaupel, 2004)

between the microvessels ($pO_2 < 2.5$ mm Hg) is marked by the light-grey, anoxia by the dark-grey zone. The profiles are calculated for the arterial end of the microvessels assuming concurrent blood flow and homogeneity within the inter-vascular space. Although the concentration of oxygen (on a molar basis) is higher than that of glucose (9 mM O_2 versus 5 mM glucose at the arterial end of a tumor microvessel), the diffusion distance for O_2 is shorter. This implies that oxygen in this tumor model is the limiting substrate for high proliferation, whereas glucose is the limiting substrate for pure cell survival. This condition is termed *diffusion-limited hypoxia* and is also known as 'chronic' hypoxia. In addition to enlarged diffusion distances, an adverse diffusion geometry (e.g. concurrent versus countercurrent tumor microvessels) can also cause hypoxia. Tumor-associated or therapy-induced anemia can contribute to the development of hypoxia (*anemic hypoxia*). This type of hypoxia is particularly intensified in tumors or tumor areas exhibiting low perfusion rates. A similar condition can be caused by carboxyhemoglobin (HbCO) formation in heavy smokers, which can lead to *toxic hypoxia*, because hemoglobin blocked by carbon monoxide (CO) can no longer transport oxygen. Very often, tumor microvessels are perfused (at least transiently) by plasma only (Kimura *et al.*, 1996). Where this occurs, hypoxia develops very rapidly around these vessels because only a few tumor cells at the arterial end can be adequately supplied under the given conditions (*hypoxemic hypoxia*). There is abundant evidence for the existence of substantial heterogeneity in the development and extent of tumor hypoxia due to pronounced intra-tumor (and inter-tumor) variability in vascularity and perfusion rates (Vaupel, Kallinowski and Okunieff, 1989; Vaupel, Briest and Höckel, 2002a).

While normal tissues can physiologically compensate for these O_2 deficiency states, locally advanced tumors (or at least larger tumor areas) cannot adequately counteract the restriction in O_2 supply and thus the development of hypoxia. In normal tissues, ischemia can (primarily) be compensated by an increase in the O_2 extraction from the blood, and anemia by a rise in local blood flow rate.

2.8 Tumor pH

Under many conditions it has been confirmed that the intracellular pH (pH_i) in tumor cells is neutral to alkaline as long as tumors are not oxygen and energy deprived (Vaupel, Kallinowski and Okunieff, 1989; Vaupel, Schaefer and Okunieff, 1994). Tumor cells have efficient mechanisms for exporting protons into the extracellular space, which represents the acidic compartment in tumors. Cellular pH regulation is mainly accomplished by a Na^+/H^+-exchanger H(NHE1), which is oncogenei-dependent and can be activated by a series of growth factors also involved in tumor angiogenesis (Orive *et al.*, 2003).

For this reason, a pH gradient exists across the cell membrane in tumors ($pH_i > pH_e$, Figure 2.8). Interestingly, this gradient is the reverse of that found in normal tissues, where pH_i is lower than pH_e (for reviews see Vaupel, Kallinowski and Okunieff, 1989; Griffiths, 1991; Vaupel, 1992).

Cancer cells intensively split glucose to lactic acid, which is one major reason for tumor acidification (see Table 2.4). Lactic acid production and metabolic acidosis not only lead to substantial proton accumulation but also to elevated respiratory quotients (RQ = CO_2 output/O_2 uptake) >1.5 in tumors due to an intensified CO_2 release according to the equation

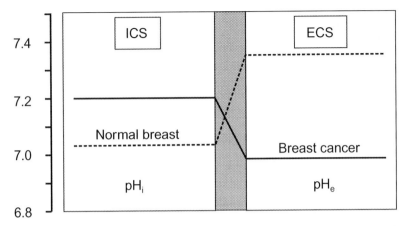

Figure 2.8 Schematic representation of pH gradients between the intracellular space (ICS) and the extracellular space (ECS) of normal breast tissue and in breast cancer. pH_i = intracellular pH, pH_e = extracellular pH

Table 2.4 Parameters characterizing the metabolic microenvironment of locally advanced human tumors

Parameter	Mean level	Tumor entity	Ref.
Glucose concentration ($\mu mol\,g^{-1}$)	1.0 ± 0.4[a] 0.3 ± 0.2[b]	Rectal adenocarcinomas	(Walenta et al., 2003)
	2.4 ± 1.3[a] 2.2 ± 1.0[b]	Uterine cervical cancers	(Walenta et al., 2000)
Lactate concentration ($\mu mol\,g^{-1}$)	4.7 ± 1.5[a] 12.3 ± 3.3[b]	Head & neck cancers	(Walenta et al., 1997)
	6.3 ± 2.8[a] 10.0 ± 2.9[b]	Uterine cervical cancers	(Walenta et al., 2000)
	8.0 ± 3.7[a] 8.6 ± 4.1[b]	Rectal adenocarcinomas	(Walenta et al., 2003)
ATP concentration ($\mu mol\,g^{-1}$)	1.0 ± 0.5[a] 0.9 ± 0.4[b]	Rectal adenocarcinomas	(Walenta et al., 2003)
	0.9 ± 0.4[a] 0.8 ± 0.5[b]	Uterine cervical cancers	(Walenta et al., 2000)
Extracellular pH	6.60–6.98	Various tumors	(Vaupel, Kallinowski and Okunieff, 1989)
pO_2 (mm Hg)	$3–15$[c] $6–14$[c] $6–17$[c]	Breast cancers Uterine cervical cancers Head & neck cancers	(Vaupel et al., 2003a) (Vaupel et al., 2002b) (Becker et al., 2000)

[a] Non-metastatic, [b] metastatic (values are means ± SD).
[c] Median pO_2 is dependent on hemoglobin level.

$$H^+ + HCO_3^- \xrightarrow{\text{CA}} H_2O + CO_2$$

Hypoxia-induced upregulation of the enzyme carbonic anhydrase (CA) is thus a meaningful physiological adaptation. Experimental evidence for the occurrence of this reaction are the very high CO_2 partial pressures and low bicarbonate concentrations found in the interstitial fluid of solid tumors (Gullino, 1970). Since the total CO_2 output is greater than the metabolic formation of CO_2 (from substrate oxidation), the RQ can rise above 1.5.

Other relevant pathogenetic mechanisms yielding an intensified tissue acidosis are based on substantial ATP hydrolysis, glutaminolysis, ketogenesis and metabolic CO_2 production (Vaupel, 1994).

2.9 The 'crucial Ps' characterizing the hostile metabolic microenvironment of solid tumors

Applying quantitative imaging bioluminescence, Walenta *et al.* (1997, 2000, 2003, Walenta and Mueller-Klieser, 2004) have provided clinical evidence that lactate accumulation mirrors malignant potential in squamous cell carcinomas of the uterine cervix and of the head and neck, and in colorectal adenocarcinomas. In Figure 2.9, cryosections were used for metabolic imaging of lactate, glucose and ATP using calibrated bioluminescence in color code. Two adjacent sections were stained with hematoxylin/eosin (HE) and for cytokeratin (CK) to identify viable tumor areas. Before sectioning, the biopsy was punctured twice with a fine needle generating two pin holes in each section allowing an exact overlay of the serial sections. This procedure enables a correlation of the different metabolites with each other and with the histological structure from which the metabolic signal originates. Concentrations of lactate in viable tumor areas exhibited pronounced intra- and inter-tumor differences compared to glucose and ATP, although tumor glucose levels correlated inversely with lactate concentrations (Walenta and Mueller-Klieser, 2004).

Production of lactate due to a high glycolytic flux is one of the conditions characterizing the hostile metabolic microenvironment of solid tumors. Other 'crucial Ps' are listed in Table 2.5. These parameters, together with some other conditions not mentioned here, may be – directly or indirectly – responsible for changes in the proteome and genome, selection for more aggressive cells, tumor progression and acquired treatment resistance (Nowell, 1976; Giaccia, 1996; Höckel *et al.*, 1996; Reynolds, Rockwell and Glazer, 1996; Yuan and Glazer, 1998; Rofstad, 2000; Stubbs *et al.*, 2000; Yuan *et al.*, 2000; Vaupel and Höckel, 2000, 2002; Brizel *et al.*, 2001; Höckel and Vaupel, 2001; Vaupel, Thews and Höckel, 2001; Vaupel, Mayer and Höckel, 2004; Coleman, Mitchell and Camphausen, 2002; Evans and Koch, 2003; Okunieff *et al.*, 2003; Subarsky and Hill, 2003).

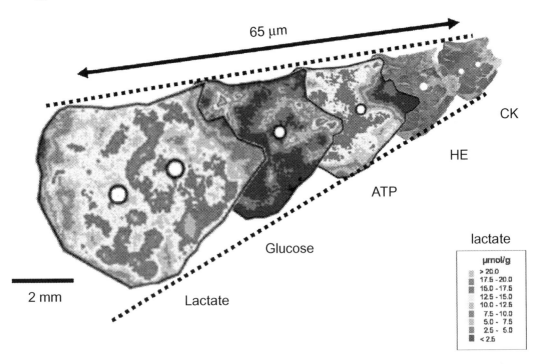

Figure 2.9   Sequence of serial cryosections through a human squamous cell carcinoma of the head and neck (HNSCC) (courtesy of Professor W. Mueller-Klieser and Dr. S. Walenta, Institute of Physiology and Pathophysiology, University of Mainz) (A color reproduction of this figure can be viewed in the color plate section.)

Table 2.5   The 'crucial Ps' characterizing the hostile (metabolic) microenvironment of solid tumors

1.	Perfusion inadequacies and vascular chaos	
2.	Perfusion heterogeneities	
3.	Permeability of tumor microvessels	
4.	Pressure of interstitial fluid	increase
5.	Partial volume of interstitial space	
6.	Production of lactate	
7.	Partial pressure of CO_2 (pCO_2)	
8.	Paucity of nutrients (e.g. glucose)	intensify
9.	Paucity of bicarbonate (HCO_3^-)	
10.	Partial pressure of oxygen (pO_2)	
11.	Production of high-energy compounds	decrease
12.	pH of extracellular compartment	

Acknowledgment

The valuable assistance of Dr. Debra K. Kelleher in preparing this manuscript is greatly appreciated.

References

Baronzio, G., Freitas, I. and Kwaan, H.C. (2003). Tumor microenvironment and hemorheological abnormalities. *Semin Thrombosis Hemostasis* **29**, 489–497.

Becker, A., Stadler, P., Lavey, R.S., Hänsgen, G., Kuhnt, T., Lautenschläger, C., Feldmann, H.J., Molls, M. and Dunst, J. (2000). Severe anemia is associated with poor tumor oxygenation in head and neck squamous cell carcinomas. *Int J Radiat Oncol Biol Phys* **46**, 459–466.

Brem, S., Brem, H., Folkman, J., Finkelstein, D. and Platz, A. (1976). Prolonged tumor dormancy by prevention of neovascularization in the vitreous. *Cancer Res* **36**, 2807–2812.

Brizel, D.M., Schroeder, T., Scher, R.L., Walenta, S., Clough, R.W., Dewhirst, M.W. and Mueller-Klieser, W. (2001). Elevated tumor lactate concentrations predict for an increased risk of metastases in head-and-neck cancer. *Int J Radiat Oncol Biol Phys* **51**, 349–353.

Carmeliet, P. and Jain, R.K. (2000). Angiogenesis in cancer and other diseases. *Nature* **407**, 249–257.

Coleman, C.N., Mitchell, J.B. and Camphausen, K. (2002). Tumor hypoxia: chicken, egg, or a piece of the farm? *J Clin Oncol* **20**, 610–615.

Ellis, L.M., Liu, W., Ahmad, S.A., Fan, F., Jung, Y.D., Shaheen, R.M. and Reinmuth, N. (2001). Overview of angiogenesis: biologic implications for antiangiogenic therapy. *Semin Oncol* **28**, 94–104.

Evans, S.M. and Koch, C.J. (2003). Prognostic significance of tumor oxygenation in humans. *Cancer Lett* **195**, 1–16.

Giaccia, A.J. (1996). Hypoxic stress proteins: survival of the fittest. *Semin Radiat Oncol* **6**, 46–58.

Gillies, R.J., Schornack, P.A., Secomb, T.W. and Raghunand, N. (1999). Causes and effects of heterogeneous perfusion in tumors. *Neoplasia* **1**, 197–207.

Griffiths, J.R. (1991). Are cancer cells acidic? *Br J Cancer* **64**, 425–427.

Gullino, P.M. (1970). Techniques for the study of tumor physiopathology. In *Methods in Cancer Research* (Vol. 5), H. Busch (ed.). Academic Press, New York, pp. 45–91.

Hanahan, D. and Weinberg, R.A. (2000). The hallmarks of cancer. *Cell* **100**, 57–70.

Hirst, D.G. and Flitney, F.W. (1997). The physiological importance and therapeutic potential of nitric oxide in the tumour-associated vasculature. In *Tumour Angiogenesis*, R. Bicknell, C.E. Lewis and N. Ferrara (eds). Oxford University Press, Oxford, pp. 153–167.

Höckel, M., Schlenger, K., Aral, B., Mitze, M., Schäffer, U. and Vaupel, P. (1996). Association between tumor hypoxia and malignant progression in advanced cancer of the uterine cervix. *Cancer Res* **56**, 4509–4515.

Höckel, M. and Vaupel, P. (2001). Tumor hypoxia: definitions and current clinical, biologic and molecular aspects. *J Natl Cancer Inst* **93**, 266–276.

Jain, R.K. (1994). Barriers to drug delivery in solid tumors. *Sci Am* **271**, 58–65.

Jussila, L. and Alitalo, K. (2002). Vascular growth factors and lymphangiogenesis. *Physiol Rev* **82**, 673–700.

Kerbel, R.S. (2000). Tumor angiogenesis: past, present and the near future. *Carcinogenesis* **21**, 505–515.

Kimura, H., Braun, R.D., Ong, E.T., Hsu, R., Secomb, T.W., Papahadjopoulos, D., Hong, K. and Dewhirst, M. (1996). Fluctuations in red cell flux in tumor microvessels can lead to transient hypoxia and reoxygenation in tumor parenchyma. *Cancer Res* 56, 5522–5528.

Konerding, M.A., Fait, E. and Gaumann, A. (2001). 3D microvascular architecture of pre-cancerous lesions and invasive carcinomas of the colon. *Br J Cancer* 84, 1354–1362.

McDonald, D.M., Munn, L. and Jain, R.K. (2000). Vasculogenic mimicry: how convincing, how novel, and how significant? *Am J Pathol* 156, 383–388.

Milosevic, M., Fyles, A., Hedley, D. and Hill, R. (2004). The human tumor microenvironment: invasive (needle) measurement of oxygen and interstitial fluid pressure. *Semin Radiat Oncol* 14, 249–258.

Nowell, P.C. (1976). The clonal evolution of tumor cell populations. *Science* 194, 23–28.

Okunieff, P., Ding, I., Vaupel, P. and Höckel, M. (2003). Evidence for and against hypoxia as the primary cause of tumor aggressiveness. *Adv Exp Med Biol* 510, 69–75.

Orive, G., Reshkin, S.J., Harguindey, S. and Pedraz, J.L. (2003). Hydrogen ion dynamics and the Na^+/H^+ exchanger in cancer angiogenesis and antiangiogenesis. *Br J Cancer* 89, 1395–1399.

Padera, T.P., Kadambi, A., di Tomaso, E., Carreira, C.M., Brown, E.B., Boucher, Y., Choi, N.C., Mathisen, D., Wain, J., Mark, E.J., Munn, L.L. and Jain, R.K. (2002). Lymphatic metastasis in the absence of functional intratumor lymphatics. *Science* 296, 1883–1886.

Papetti, M. and Herman, I.M. (2002). Mechanisms of normal and tumor-derived angiogenesis. *Am J Physiol Cell Physiol* 282, C947-C970.

Patan, S., Munn, L.L. and Jain, R.K. (1996). Intussusceptive microvascular growth in a human colon adenocarcinoma xenograft: a novel mechanism of tumor angiogenesis. *Microvasc Res* 51, 260–272.

Pugh, C.W. and Ratcliffe, P.J. (2003). Regulation of angiogenesis by hypoxia: role of the HIF system. *Nature Med* 9, 677–684.

Reynolds, T.Y., Rockwell, S. and Glazer, P.M. (1996). Genetic instability induced by the tumor microenvironment. *Cancer Res* 56, 5754–5757.

Ribatti, D., Vacca, A. and Dammacco, F. (2003). New non-angiogenesis dependent pathways for tumour growth. *Eur J Cancer* 39, 1835–1841.

Rofstad, E.K. (2000). Microenvironment-induced cancer metastasis. *Int J Radiat Biol* 76, 589–605.

Ruoslahti, E. (2002). Specialization of tumour vasculature. *Nature Rev Cancer* 2, 83–90.

Semenza, G.L. (2000). HIF-1: using two hands to flip the angiogenic switch. *Cancer Metab Rev* 19, 59–65.

Shweiki, D., Neeman, M., Itin, A. and Keshet, E. (1995). Induction of vascular endothelial growth factor expression by hypoxia and by glucose deficiency in multicell spheroids: implications for tumor angiogenesis. *Proc Natl Acad Sci USA* 92, 768–772.

Sivridis, E., Giatromanolaki, A. and Koukourakis, M.I. (2003). The vascular network of tumours – what is it not for? *J Pathol* 201, 173–180.

Stubbs, M., McSheehy, P.M.J., Griffiths, J.R. and Bashford, C.L. (2000). Causes and consequences of tumour acidity and implications for treatment. *Mol Med Today* 6, 15–19.

Subarsky, P. and Hill, R.P. (2003). The hypoxic tumour microenvironment and metastatic progression. *Clin Exp Metastasis* 20, 237–250.

Vaupel, P. (1992). Physiological properties of malignant tumours. *NMR Biomed* 5, 220–225.

Vaupel, P.W. (1994). *Blood Flow, Oxygenation, Tissue pH Distribution, and Bioenergetic Status of Tumors*, Lecture 23, Ernst Schering Research Foundation.

Vaupel, P. (2004). Tumor microenvironmental physiology and its implications for radiation oncology. *Semin Radiat Oncol* 14, 198–206.

Vaupel, P., Briest, S. and Höckel, M. (2002a). Hypoxia in breast cancer: pathogenesis, characterization and biological/therapeutic implications. *Wien Med Wschr* **152**, 334–342.

Vaupel, P. and Höckel, M. (2000). Blood supply, oxygenation status and metabolic micromilieu of breast cancers: characterization and therapeutic relevance. *Int J Oncol* **17**, 869–879.

Vaupel, P. and Höckel, M. (2002). Tumor hypoxia and therapeutic resistance. In *Recombinant Human Erythropoietin (rhEPO) in Clinical Oncology*, M.R. Nowrousian (ed.). Springer, Berlin, pp. 127–146.

Vaupel, P., Kallinowski, F. and Okunieff, P. (1989). Blood flow, oxygen and nutrient supply, and metabolic microenvironment of human tumors: a review. *Cancer Res* **49**, 6449–6465.

Vaupel, P. and Kelleher, D.K. (eds). (1999). *Tumor Hypoxia*, Wissenschaftliche Verlagsgesellschaft, Stuttgart.

Vaupel, P., Mayer, A., Briest, S. and Höckel, M. (2003a). Oxygenation gain factor: a novel parameter characterizing the association between hemoglobin level and the oxygenation status of breast cancers. *Cancer Res* **63**, 7634–7637.

Vaupel, P., Mayer, A. and Höckel, M. (2004). Tumor hypoxia and malignant progression. *Methods Enzymol* **381**, 335–354.

Vaupel, P., Schaefer, C. and Okunieff, P. (1994). Intracellular acidosis in murine fibrosarcomas coincides with ATP depletion, hypoxia, and high levels of lactate and total P_i. *NMR Biomed* **7**, 128–136.

Vaupel, P., Thews, O. and Hoeckel, M. (2001). Treatment resistance of solid tumors: role of hypoxia and anemia. *Med Oncol* **18**, 243–259.

Vaupel, P., Thews, O., Kelleher, D.K. and Konerding, M.A. (2003b). O_2 extraction is a key parameter determining the oxygenation status of malignant tumors and normal tissues. *Int J Oncol* **22**, 795–798.

Vaupel, P., Thews, O., Mayer, A., Höckel, S. and Höckel, M. (2002b). Oxygenation status of gynecologic tumors: what is the optimal hemoglobin level? *Strahlenther Onkol* **178**, 727–731.

Walenta, S., Chau, T.-V., Schroeder, T., Lehr, H.-A., Kunz-Schughart, L.A., Fuerst, A. and Mueller-Klieser, W. (2003). Metabolic classification of human rectal adenocarcinomas: a novel guideline for clinical oncologists? *J Cancer Res Clin Oncol* **129**, 321–326.

Walenta, S. and Mueller-Klieser, W.F. (2004). Lactate: mirror and motor of tumor malignancy. *Semin Radiat Oncol* **14**, 267–274.

Walenta, S., Salameh, A., Lyng, H., Evensen, J.F., Mitze, M., Rofstad, E.K. and Mueller-Klieser, W. (1997). Correlation of high lactate levels in head and neck tumors with incidence of metastasis. *Am J Pathol* **150**, 409–415.

Walenta, S., Wetterling, M., Lehrke, M., Schwickert, G., Sundfor, K., Rofstad, E.K. and Mueller-Klieser, W. (2000). High lactate levels predict likelihood of metastases, tumor recurrence, and restricted patient survival in human cervical cancers. *Cancer Res* **60**, 916–921.

Yancopoulos, G.D., Davis, S., Gale, N.W., Rudge, J.S., Wiegand, S.J. and Holash, J. (2000). Vascular-specific growth factors and blood vessel formation. *Nature* **407**, 242–248.

Yuan, J. and Glazer, P.M. (1998). Mutagenesis induced by the tumor microenvironment. *Mutation Res* **400**, 439–446.

Yuan, J., Narayanan, L., Rockwell, S. and Glazer, P.M. (2000). Diminished DNA repair and elevated mutagenesis in mammalian cells exposed to hypoxia and low pH. *Cancer Res* **60**, 4372–4376.

3

The Role of Microvasculature in Metastasis Formation

Oliver Stoeltzing and **Lee M. Ellis**

Abstract

The development of a microvascular network within tumours, also termed tumour angiogenesis, is an essential process for the development and outgrowth of cancer metastases. Metastases develop through a series of interlinked steps, each of which is essential for the establishment and progression of a metastatic lesion. After an initial phase of extensive tumour cell proliferation in the primary lesion and creation of an extensive vascularization network from pre-existing vessels (vessel cooption), tumour cells may elicit the ability to invade the extracellular matrix for entering the bloodstream, lymphatic channels, or both. However, similarly to the primary lesion, metastatic lesions must establish a sufficient microvascular network at an organ site (which in addition displays a different microenvironment compared to the primary lesion), in order to facilitate their outgrowth. This chapter provides a comprehensive overview on factors regulating the complex process of tumour angiogenesis and metastases formation, with respect to various solid malignancies.

Keywords

angiogenesis, microvasculature, VEGF, cancer, metastasis

3.1 Introduction

Metastases develop through a series of interlinked steps, each of which is essential for the establishment and progression of a metastatic lesion. Two major early steps in the formation of distant metastases are: (a) proliferation of tumor

Vascular-targeted Therapies in Oncology   Edited by Dietmar W. Siemann
© 2006 John Wiley & Sons, Ltd.

cells in the *primary* lesion and (b) creation of an extensive vascularization network from pre-existing vessels (vessel co-option) plus development of intra-tumoral neo-vessels (angiogenesis). As a third step, tumor cells must eventually develop the ability to invade the extracellular matrix (ECM) in order to facilitate access to the bloodstream, lymphatic channels or both. Once tumor cells have spread to a metastatic organ site (such as liver, lung etc.) and attached to or 'trans-vaded' through the ECM, the process of angiogenesis is again implicated in the development of a sufficient microvasculature within tumor metastases in order to support their progressive growth. In Figure 3.1, the tumor microenvi-ronment mainly consists of tumor cells (T), endothelial cells (E), pericytes (P), immune cells and stromal cells (S). Growth factors and cytokines may be released by tumor cells that exhibit their effects – after binding to the respective receptor – either on other cells (such as EC, pericytes) or on the tumor cells themselves (autocrine effect). A complex interaction of these cell types modu-lates the angiogenic process, leading to development of an 'organ-site' specific neoplastic microvasculature. New approaches of anticancer therapies are cur-rently under development – many of them already being investigated in phase

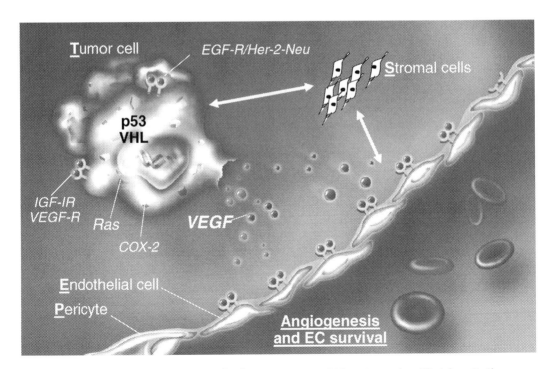

Figure 3.1 Schematic interaction of cell compartments within a tumor (modified from ImClone Systems, NY)

III clinical trials, which focus on directly targeting tumor biology and interference with the neoplastic angiogenic processes. The aspect of neoplastic microvasculature and angiogenesis represents an important parameter of tumor biology, so that impairing this process with modern molecular targeted agents may inhibit tumor growth and metastatic spread. Therefore, a profound understanding of the biology of metastasis and their microvasculature is essential for the development of successful innovative cancer therapeutics.

In general, angiogenesis is essential for solid malignancies (including tumor metastases) to grow beyond 1–2 mm in size, when oxygen diffusion alone is no longer sufficient to maintain adequate tissue oxygenation (Folkman, 1992, 1995). The process of non-neoplastic angiogenesis is regulated by numerous pro- and anti-angiogenic factors that function in a dynamic and absolutely coordinated manner to lead to a mature and functional vascular network. However, tumor angiogenesis is much less coordinated and the result of an overall net gain in pro-angiogenic stimuli. This net gain may be achieved through either an increase in the expression of pro-angiogenic molecules, or a significant decrease in the expression of anti-angiogenic molecules, or a combination thereof. In neoplastic lesions, this process is more accurately defined as a combination of angiogenesis and vasculogenesis in which the main blood supply is derived from pre-existing vessels (Fidler *et al.*, 2000) but circulating endothelial cell (EC) precursors may also contribute to the growing vascular network (Monestiroli *et al.*, 2001).

The abnormal vascularization in tumors (i.e. high vessel density within tumors) and increased expression of certain angiogenic factors in various human cancers have been associated with tumor progression and poor outcome (Ikeda *et al.*, 1999; Kitadai *et al.*, 1998; Kondo *et al.*, 2000; Maeda *et al.*, 1995; Takahashi *et al.*, 1995; Ushijima *et al.*, 2001). One of the best characterized angiogenic factors, and one that has been associated with angiogenesis and metastasis in many cancer systems (Duque *et al.*, 1999; Kido *et al.*, 2001; Maeda *et al.*, 1995; Takahashi *et al.*, 1995; Yuan *et al.*, 2000), is vascular endothelial growth factor (VEGF), also known as vascular permeability factor (Dvorak *et al.*, 1995; Senger *et al.*, 1986, 1993). VEGF is also a potent EC mitogen and with its ability to mediate EC survival it facilitates angiogenesis in tumors even under adverse conditions such as hypoxia or an acidic milieu (Gerber *et al.*, 1998; Keck *et al.*, 1989; Leung *et al.*, 1989; Plouet, Schilling and Gospodarowicz, 1989). *In vivo*, VEGF also increases vascular permeability (by 50 000 times that of histamine, the 'gold standard' for induction of permeability) and may contribute to the formation of ascites or pleural effusion in patients with cancer (Kraft *et al.*, 1999; Nagy *et al.*, 1995; Senger *et al.*, 1983, 1986; Xu *et al.*, 2000; Zebrowski *et al.*, 1999). Many other factors have been implicated in the regulation of EC proliferation and survival as well, including angiopoietins, fibroblast growth factors (FGFs), epidermal growth factor (EGF), interleukin (IL)-8, platelet-derived growth factor (PDGF), platelet-derived EC growth factor (PD-ECGF, also known as thymidine phosphorylase) and hepatocyte growth factor (HGF) (reviewed by Yancopoulos *et al.* (2000)). The angiopoietins act specifically on ECs through the EC receptor Tie-2 (Tek), whereas other growth factors (e.g. PDGF, EGF or bFGF) also bind to receptors on other types of cell, including cancer cells. In addition, some VEGF receptors (i.e. VEGF-R1 and VEGF-R2) that once were considered endothelial cell specific are also found to be expressed on certain tumor cells (Zhang *et al.*, 2002).

For the development of angiogenesis targeting strategies, it has to be realized that tumor angiogenesis is not regulated by a single angiogenic molecule but rather depends on the cooperation and integration of various factors that act in a coordinated fashion (reviewed by Carmeliet and Jain (2000)). However, the most tightly regulated angiogenic factor is VEGF. Because VEGF is of universal importance in tumor angiogenesis of primary and metastatic tumors, this chapter focuses on the mechanisms that regulate VEGF expression in tumor cells and discusses the role of microvasculature in metastasis formation of various cancer entities.

3.2   Regulators of angiogenesis in solid tumors

The regulation of angiogenesis in solid malignancies is a complex process that involves differential expression of certain pro-angiogenic and anti-angiogenic factors and molecules in tumors. In addition, there is great heterogeneity among tumor entities in regards to angiogenesis and involved molecular regulators of tumor progression. However, one of the most common factors involved in tumor angiogenesis and subsequent metastasis formation is the vascular endothelial growth factor (VEGF). The function and regulation of VEGF and its receptors has been extensively studied over the past decades, eventually leading to the development of promising molecular targeted treatment strategies for patients with cancer. This section will focus on the role of the VEGF/VEGF-R system in cancer angiogenesis and describe the most common regulation pathways of relevant proangiogenic factors.

Vascular endothelial growth factors (VEGFs) and their receptors

The VEGF family currently comprises six secreted glycoproteins designated VEGF-A, VEGF-B, VEGF-C, VEGF-D, VEGF-E and placental growth factor (PlGF) (Ferrara and Davis-Smyth, 1997). In Figure 3.2, VEGFs (A–E) and their receptors are shown. Importantly, VEGFR-2 function can be enhanced by a simultaneous binding of a VEGF165 molecule to NRP-1 and VEGFR-2 via different binding sites (paracrine effect) (shown). The NRP-1 receptor may also be on another cell (i.e. tumor cell) presenting bound VEGF165 to an EC VEGFR-2

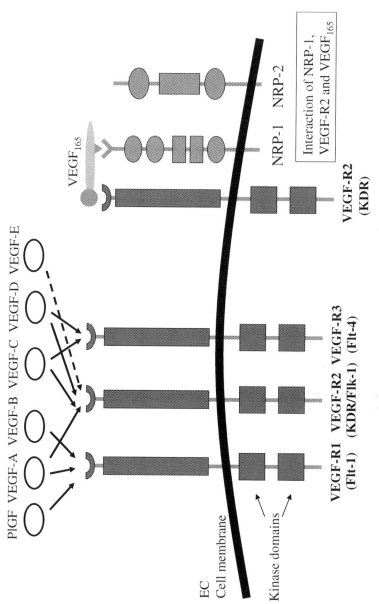

Figure 3.2 VEGFs and their receptors plus co-receptors

to the counter cell (juxtacrine effect) (not shown). The importance of the NRP-2 receptor as co-receptor for VEGF-R has not been well defined yet. The best characterized of the VEGF family members is VEGF-A (referred to as VEGF in this chapter), a 34–50 kDa homodimeric glycoprotein that is expressed in various isoforms secondary to alternative exon splicing that leads to mature 121-, 165-, 189- and 206-amino-acid proteins (Houck et al., 1991). $VEGF_{121}$ and $VEGF_{165}$ are secreted by cells, whereas the larger isoforms ($VEGF_{189}$ and $VEGF_{206}$) are associated with the cell surface and sequestered in the extracellular matrix (ECM) (Houck et al., 1991). $VEGF_{165}$ also has intermediary properties, as a significant fraction remains bound to the cell surface and ECM (Park et al., 1993). $VEGF_{165}$ is a 45 kDa glycoprotein with a heparin-binding domain (Ferrara and Henzel, 1989). $VEGF_{121}$ is an acidic polypeptide that does not bind heparin, whereas $VEGF_{189}$ and $VEGF_{206}$ are highly basic and bind to heparin with high affinity. Loss of the heparin-binding domain on VEGF has been shown to result in a significant reduction of mitogenic activity (Keyt et al., 1996). The ECM-bound isoforms can be released in a diffusible form by plasmin cleavage at the C-terminus, which generates a bioactive fragment. Some less commonly expressed splice variants ($VEGF_{145}$, $VEGF_{183}$) have also been reported (Neufeld et al., 1999). $VEGF_{165}$ is the predominant isoform and is commonly overexpressed in a variety of human solid tumors. Mouse embryos lacking a single VEGF allele demonstrate growth inhibition and impaired angiogenesis with degeneration of ECs, and they die between day 11 and day 12 of gestation (Ferrara et al., 1996). Recent studies suggest that expression patterns of certain VEGF isoforms are tissue specific, implying that these isoforms have specific roles in development and probably in tumor angiogenesis as well (Cheung et al., 1998).

The VEGFs mediate their function via high-affinity binding to receptor tyrosine kinases that are predominantly expressed on ECs. However, recent evidence suggests that some of these receptors may also be expressed on tumor cells (Neuchrist et al., 2003), bone-marrow-derived ECs (Hattori et al., 2001), or lymphatic ECs (Partanen et al., 2000). The current nomenclature lists three VEGF receptors (VEGFRs): VEGFR-1 (also known as Flt-1), VEGFR-2 (Flk-1 or KDR; Flk-1 is the murine homolog of KDR) and VEGFR-3 (Flt-4). Two co-receptors for VEGFR-2, neuropilin-1 and neuropilin-2, have also been discovered. These neuropilin receptors (NRPs) are expressed on numerous cell types, including cancer cells, and have been implicated in the regulation of the binding affinity of $VEGF_{165}$ to VEGFR-2; as such, they contribute to augmenting VEGFR function without transmitting intracellular signals by themselves (Parikh et al., 2004; Soker et al., 2002). However, NRPs may significantly regulate growth and vascularization of solid malignancies (Parikh et al., 2004).

The ligand specificities of the above-mentioned VEGFRs differ and are illustrated in Figure 3.2. Upon activation, VEGFRs mediate specific functions in vitro and in vivo. In adults, VEGFR-1 and VEGFR-2 are expressed mainly in the vascular endothelium, whereas VEGFR-3 is restricted largely to the lymphatic endothelium. VEGFR-1 seems to be important for EC migration and differentiation, whereas VEGFR-2 activation enhances EC survival and proliferation and increases vascular permeability (Dvorak *et al.*, 1995). VEGFR-3 has been shown to be involved in lymphangiogenesis and lymphatic metastasis (Achen *et al.*, 1998).

In the following sections, we describe important mediators of VEGF expression in tumor cells, followed by a brief description of some other factors involved in neoplastic angiogenesis and microvasculature function.

Regulation of VEGF expression in tumors

The direct effect of growth factors and their receptors on tumor growth has been recognized for more than two decades now. However, their implication in tumor angiogenesis by regulating the expression of certain angiogenic molecules has only recently been discovered. Since VEGF has been identified as one of the crucial regulators of tumor angiogenesis, an abundant numbers of studies have been conducted to investigate the mechanisms of VEGF regulation in normal and malignant tissues, respectively. It is now realized that multiple factors and signaling pathways contribute to a very complex regulation pathway of VEGF expression. In Figure 3.3, common pathways involved in the regulation of VEGF expression in cancer cells are shown. Activation of certain growth factor receptor tyrosine kinases (RTK) or oncogene activation (Her2, Src) may lead to phosphorylation of signaling intermediates such as MAPK, PI-3K, STAT3 and P38, respectively. In addition, Ras function and its constitutive activation has been shown to be an important mediator of a Ras–Raf–MEK signaling cascade implicated in constitutive MAPK activation and consecutive VEGF expression. MAPK mainly mediates proangiogenic gene expression through transcription factors such as HIF-1α, Nf-κB and AP-1, which bind to a certain region within the *VEGF* promoter. Besides the involvement of certain oncogenes (and loss of tumor suppressor gene function), multiple growth factors, cytokines and transcriptional activators have been identified as critical modulators of VEGF expression. Some of the most important regulatory systems are discussed below.

Growth factors and cytokines

Epidermal growth factor receptor family

Among the best studied growth factor receptor systems is that of the EGF receptor family, which comprises four homologous receptors: the epidermal growth factor receptor (EGFR, also called HER1 or ErbB1), ErbB2 (HER2/neu), ErbB3 (HER3) and ErbB4 (HER4) (reviewed by Klapper *et al.* (2000)).

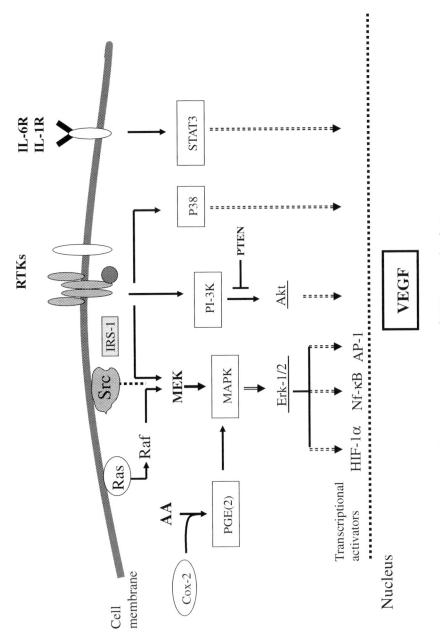

Figure 3.3   Regulators of VEGF expression in tumors

The EGFR (ErbB1) system is implicated in VEGF regulation and angiogenesis, which has been validated for several tumor systems, such as colon carcinoma, pancreatic cancer, gastric cancer, glioblastoma multiforme, non-small cell lung cancer and renal cell carcinoma (reviewed by Arteaga, Chinratanalab and Carter (2001)). In experimental models, inhibition of EGFR function by receptor tyrosine kinase (RTK) inhibitors or selective EGFR antibodies led to a significant reduction of VEGF expression, angiogenesis, and tumor growth in mice.

Second, the constitutively active receptor tyrosine kinase HER2/neu (ErbB2) is also known to induce VEGF and angiogenesis in tumors (Kumar and Yarmand-Bagheri, 2001). Studies of NIH 3T3 fibroblasts that had been transformed with mutant HER2/neu demonstrated significant induction of VEGF expression, and the magnitude of this effect was further elevated by exposure to hypoxia (Petit *et al.*, 1997). Laughner and colleagues subsequently showed that HER2/neu overexpression in mouse 3T3 cells led to increased activity of hypoxia-inducible factor 1α (HIF-1α) and consecutively VEGF expression in these cells (Laughner *et al.*, 2001). Their finding that heregulin stimulation led to HER2/neu transactivation in MCF-7 breast cancer cells suggested that similar mechanisms were also present in cancer cells that eventually up-regulate VEGF (Laughner *et al.*, 2001). As the HER2/neu receptor system has been implicated in the progression and angiogenesis of human breast cancer (and possibly lung or colon cancer as well), the development of neutralizing antibodies to HER2/neu has become a major focus in molecular cancer research. However, HER2/neu seems to be mostly relevant in the molecular pathology of breast cancer, as the majority of studies regarding VEGF regulation and its subsequent suppression by administration of various antibodies to HER-2/neu, have been conducted in preclinical breast cancer models. Petit *et al.* showed that treatment of the HER2/neu-positive human breast cancer cell line SKBR-3 with a specific neutralizing anti-HER2/neu monoclonal antibody (4D5) resulted in a dose-dependent reduction of VEGF protein expression in these cells (Petit *et al.*, 1997). In addition, the HER2/neu system may also regulate the expression of VEGF family members other than VEGF-A in human breast cancer; specifically, Yang *et al.* reported that HER2/neu expression correlated with VEGF-C and VEGF-D expression in human breast cancer specimens, as measured by immunohistochemical analysis (Yang *et al.*, 2002). HER2/neu may therefore contribute to the development of pro-angiogenic and pro-lymphangiogenic changes in the tumor microenvironment in a variety of types of cancer in humans.

Various ErbB family receptors elicit the ability to heterodimerize upon activation, which leads to significant increases in VEGF levels in cancer cells. For example, activation of the ErbB4 receptor system by its ligand heregulin-β1 has been shown to be an important mediator of VEGF expression in breast and lung cancer cells (Yen *et al.*, 2000). In these experiments, Yen *et al.* used a panel of human breast and lung cancer cell lines that either constitutively overexpressed ErbB2, or that were engineered to stably overexpress the ErbB2 receptor. The authors demonstrated hereby that heregulin induced VEGF secretion in most cancer cell lines but not in normal human mammary or bronchial primary cells (Yen *et al.*, 2000). This observation supports the concept of a relevant functional interplay in cancer cells between HER2 and other ErbB receptor systems such as ErbB3 and ErbB4 (reviewed by Arteaga, Chinratanalab and Carter (2001)). These findings indicate that the HER2 system is an important target for direct and indirect therapy of tumor angiogenesis, and clinical trials of inhibiting HER2 are currently ongoing.

Insulin-like growth factor-I receptor system

The insulin-like growth factor-I receptor (IGF-IR) is often overexpressed in a variety of human cancers, and its overexpression has been associated with aggressive disease and formation of metastases. Activation of IGF-IR by its major ligands, IGF-I and IGF-II (and insulin to a much lesser degree), initiates intracellular signaling, mainly via the mitogen-activated protein kinase (MAPK, also known as Erk1/2) and phosphatidylinositol 3′-kinase (PI-3K)/Akt pathways and downstream activation of transcription factors such as HIF-1α and nuclear factor-kappaB (NF-κB) (Figure 3.3).

The main source of IGF-I is the liver, a fact of tremendous importance for the development and growth of liver metastases derived from gastrointestinal (e.g. colon or pancreas) cancers that overexpress IGF-IR (Reinmuth *et al.*, 2002; Stoeltzing *et al.*, 2003b). Recent experimental models have clearly demonstrated the importance of the IGF-IR system for mediating angiogenesis by up-regulating VEGF expression in various neoplastic (Reinmuth *et al.*, 2002; Warren *et al.*, 1996) and non-neoplastic tissues (Smith *et al.*, 1999). In the latter, Smith and colleagues demonstrated that interaction of IGF-I with IGF-IR increased retinal neovascularization by up-regulating VEGF expression in retinal endothelial cells through activation of the MAPK signaling pathway (Smith *et al.*, 1999). In this model, IGF-IR activation was necessary for VEGF to have the maximum effect in ocular angiogenesis (Smith *et al.*, 1999). In neoplastic systems, IGF-I-mediated induction of VEGF in cancer cells *in vitro* has been reported for breast cancer cells (Oh *et al.*, 2002), endometrial adenocarcinoma cells (Bermont *et al.*, 2000) and colorectal cancer cells (Reinmuth *et al.*, 2002; Warren *et al.*, 1996). However, only a few studies have addressed the role of IGF-I and IGF-IR in tumor angiogenesis (i.e. regulation of VEGF expression) in primary tumors and metastases *in vivo*. Reinmuth and colleagues from our laboratory showed that inhibition of IGF-IR function (by transfection with a dominant-negative receptor construct) reduced VEGF expression *in vitro* in two human colon carcinoma cell lines (HT29 and KM12L4), which resulted in a significant reduction of angiogenesis and hepatic colorectal tumor growth in two different *in vivo* models (Reinmuth *et al.*, 2002). Tumors from the dominant-negative IGF-IR-transfected cell lines expressed less VEGF than did tumors from control cells (Reinmuth *et al.*, 2002). The anti-angiogenic and growth-inhibitory effects of a molecular IGF-IR blockade were even more pronounced in an orthotopic model of pancreatic cancer (Stoeltzing *et al.*, 2003b). Because IGF-IR is highly homologous to the insulin receptor, targeting this particular receptor has proven difficult; however, several agents are currently being evaluated in preclinical trials.

Hepatocyte growth factor

HGF, also known as scatter factor, has recently been shown to elicit pro-angiogenic activity by up-regulating VEGF expression in a variety of cancers (Sengupta *et al.*, 2003a). HGF is the primary ligand for the c-Met protooncogene, a transmembrane receptor tyrosine kinase that is primarily expressed in epithelial tissues. Numerous studies have implicated aberrant c-Met function in the progression and metastasis of human tumors such as colorectal cancer, pancreatic carcinoma, melanoma and osteosarcoma (reviewed by Danilkovitch-Miagkova and Zbar (2002)). However, the role of HGF as a paracrine factor in regulating the expression of certain pro-angiogenic factors by tumor cells has only recently been described (Dong *et al.*, 2001). In addition, a direct effect of HGF/c-Met signaling on VEGF expression in cancer cells has been demonstrated by several groups. In glioma cells (which are often positive for c-Met), treatment with HGF resulted in enhanced secretion of VEGF protein accompanied by increased transcription of VEGF mRNA in a dose-dependent fashion (Moriyama *et al.*, 1998). Using another tumor system, Dong and colleagues investigated the association of HGF/c-Met and VEGF regulation in serum samples from patients with head and neck squamous cell carcinoma. Their results showed that increases in serum HGF levels correlated with higher serum VEGF levels in these patients (Dong *et al.*, 2001). The authors further explored the association between HGF/c-Met activation and VEGF expression by treating various head and neck squamous cell carcinoma cell lines (which often overexpress c-Met) with recombinant HGF *in vitro*. These experiments led to identification of the MAPK (Erk1/2) and PI-3K/Akt signaling pathways as being the critical mediators for VEGF up-regulation in those tumor cells. The importance of the MAPK and PI-3K pathways for mediating HGF/c-Met induced VEGF expression has also been described in ECs (Sengupta *et al.*, 2003b). However, to date it has been difficult to effectively impair c-Met function by using inhibitors specific for this receptor tyrosine kinase.

Interleukin-1β

Certain cytokines have been implicated in angiogenesis in malignant disorders through their contribution to raising VEGF levels in the particular tumor microenvironment. One such cytokine, IL-1β, has been shown to induce VEGF expression in human colon cancer cells by activating its corresponding receptor, IL-1R (Akagi *et al.*, 1999). This up-regulation of VEGF upon stimulation with

IL-1β occurred through increased promoter activity and transcriptional regulation of the VEGF gene (Akagi *et al.*, 1999). Yano and colleagues recently demonstrated that overexpressing IL-1β, by means of stable transfection, led to up-regulation of various cytokines, including VEGF, in human lung cancer cells (Yano *et al.*, 2003). In their experimental model of lung cancer, IL-1β-overexpressing cells formed significantly more lung metastases, which was associated with a higher degree of vascularization in metastases. These effects were abrogated by treatment with an antibody to IL-1β (Yano *et al.*, 2003). The IL-1/IL-1R system may contribute to VEGF expression in a variety of cell systems, and inhibition of IL-1β-induced angiogenesis by the administration of IL-1-binding antibodies is currently being investigated in other experimental models. In fact, inhibition of IL-1/IL-1R is effective in the treatment of arthritis, a disease known to depend on angiogenesis.

Interleukin-6

Another cytokine that elicits pro-angiogenic properties *in vivo* by modulating VEGF expression is IL-6. This effect is mediated by interaction of IL-6 with the alpha chain of the IL-6 receptor (IL-6R) and subsequent receptor tyrosine kinase activation. In cervical carcinomas, IL-6 has been shown to promote tumor growth *in vivo* (Wei *et al.*, 2001). Wei and associates showed that this effect was caused by increased VEGF expression and increased angiogenesis in C33A cervical tumor cells (Wei *et al.*, 2003); using gene promoters and dominant-negative transfection, they also identified the STAT3 signaling pathway as being the exclusive pathway for mediating IL-6-induced up-regulation of VEGF in those cells. IL-6 has additionally been implicated in the pathogenesis and neo-vascularization of gastric (Huang *et al.*, 2002) and pancreatic carcinomas (Masui *et al.*, 2002) by up-regulating VEGF. Masui and colleagues used immunohisto-chemical staining to demonstrate the frequent expression of the IL-6R in human pancreatic cancer specimens and showed that stimulating the pancreatic cancer cell line CFPAC-1 with IL-6 led to up-regulation of VEGF expression in those cells (Masui *et al.*, 2002). However, the significance of the IL-6/IL-6R system in the regulation of angiogenic molecules such as VEGF *in vivo* remains to be elucidated.

Hypoxia-inducible factor-1α

One of the strongest natural inducers of VEGF expression in both normal and malignant tissues is hypoxia. This induction is physiologically mediated through the activity of the transcription factor HIF-1α. Under non-hypoxic conditions, HIF-1α is rapidly ubiquitinated and degraded. This process requires a functional protein encoded by the von Hippel-Lindau (VHL) tumor suppressor gene (Krieg *et al.*, 2000). Upon exposure to low oxygen-tension levels, a very common condition in tumors (Helmlinger *et al.*, 1997), HIF-1α forms heterodimers with the constitutively expressed HIF-1β subunit (Wang *et al.*, 1995). This heterodimerization is necessary for creation of an active HIF-1 complex (the dimer of HIF-1α and HIF-1β), which subsequently translocates into the nucleus in order to bind to the consensus sequence 'hypoxia-response element' (HRE). This step eventually initiates transcriptional activity of target genes such as VEGF, erythropoietin, transferrin, endothelin-1, inducible nitric oxide synthase and IGF-II (Wang *et al.*, 1995). HIF-1α also has a pivotal role in cancer angiogenesis and metastasis and is often overexpressed in a variety of human cancers and their metastases (Zhong *et al.*, 1999). Constitutive HIF-1α activation in human cancer has been associated with high VEGF expression levels and development of a pro-angiogenic tumor microenvironment. However, this constitutive activation of HIF-1α can occur by either of two ways – through inhibition of its degradation or through an increase in its expression, or both. In addition to hypoxic regulation of HIF-1 activation, some hypoxia-independent mechanisms have also been described. Several studies have shown that genetic alterations of tumor suppressor genes (e.g. *p53*, *VHL*, *PTEN*) and oncogenes (e.g. Src, HER2/neu, H-Ras) can induce HIF-1 activity in tumor tissues, through either its overexpression or inhibition of its degradation. Further, activation of certain growth factor receptors such as IGF-IR has been shown to up-regulate HIF-1α expression, and subsequently VEGF, in human colon carcinoma cells (Fukuda *et al.*, 2002). Studies in our laboratory validated the existence of this IGF-I/IGF-IR/HIF-1α signaling pathway in pancreatic cancer cells, where HIF-1α seems to be in part constitutively activated by an IGF-IR autocrine loop (Stoeltzing *et al.*, 2003b).

Findings from these and other studies suggest that HIF-1α could be an effective molecular target for the treatment of solid malignancies. As specific inhibitors of HIF-1α are not available at this time, the effects of *in vivo* inhibition of HIF-1α function on tumor growth and angiogenesis in solid malignancies remain to be elucidated.

Nuclear transcription factors: Nf-κB and AP-1

Two transcription factors that have been identified as important regulators of VEGF expression, located at the downstream end of the signaling cascade, are NF-κB and AP-1. For a variety of target genes (e.g. VEGF) it has been validated that their expression is under the control of both factors. NF-κB is often co-activated by signaling pathways that also regulate the activity of AP-1. However, NF-κB and AP-1 are both part of signaling cascades that are often shared by activated receptors of growth factors (EGF), cytokines (interleukin-1α) or oncogenes (HER-2/neu) or that participate in cellular reactions to hypoxia (Bancroft *et al.*, 2002). Through these mechanisms, NF-κB and AP-1 can be constitutively activated and contribute to high VEGF expression levels in cancer cells (Bancroft *et al.*, 2001). Inhibition of NF-κB function by transfection with a dominant-negative construct has been shown to decrease VEGF levels and reduce angiogenesis *in vivo* (Shibata *et al.*, 2002). Interestingly, inhibition of EGFR function also decreased NF-κB activity and VEGF promoter activity in head and neck squamous cell carcinoma cells (Bancroft *et al.*, 2002). Given the fact that NF-κB is regulated by multiple signaling pathways, the development of inhibitors of NF-κB may be another promising approach for lowering VEGF levels in cancer cells.

Other factors associated with angiogenesis in tumors

Besides the implication of VEGF in neoplastic angiogenesis, some other factors have been identified as crucial regulators of endothelial cell survival and stabilization. Some factor may specifically control the survival of EC (such as angiopoietins), whereas other factors contribute to EC stability/function by either recruiting periendothelial supportive cells (pericytes) or direct interaction with endothelial cell receptors (e.g. integrins). This section provides an overview on some relevant molecules involved in tumor angiogenesis that has also led to the development of some anti-angiogenesis targeted strategies.

Angiopoietins

Angiopoietins constitute a family of angiogenic factors identified as specific for the vascular endothelium, which results from the restricted distribution of the angiopoietin tyrosine kinase receptor Tie-2 (also known as TEK) to ECs (Partanen *et al.*, 1992; Suri *et al.*, 1996). Tie-1 is an orphan receptor whose ligand has not been identified to date. Of the four currently known angiopoietins (Ang-1 to Ang-4), the best characterized are Ang-1 and Ang-2, both of which exert their biologic function through the Tie-2 receptor (Holash, Wiegand and Yancopoulos, 1999). Ang-1 may control the ability of ECs to stabilize the structure and modulate blood vessel function. It is likely that Ang-1 works in conjunction with VEGF to help stabilize vascular networks. Ang-1 functions as a survival factor, as it dose-dependently inhibited apoptosis of serum-deprived EC cultures, an effect augmented by addition of VEGF (Ellis *et al.*, 2002; Suri *et al.*, 1996). Moreover, the stabilizing effect of Ang-1 seems to be dependent on the Tie-2 receptor, since addition of a soluble form of the Tie-2, but not Tie-1 receptor, completely blocked the effects of Ang-1. Ang-1 also appears to recruit periendothelial support cells, and this interaction may be required for EC survival. This is evidenced by the fact that Ang-1 knockout embryos are able to undergo VEGF-dependent angiogenesis; however, ECs are unable to further interact with periendothelial cells.

Ang-2 is thought to antagonize the stabilizing action of Ang-1. It also binds the Tie-2 receptor but fails to induce phosphorylation, thus leading to EC destabilization. In the presence of VEGF, vessel destabilization by Ang-2 has been hypothesized to induce an angiogenic response. However, in the absence of VEGF, Ang-2 leads to vessel regression (Maisonpierre et al., 1997). In experimental models, stable overexpression led to inhibition of tumor growth and angiogenesis (Ahmad et al., 2001; Stoeltzing et al., 2002, 2003a). In addition, Ang-1 overexpression led to significant increases in pericyte coverage of tumor vessels in hepatic colon cancer metastases (Stoeltzing et al., 2003a). However, future studies are needed to further understand the importance of angiopoietins in cancer and evaluate their usefulness as targets in antiangiogenic therapy.

Platelet-derived growth factor-B (PDGF-B)

The family of PDGFs consists of four different isoforms, PDGF-A, PDGF-B, PDGF-C and PDGF-D. PDGF-A and B can form homodimers and heterodimers by disulfide bonding, whereas the recently discovered PDGF-C and PDGF-D isoforms (Cao et al., 2002) seem to be expressed only as homodimers. PDGF-A and B bind to homo- or heterodimers of PDGF-receptor (PDGFR-) α or PDGFR-β proteins on the cell surface (Bergsten et al., 2001). PDGFs promote angiogenesis in vivo by regulating EC survival and pericyte (vascular smooth muscle cell) recruitment (Guo et al., 2003; Reinmuth et al., 2001). PDGFs can also regulate angiogenesis indirectly by inducing VEGF in some types of cell. Stimulation of pericytes with recombinant PDGF-BB may increase VEGF expression by up-regulating its transcription, an effect mediated by the PI-3K/Akt signaling pathway (Reinmuth et al., 2001). This paracrine mechanism of VEGF secretion has important implications for the survival of ECs in vivo. Overexpression of PDGF-B and PDGFR-β in human gliomas has been shown to be responsible for recruiting pericytes to vessels (Guo et al., 2003). Overexpression of PDGF-B in glioma cells seems to enhance the formation of intracranial gliomas by stimulating VEGF expression in neovessels and by attracting vessel-associated pericytes (Guo et al., 2003).

In cells derived from neurofibromas, PDGF-BB can directly induce VEGF expression, an effect mediated by the MAPK signaling pathway; this mechanism seems to underlie the molecular pathology of highly vascularized neurofibromas (Kotsuji-Maruyama et al., 2002). The PDGFR system has become a promising target for anti-angiogenic regimens, as shown by Shaheen and associates in 2001 (Shaheen et al., 2001) and Bergers et al. in 2003 (Bergers et al., 2003). These investigators demonstrated that adding inhibition of PDGFR activity to inhibitors of VEGFR activity enhanced the anti-angiogenic effect in vivo. Clinical trials of dual-kinase inhibitors to both VEGFR and PDGFR are ongoing.

Interleukin-8 (IL-8)

The pro-inflammatory molecule IL-8 belongs to a large family of chemokines, which was initially described as a neutrophil chemoattractant (Matsushima, Baldwin and Mukaida, 1992). IL-8 is expressed in many different cell types, including several human cancer cell lines. In *in vitro* studies, IL-8 has been proven to promote cell proliferation and growth of tumor cells in an autocrine manner (Arenberg *et al.*, 1996). In addition, IL-8 acts as a pro-angiogenic factor by inducing proliferation and chemotaxis of ECs (Kasahara *et al.*, 1991). The pro-angiogenic effect of IL-8 has also been recognized in experimental models of pancreatic cancer (Bruns *et al.*, 2000; Shi *et al.*, 1999) and melanoma (Huang *et al.*, 2000). However, IL-8 does not seem to be constitutively up-regulated in cancer cells; its overexpression occurs rather upon unspecific stimulation (growth factors; hypoxia) and in orchestration with up-regulation of other angiogenic molecules (such as VEGF and bFGF).

Integrins

The integrins are cell surface receptors and represent a large family of cell adhesion receptors. They are heterodimeric transmembrane receptor complexes, composed of non-covalently bound α and β chains. At present, 18 α and eight β subunits are known, forming 24 different $\alpha\beta$ heterodimers and thereby defining ligand specificities (reviewed by Hynes (1992) and Ivaska and Heino (2000)). Integrins can mediate cellular adhesion to ECM proteins and to adjacent cells. Beyond this cell adhesion function, integrins have recently been identified as being involved in crucial intracellular signaling pathways. Despite lacking cytoplasmic kinase activity, they may contribute to EC survival, migration (adhesion) and proliferation (angiogenesis), respectively. Ligands for integrins include fibronectin, collagen and vitronectin as components of the ECM. Certain integrins can also bind to soluble ligands such as fibrinogen or to counter-receptors such as intracellular adhesion molecules on adjacent cells. In addition, they are able to enhance the receptor function of VEGFR-2 (Miyamoto *et al.*, 1996; Soldi *et al.*, 1999).

In particular, the integrins $\alpha_V\beta_3$ and $\alpha_V\beta_5$ (and potentially $\beta1$ integrin complexes) play a major role in angiogenesis (Friedlander *et al.*, 1996; Senger *et al.*, 1997). The interaction of $\alpha_V\beta_3$ and the ECM has been identified as a crucial event for EC survival in nascent vessels (Brooks, Clark and Cheresh, 1994). Therefore, antagonists and small neutralizing peptides to these receptors have been developed as a potential antiangiogenic strategy. To date, the integrin $\alpha_V\beta_3$ seems to be the dominant integrin involved in angiogenesis. Although it is only minimally expressed in quiescent blood vessels, it is significantly up-regulated during angiogenesis *in vivo* (Brooks, Clark and Cheresh, 1994). Further, $\alpha_V\beta_3$ is involved in activation of VEGFR-2 by enhancing its mitogenic potential after binding to VEGF-165. Inhibition of $\alpha_V\beta_3$ function by an anti-β_3 integrin mono-clonal antibody leads to decreased tyrosine phosphorylation of VEGFR-2, reducing activation of downstream signals and diminishing biologic effects triggered by VEGF-165 (Soldi *et al.*, 1999). Interestingly, hypoxic conditions, as present in the center of the tumor, seem to regulate the expression of $\alpha_V\beta_3$ as well. ECs cultured under hypoxic conditions showed increased attachment to fibrinogen, a process that is mediated by $\alpha_V\beta_3$, and up-regulated expression of $\alpha_V\beta_3$. In contrast, the expression of $\alpha_V\beta_5$ was not affected by this process (Walton *et al.*, 2000).

3.3 Angiogenesis and metastasis formation

As mentioned briefly in the introduction, metastases develop through a series of sequential and interlinked steps, each of which is essential for the establish-ment and progression of a metastatic lesion. Two major early steps in the for-mation of distant metastases are proliferation of tumor cells in the primary lesion and creation of an extensive vascularization network from pre-existing vessels (vessel cooption). As a third step, tumor cells must also invade the extra-cellular matrix (ECM) to enter the bloodstream, lymphatic channels or both. The process of invasion is supported by a reduction in cell-to-cell adhesion, an increase in cell motility, and the secretion of ECM-degrading enzymes such as matrix metalloproteinases, cathepsins and plasminogen activators (Fidler, 1995). After entry into the circulation, tumor cells can form aggregates with leukocytes and platelets, thereby increasing the probability of their forming tumor emboli in distant capillary beds. Tumor cells can attach to the vascular endothelium, induce endothelial retraction and subsequently bind to glycoproteins of the basement membrane by specific cell-surface receptors. Subsequently, some tumor cells extravasate into the parenchyma at a metastatic organ site. Further prolif-eration within the organ parenchyma is controlled by the interplay of growth stimulatory and inhibitory factors in the local organ microenvironment. Only metastatic cells that express adequate amounts of the receptors that correspond to locally produced growth stimulatory factors will grow (Fidler, 1995). For the next step, the production of macroscopically detectable lesions, the metastases must develop an adequate vascular network (Fidler and Ellis, 1994). Interest-ingly, results from a recent study suggested that metastatic cells may also form tumors invasion independently, but in dependence on angiogenesis (Sugino *et al.*, 2002).

  Therefore, angiogenesis is not only an essential process for outgrowth of the primary tumor lesions, and the basis for hematogenous tumor cell dissemina-tion, it is also required for the growth and establishment of distant metastases. This section will describe the influence of an organ microenvironment on tumor angiogenesis plus the relevance of angiogenesis for metastases formation in various cancer entities (solid tumors).

Role of tumor micro-environment in angiogenesis

For future vascular targeting strategies, it is important to realize that tumor vasculature in primary tumor lesions will be distinct from that observed in their metastases. The organ microenvironment at the metastatic organ site plays a substantial role in the development of a microvasculature in tumor metastases. In addition, the organ preference for metastatic colonization is influenced by communication between the circulating tumor cell and the target host tissue.

The effect of an organ microenvironment on tumor biology has been recognized for more than 100 years, since Paget's 'seed and soil' hypothesis. It has now been generally accepted that microenvironment influences tumor biology. Significant discrepancies in vascularization, growth rate, metastatic potential and efficacy of systemic treatment between ectopic and orthotopic tumors have been reported in experimental studies (Fidler, 1995; Kitadai et al., 1995; Paget, 1989). The tumor cell's microenvironment is composed of heterogeneous cells as well as the extracellular matrix (ECM). Each component of the microenvironment can interact with the others and with the tumor cell. Since angiogenesis is essential for metastasis formation and growth (Fidler and Ellis, 1994; Folkman, 1990), site-specific microenvironmental regulation of angiogenesis is one of the most important determinants of the organ preference of metastases. The microenvironment not only consists of organ-specific cells such as hepatocytes, but also endothelial cells, pericytes, inflammatory cells, fibroblasts and the ECM. The observation that blood vessel growth is controlled by the microenvironment rather than by some intrinsic genetic endothelial program is also supported by transplantation studies in the quail chick system (Pardanaud et al., 1987). Endothelial cells lose organ-specific characteristics when they are isolated from the organ environment and cultured in vitro (Jung et al., 2000; Takahashi et al., 1995). These studies highlight the importance of understanding the biological heterogeneity of tumor angiogenesis and the redundancy of angiogenic factor expression in specific organ microenvironments.

Tumor vascularization in metastases

The importance of tumor angiogenesis and development of a microvasculature in metastases has been well recognized and intensively studied over the past decades. Microvessel density, vessel structure and microvessel function in metastatic lesions may differ widely among tumor types and organ sites, due to differences in tumor microenvironment and biological behavior of the primary tumor entity. In order to investigate neoplastic vascularization and vessel function in human (and mouse) primary and metastatic tumor tissues, various approaches and methods have been applied, including immunohistochemical analyses, ultrastructural analyses (electron microscopy), fluorescent in vivo imaging of tumor vessels and many other experimental models of angiogenesis (reviewed by Staton *et al.* (2004)).

To study angiogenesis in human tumor specimens using current technology, it is necessary to obtain tissue for histological evaluation. The standard for evaluation of vascularization in a human tumor specimen is to highlight the tumor endothelium with antibodies that differentiate ECs from other cells within the tumor. For this purpose, endothelial-specific antibodies such as FVIII-RA, CD31/PECAM-1, VE-cadherin and CD34 have been used in immunohistochemical staining procedures. However, the second, and much more difficult, step is the rating and appropriate interpretation of stained tumor sections. One of the most common parameters for rating tumor angiogenesis is calculation of microvessel density (MVD), which was considered to be the 'gold standard'. Various methods and guidelines for determining MVD in tumors have been described, based on the initial method reported by Weidner *et al.* (Takahashi *et al.*, 1996; Weidner *et al.*, 1991). For example vessels may be counted by choosing the five most vascularized areas in a tumor and counting the vessels in these areas under higher magnification. Vessels can also be quantified using image analysis (densitometry: vessel area as parameter of functional vascular volume) or vessel density can be graded on a scale 0+ to 3+, with being 3+ the most vascular. In addition, the degree of angiogenesis can be assessed by counting numbers of branch-points or measuring inter-capillary distance. In the era of anti-angiogenic therapy, it has become even more difficult to objectively assess tumor vascularization. Due to effects such as tumor shrinkage, reduction of interstitial pressure and 'vessel normalization' by an anti-angiogenic and anti-neoplastic therapy regimen, the simple determination of MVD may not reflect these profound changes. Further studies are required to identify optimal biomarkers for monitoring tumor angiogenesis in patients receiving anti-angiogenic therapy.

This section gives an overview on studies that provide evidence for the role of the microvasculature in metastases formation of solid malignancies.

Gastrointestinal cancers

The survival of tumors and thus their metastases are dependent upon creation of a sufficient vascular network. Several growth factors and cytokines have been identified that regulate angiogenesis in cancers of the gastrointestinal tract (reviewed by Reinmuth *et al.* (2003)). However, abundant studies have predominantly correlated increased expression of VEGF in primary tumors of gastrointestinal cancer entities (i.e. gastric, pancreatic and colorectal cancer) with angiogenesis and subsequent metastasis.

For gastric cancer, several investigators have demonstrated that microvessel density is associated with tumor progression and poor prognosis. In an early study, Maeda and colleagues reported on 124 gastric cancer specimens and showed that increasing MVD correlated with lymph node metastasis, hepatic metastasis and poor prognosis (Maeda *et al.*, 1995). Similar findings were reported by another group, investigating MVD in intestinal type gastric cancer (Araya *et al.*, 1997). An elevated vascularization and MVD in gastric tumors has been associated with increased vascular invasion (Maehara *et al.*, 2000), tumor size plus lymph node metastasis (Xiangming *et al.*, 1998) and poor prognosis. In a recent study, Du and colleagues investigated MVD and VEGF expression in gastric cancer and esophageal cancers. Again, tumor vascularization, as reflected by MVD, was correlated to metastasis development (Du *et al.*, 2003). Interestingly, the histologic classification of gastric cancer, i.e. diffuse-type versus intestinal-type cancer, may also have an influence on the angiogenic phenotype of these tumors. Takahashi *et al.* demonstrated that vessel counts (and VEGF expression) were significantly higher in intestinal-type tumors than in the diffuse type (Takahashi *et al.*, 1996).

In colorectal cancers, the role of VEGF and microvasculature in primary tumors has been studied most comprehensively. Results from these studies led to the development of new angiogenesis targeting strategies, such as the treatment of patients with specific antibodies to VEGF (bevacizumab). Increased microvessel density in colorectal tumors has been linked to hematogenous metastasis (Vermeulen *et al.*, 1999) and tumor progression (Takebayashi *et al.*, 1996). The liver is the most common site for development of colorectal metastases. Most metastatic tumors in the liver are supplied by the hepatic artery, although the portal blood flow may contribute to the tumor blood supply to varying degrees. Few reports are available on tumor vessel origin and vascularization of liver metastasis (Gervaz *et al.*, 2000; Terayama *et al.*, 1996a, 1996b). Terayama *et al.* used immunohistochemical analysis to study the diameter of tumor vessels in human tumor specimens. Angiogenesis of liver metastases progressed in a stepwise fashion as the metastases grew and as capillaries appeared in sinusoidal endothelium around the metastases (Terayama *et al.*, 1996a, 1996b). However, it is interesting to note that colorectal liver metastases may develop a vascular network that is less dependent on VEGF expression. In an experimental study, it has been verified that human colon cancer cells growing in the cecum of nude mice produced more VEGF than did cells in the liver (intermediate) or in the subcutis (lowest) (Jung *et al.*, 2000). In another study of primary colon cancer and hepatic metastases from 17 patients who had tumors removed from both sites, it has been found that 11 of 17 patients had higher VEGF levels in the primary tumor than in the liver metastases. In contrast, bFGF expression was roughly equal at the primary and the metastatic sites (Jung *et al.*, 2000).

Similar reports on angiogenesis and metastasis formation are available for pancreatic cancer (adenocarcinoma) (Linder *et al.*, 2001). Increased microvessel density has been shown to contribute to progressive disease, metastasis formation and poor prognosis for patients (Ikeda *et al.*, 1999; Linder *et al.*, 2001).

In experimental models, creation of aggressively growing pancreatic cancer cell lines led to the establishment of highly vascularized tumors (increased VEGF expression) and metastases (Bruns *et al.*, 2000; Sato *et al.*, 2000). Besides loco regional lymph nodes, liver is the most common site for metastasis formation.

Breast cancer

Axillary lymph node status is the most important prognostic factor in operable breast cancer, but experimental and clinical evidence suggests that the process of metastasis is also angiogenesis dependent (Hayes, 1994; Weidner *et al.*, 1991). Various angiogenic growth factors and cytokines induce neovascularization in breast cancer, namely members of the vascular endothelial growth factor (VEGF) gene families (Gunningham *et al.*, 2001; Kim *et al.*, 2004a; Rajesh *et al.*, 2004). The expression of these molecules may also be regulated by certain oncogenes such as Her-2/neu and Src (see above). Comparably to colorectal cancer, a tremendous amount of studies have been published on the relation of angiogenesis and metastasis formation in human breast cancer. Again, a strong correlation has been found between VEGF expression and increased tumor microvasculature, malignancy, and metastasis in breast cancer. Relevant metastatic organ sites for breast cancer metastasis formation include the brain, the bone (discussed under prostate cancer), the liver and the lung (discussed under NSCLC). In a recent report, Kim and colleagues demonstrated that VEGF plus IL-8 are predominant promoters of vascularization in brain metastases of human breast cancer tumors (Kim *et al.*, 2004a). In their study, the authors selected variant human metastatic breast cancer cells by re-culturing cells after three cycles of orthotopic implantation. Subsequently, the metastasis-selected cells showed increased potential for experimental brain metastasis and mice injected with these cells had significantly shorter mean survival than mice injected with the original cell line. In addition, brain metastatic lesions of the selected variants contained significantly more CD31-positive blood vessels (MVD) than metastases of the non-selected cell line. The variants selected from brain metastases released significantly more VEGF-A and IL-8 into culture supernatants than the original cell line, when cultured under non-hypoxic conditions (Kim *et al.*, 2004a). In addition to VEGF and cytokines, the activation of hormone receptors (estrogen receptor) may also contribute to significant angiogenesis in brain tumors, as early investigations by Schackert *et al.* demonstrated (Schackert *et al.*, 1989).

Prostate cancer

The process and implication of angiogenesis in prostate cancer growth has been the focus of many investigations over the past decade. Similar to other solid

malignancies, VEGF seems here to be one of the driving forces for tumor vascularization and metastasis formation, in conjunction with hormones and
growth factors (Balbay *et al.*, 1999; Chevalier *et al.*, 2002; Inoue *et al.*, 2000).
The bone is one of the preferred metastatic sites of prostate cancer and VEGF
is thought to be a promoter of bone metastasis formation in this tumor type.
However, the growth of metastatic prostate cancer cells in the bone involves an
intimate interaction between the tumor cells and various elements of the bone
microenvironment, resulting in increased rate of bone turnover and rapid tumor
growth. Evidence of an angiogenesis-dependent growth of prostate cancer bone
tumors is provided at least by two recent studies (Kim *et al.*, 2004b; Uehara
et al., 2003). Both Uehara *et al.* and Kim *et al.* demonstrated that interference
with either the PDGFR or EGFR system, or the combination of both, significantly reduces angiogenesis and growth of bone metastases. The authors additionally showed selective apoptosis of tumor endothelial cells upon this treatment
with RTKs to EGFR or PDGFR, suggesting that neoplastic vascularization in
bone metastases is an essential process for further progression and spread (Kim
et al., 2004b; Uehara *et al.*, 2003).

Lung cancer (NSCLC)

Lung cancer is the most common cause of death by malignancy in industrial-
ized countries. Only a few patients can be cured or an acceptable long-term
survival achieved. This poor prognosis is in part related to certain molecular
characteristics of tumors. In this section, the role of angiogenesis in growth
and progression of non-small-cell lung cancer will be described. The implication of microvessel density on the survival of patients with NSCLC has been
investigated in many studies. A recently published meta-analysis by Meert *et
al.* clearly supported the hypothesis that increased tumor vascularization of
primary NSCLC correlates with progression and poor prognosis (Meert *et al.*,
2002). The authors analyzed 32 reported studies on MVD analyses of human
cancer tissues (NSCLC), which had been stained with either FVIII, CD34 or
CD31, and concluded that high MVD (reflecting tumor angiogenesis) would
contribute to poor survival of surgically treated patients (Meert *et al.*,
2002).

In non-small-cell lung carcinomas, most reports show an association between
neovascularization and VEGF expression as well as the presence of metastases,
although a few reports do not agree with these findings (Fontanini *et al.*, 1997).
Although small cell lung cancers (SCLCs) may elicit a higher degree of vascularization, a clear correlation of VEGF expression and angiogenesis has been
shown only for NSCLC (Stefanou *et al.*, 2004). In addition to VEGF, certain
cytokines like IL-8 may also promote neovascularization in NSCLC (Yuan
et al., 2002), and activation growth factor receptors of the EGF family
(Galligioni and Ferro, 2001; Nguyen and Schrump, 2004).

The lung is a common organ site for the establishment of secondary malignancies derived from gastrointestinal and extra-intestinal cancers. Interestingly, it has been reported that metastatic tumor growth in the lung does not even require an invasion of tumor cells into lung parenchyma, but rather depends on angiogenesis (Sugino *et al.*, 2002). Sugino *et al.* showed that tumor cells, which express certain angiogenic profiles, were able to establish intravascular tumor growth in the lung without penetration of the vascular wall (Sugino *et al.*, 2002). This suggests that, in addition to primary tumor growth of NSCLC (and SCLC), neovascularization is required for metastatic tumor growth in the lung or lung capillaries.

3.4 Summary

Tumor angiogenesis is an essential process for the development and outgrowth of metastatic lesions at organ sites remote from the primary tumor. Only by establishing a sufficient microvascular network will, metastases be able to survive, grow and spread. However, it is important to realize that the organ microenvironment significantly impacts the angiogenic process in metastases, leading to substantial differences in vascular morphology, vascular function and molecular profiles of tumor endothelial cells. The aspects 'angiogenesis' and 'neoplastic microvasculature' represent important parameters of tumor biology. Therefore, it seems very promising to specifically target neoplastic microvasculature in order to obtain a relevant biologic effect in tumors. Impairing the microvasculature function in primary tumors and their metastases by using modern molecular targeted agents may significantly inhibit growth and metastatic spread. A profound understanding of the biology of metastases and their microvasculature is essential for the development of successful innovative cancer therapeutics.

References

Achen, M.G., Jeltsch, M., Kukk, E., Makinen, T., Vitali, A., Wilks, A.F., Alitalo, K. and Stacker, S.A. (1998). Vascular endothelial growth factor D (VEGF-D) is a ligand for the tyrosine kinases VEGF receptor 2 (Flk1) and VEGF receptor 3 (Flt4). *Proc Natl Acad Sci USA* **95**, 548–553.

Ahmad, S.A., Liu, W., Jung, Y.D., Fan, F., Wilson, M., Reinmuth, N., Shaheen, R.M., Bucana, C.D. and Ellis, L.M. (2001). The effects of angiopoietin-1 and -2 on tumor growth and angiogenesis in human colon cancer. *Cancer Res*, **61**, 1255–1259.

Akagi, Y., Liu, W., Xie, K., Zebrowski, B., Shaheen, R.M. and Ellis, L.M. (1999). Regulation of vascular endothelial growth factor expression in human colon cancer by interleukin-1beta. *Br J Cancer* **80**, 1506–1511.

Araya, M., Terashima, M., Takagane, A., Abe, K., Nishizuka, S., Yonezawa, H., Irinoda, T., Nakaya, T. and Saito, K. (1997). Microvessel count predicts metastasis and prognosis in patients with gastric cancer. *J Surg Oncol* **65**, 232–236.

Arenberg, D.A., Kunkel, S.L., Polverini, P.J., Glass, M., Burdick, M.D. and Strieter, R.M. (1996). Inhibition of interleukin-8 reduces tumorigenesis of human non-small cell lung cancer in SCID mice. *J Clin Invest* **97**, 2792–2802.

Arteaga, C.L., Chinratanalab, W. and Carter, M.B. (2001). Inhibitors of HER2/neu (erbB-2) signal transduction. *Semin Oncol* **28**, 30–35.

Balbay, M.D., Pettaway, C.A., Kuniyasu, H., Inoue, K., Ramirez, E., Li, E., Fidler, I.J. and Dinney, C.P. (1999). Highly metastatic human prostate cancer growing within the prostate of athymic mice overexpresses vascular endothelial growth factor. *Clin Cancer Res* **5**, 783–789.

Bancroft, C.C., Chen, Z., Dong, G., Sunwoo, J.B., Yeh, N., Park, C. and Van Waes, C. (2001). Coexpression of proangiogenic factors IL-8 and VEGF by human head and neck squamous cell carcinoma involves coactivation by MEK-MAPK and IKK-NF-kappaB signal pathways. *Clin Cancer Res* **7**, 435–442.

Bancroft, C.C., Chen, Z., Yeh, J., Sunwoo, J.B., Yeh, N.T., Jackson, S., Jackson, C. and Van Waes, C. (2002). Effects of pharmacologic antagonists of epidermal growth factor receptor, PI3K and MEK signal kinases on NF-kappaB and AP-1 activation and IL-8 and VEGF expression in human head and neck squamous cell carcinoma lines. *Int J Cancer* **99**, 538–548.

Bergers, G., Song, S., Meyer-Morse, N., Bergsland, E. and Hanahan, D. (2003). Benefits of targeting both pericytes and endothelial cells in the tumor vasculature with kinase inhibitors. *J Clin Invest* **111**, 1287–1295.

Bergsten, E., Uutela, M., Li, X., Pietras, K., Ostman, A., Heldin, C.H., Alitalo, K. and Eriksson, U. (2001). PDGF-D is a specific, protease-activated ligand for the PDGF beta-receptor. *Nat Cell Biol* **3**, 512–516.

Bermont, L., Lamielle, F., Fauconnet, S., Esumi, H., Weisz, A. and Adessi, G.L. (2000). Regulation of vascular endothelial growth factor expression by insulin-like growth factor-I in endometrial adenocarcinoma cells. *Int J Cancer* **85**, 117–123.

Brooks, P.C., Clark, R.A. and Cheresh, D.A. (1994). Requirement of vascular integrin alpha v beta 3 for angiogenesis. *Science* **264**, 569–571.

Bruns, C.J., Harbison, M.T., Davis, D.W., Portera, C.A., Tsan, R., McConkey, D.J., Evans, D.B., Abbruzzese, J.L., Hicklin, D.J. and Radinsky, R. (2000). Epidermal growth factor receptor blockade with C225 plus gemcitabine results in regression of human pancreatic carcinoma growing orthotopically in nude mice by antiangiogenic mechanisms. *Clin Cancer Res* **6**, 1936–1948.

Cao, R., Brakenhielm, E., Li, X., Pietras, K., Widenfalk, J., Ostman, A., Eriksson, U. and Cao, Y. (2002). Angiogenesis stimulated by PDGF-CC, a novel member in the PDGF family, involves activation of PDGFR-alphaalpha and -alphabeta receptors. *FASEB J* **16**, 1575–1583.

Carmeliet, P. and Jain, R.K. (2000). Angiogenesis in cancer and other diseases. *Nature* **407**, 249–257.

Cheung, N., Wong, M.P., Yuen, S.T., Leung, S.Y. and Chung, L.P. (1998). Tissue-specific expression pattern of vascular endothelial growth factor isoforms in the malignant transformation of lung and colon. *Hum Pathol* **29**, 910–914.

Chevalier, S., Defoy, I., Lacoste, J., Hamel, L., Guy, L., Begin, L.R. and Aprikian, A.G. (2002). Vascular endothelial growth factor and signaling in the prostate: more than angiogenesis. *Mol Cell Endocrinol* **189**, 169–179.

Danilkovitch-Miagkova, A. and Zbar, B. (2002). Dysregulation of Met receptor tyrosine kinase activity in invasive tumors. *J Clin Invest* **109**, 863–867.

Dong, G., Chen, Z., Li, Z.Y., Yeh, N.T., Bancroft, C.C. and Van Waes, C. (2001). Hepatocyte growth factor/scatter factor-induced activation of MEK and PI3K signal pathways contributes to expression of proangiogenic cytokines interleukin-8 and vascular endothelial growth factor in head and neck squamous cell carcinoma. *Cancer Res* **61**, 5911–5918.

Du, J.R., Jiang, Y., Zhang, Y.M. and Fu, H. (2003). Vascular endothelial growth factor and microvascular density in esophageal and gastric carcinomas. *World J Gastroenterol* **9**, 1604–1606.

Duque, J.L., Loughlin, K.R., Adam, R.M., Kantoff, P.W., Zurakowski, D. and Freeman, M.R. (1999). Plasma levels of vascular endothelial growth factor are increased in patients with metastatic prostate cancer. *Urology* **54**, 523–527.

Dvorak, H.F., Detmar, M., Claffey, K.P., Nagy, J.A., van de Water, L. and Senger, D.R. (1995). Vascular permeability factor/vascular endothelial growth factor: an important mediator of angiogenesis in malignancy and inflammation. *Int Arch Allergy Immunol* **107**, 233–235.

Ellis, L.M., Ahmad, S., Fan, F., Liu, W., Jung, Y.D., Stoeltzing, O., Reinmuth, N. and Parikh, A.A. (2002). Angiopoietins and their role in colon cancer angiogenesis. *Oncology (Huntingt)* **16**, 31–35.

Ferrara, N., Carver-Moore, K., Chen, H., Dowd, M., Lu, L., O'Shea, K.S., Powell-Braxton, L., Hillan, K.J. and Moore, M.W. (1996). Heterozygous embryonic lethality induced by targeted inactivation of the VEGF gene. *Nature* **380**, 439–442.

Ferrara, N. and Davis-Smyth, T. (1997). The biology of vascular endothelial growth factor. *Endocr Rev* **18**, 4–25.

Ferrara, N. and Henzel, W.J. (1989). Pituitary follicular cells secrete a novel heparin-binding growth factor specific for vascular endothelial cells. *Biochem Biophys Res Commun* **161**, 851–858.

Fidler, I.J. (1995). Critical factors in the biology of human cancer metastasis. *Am Surg* **61**, 1065–1066.

Fidler, I.J. and Ellis, L.M. (1994). The implications of angiogenesis for the biology and therapy of cancer metastasis. *Cell* **79**, 185–188.

Fidler, I.J., Singh, R.K., Yoneda, J., Kumar, R., Xu, L., Dong, Z., Bielenberg, D.R., McCarty, M. and Ellis, L.M. (2000). Critical determinants of neoplastic angiogenesis. *Cancer J* **6** (Suppl. 3), S225–S236.

Folkman, J. (1990). What is the evidence that tumors are angiogenesis dependent? *J Natl Cancer Inst* **82**, 4–6.

Folkman, J. (1992). The role of angiogenesis in tumor growth. *Semin Cancer Biol* **3**, 65–71.

Folkman, J. (1995). Angiogenesis in cancer, vascular, rheumatoid and other disease. *Nat Med* **1**, 27–31.

Fontanini, G., Vignati, S., Boldrini, L., Chine, S., Silvestri, V., Lucchi, M., Mussi, A., Angeletti, C.A. and Bevilacqua, G. (1997). Vascular endothelial growth factor is associated with neovascularization and influences progression of non-small cell lung carcinoma. *Clin Cancer Res* **3**, 861–865.

Friedlander, M., Theesfeld, C.L., Sugita, M., Fruttiger, M., Thomas, M.A., Chang, S. and Cheresh, D.A. (1996). Involvement of integrins alpha v beta 3 and alpha v beta 5 in ocular neovascular diseases. *Proc Natl Acad Sci USA* **93**, 9764–9769.

Fukuda, R., Hirota, K., Fan, F., Jung, Y.D., Ellis, L.M. and Semenza, G.L. (2002). Insulin-like growth factor 1 induces hypoxia-inducible factor 1-mediated vascular endothelial growth factor expression, which is dependent on MAP kinase and phosphatidylinositol 3-kinase signaling in colon cancer cells. *J Biol Chem* **277**, 38205–38211.

Galligioni, E. and Ferro, A. (2001). Angiogenesis and antiangiogenic agents in non-small cell lung cancer. *Lung Cancer* **34** (Suppl. 4), S3–S7.

Gerber, H.P., McMurtrey, A., Kowalski, J., Yan, M., Keyt, B.A., Dixit, V. and Ferrara, N. (1998). Vascular endothelial growth factor regulates endothelial cell survival through the phosphatidylinositol 3′-kinase/Akt signal transduction pathway. Requirement for Flk-1/KDR activation. *J Biol Chem* **273**, 30336–30343.

Gervaz, P., Scholl, B., Mainguene, C., Poitry, S., Gillet, M. and Wexner, S. (2000). Angiogenesis of liver metastases: role of sinusoidal endothelial cells. *Dis Colon and Rectum* **43**, 980–986.

Gunningham, S.P., Currie, M.J., Han, C., Robinson, B.A., Scott, P.A., Harris, A.L. and Fox, S.B. (2001). VEGF-B expression in human primary breast cancers is associated with lymph node metastasis but not angiogenesis. *J Pathol* **193**, 325–332.

Guo, P., Hu, B., Gu, W., Xu, L., Wang, D., Huang, H.J., Cavenee, W.K. and Cheng, S.Y. (2003). Platelet-derived growth factor-B enhances glioma angiogenesis by stimulating vascular endothelial growth factor expression in tumor endothelia and by promoting pericyte recruitment. *Am J Pathol* **162**, 1083–1093.

Hattori, K., Muta, M., Toi, M., Iizasa, H., Shinsei, M., Terasaki, T., Obinata, M., Ueda, M. and Nakashima, E. (2001). Establishment of bone marrow-derived endothelial cell lines from ts-SV40 T-antigen gene transgenic rats. *Pharm Res* **18**, 9–15.

Hayes, D.F. (1994). Angiogenesis and breast cancer. *Hematol Oncol Clin North Am* **8**, 51–71.

Helmlinger, G., Yuan, F., Dellian, M. and Jain, R.K. (1997). Interstitial pH and pO2 gradients in solid tumors in vivo: high-resolution measurements reveal a lack of correlation. *Nat Med* **3**, 177–182.

Holash, J., Wiegand, S.J. and Yancopoulos, G.D. (1999). New model of tumor angiogenesis: dynamic balance between vessel regression and growth mediated by angiopoietins and VEGF. *Oncogene* **18**, 5356–5362.

Houck, K.A., Ferrara, N., Winer, J., Cachianes, G., Li, B. and Leung, D.W. (1991). The vascular endothelial growth factor family: identification of a fourth molecular species and characterization of alternative splicing of RNA. *Mol Endocrinol* **5**, 1806–1814.

Huang, S., DeGuzman, A., Bucana, C.D. and Fidler, I.J. (2000). Nuclear factor-kappaB activity correlates with growth, angiogenesis, and metastasis of human melanoma cells in nude mice. *Clin Cancer Res* **6**, 2573–2581.

Huang, S.P., Wu, M.S., Wang, H.P., Yang, C.S., Kuo, M.L. and Lin, J.T. (2002). Correlation between serum levels of interleukin-6 and vascular endothelial growth factor in gastric carcinoma. *J Gastroenterol Hepatol* **17**, 1165–1169.

Hynes, R.O. (1992). Integrins: versatility, modulation, and signaling in cell adhesion. *Cell* **69**, 11–25.

Ikeda, N., Adachi, M., Taki, T., Huang, C., Hashida, H., Takabayashi, A., Sho, M., Nakajima, Y., Kanehiro, H., Hisanaga, M., Nakano, H. and Miyake, M. (1999). Prognostic significance of angiogenesis in human pancreatic cancer. *Br J Cancer* **79**, 1553–1563.

Inoue, K., Slaton, J.W., Eve, B.Y., Kim, S.J., Perrotte, P., Balbay, M.D., Yano, S., Bar-Eli, M., Radinsky, R., Pettaway, C.A. and Dinney, C.P. (2000). Interleukin 8 expression regulates tumorigenicity and metastases in androgen-independent prostate cancer. *Clin Cancer Res* **6**, 2104–2119.

Ivaska, J. and Heino, J. (2000). Adhesion receptors and cell invasion: mechanisms of integrin-guided degradation of extracellular matrix. *Cell Mol Life Sci* **57**, 16–24.

Jung, Y.D., Ahmad, S.A., Akagi, Y., Takahashi, Y., Liu, W., Reinmuth, N., Shaheen, R.M., Fan, F. and Ellis, L.M. (2000). Role of the tumor microenvironment in mediating response to anti-angiogenic therapy. *Cancer and Metastasis Rev* **19**, 147–157.

Kasahara, T., Mukaida, N., Yamashita, K., Yagisawa, H., Akahoshi, T. and Matsushima, K. (1991). IL-1 and TNF-alpha induction of IL-8 and monocyte chemotactic and activating factor (MCAF) mRNA expression in a human astrocytoma cell line. *Immunology* **74**, 60–67.

Keck, P.J., Hauser, S.D., Krivi, G., Sanzo, K., Warren, T., Feder, J. and Connolly, D.T. (1989). Vascular permeability factor, an endothelial cell mitogen related to PDGF. *Science* **246**, 1309–1312.

Keyt, B.A., Berleau, L.T., Nguyen, H.V., Chen, H., Heinsohn, H., Vandlen, R. and Ferrara, N. (1996). The carboxyl-terminal domain (111–165) of vascular endothelial growth factor is critical for its mitogenic potency. *J Biol Chem* **271**, 7788–7795.

Kido, S., Kitadai, Y., Hattori, N., Haruma, K., Kido, T., Ohta, M., Tanaka, S., Yoshihara, M., Sumii, K., Ohmoto, Y. and Chayama, K. (2001). Interleukin 8 and vascular endothelial growth factor – prognostic factors in human gastric carcinomas? *Eur J Cancer* **37**, 1482–1487.

Kim, L.S., Huang, S., Lu, W., Lev, D.C. and Price, J.E. (2004a). Vascular endothelial growth factor expression promotes the growth of breast cancer brain metastases in nude mice. *Clin Exp Metastasis* **21**, 107–118.

Kim, S.J., Uehara, H., Yazici, S., Langley, R.R., He, J., Tsan, R., Fan, D., Killion, J.J. and Fidler, I.J. (2004b). Simultaneous blockade of platelet-derived growth factor-receptor and epidermal growth factor-receptor signaling and systemic administration of paclitaxel as therapy for human prostate cancer metastasis in bone of nude mice. *Cancer Res* **64**, 4201–4208.

Kitadai, Y., Ellis, L.M., Takahashi, Y., Bucana, C.D., Anzai, H., Tahara, E. and Fidler, I.J. (1995). Multiparametric in situ messenger RNA hybridization analysis to detect metastasis-related genes in surgical specimens of human colon carcinomas. *Clin Cancer Res* **1**, 1095–1102.

Kitadai, Y., Haruma, K., Tokutomi, T., Tanaka, S., Sumii, K., Carvalho, M., Kuwabara, M., Yoshida, K., Hirai, T., Kajiyama, G. and Tahara, E. (1998). Significance of vessel count and vascular endothelial growth factor in human esophageal carcinomas. *Clin Cancer Res* **4**, 2195–2200.

Klapper, L.N., Kirschbaum, M.H., Sela, M. and Yarden, Y. (2000). Biochemical and clinical implications of the ErbB/HER signaling network of growth factor receptors. *Adv Cancer Res* **77**, 25–79.

Kondo, Y., Arii, S., Mori, A., Furutani, M., Chiba, T. and Imamura, M. (2000). Enhancement of angiogenesis, tumor growth, and metastasis by transfection of vascular endothelial growth factor into LoVo human colon cancer cell line. *Clin Cancer Res* **6**, 622–630.

Kotsuji-Maruyama, T., Imakado, S., Kawachi, Y. and Otsuka, F. (2002). PDGF-BB induces MAP kinase phosphorylation and VEGF expression in neurofibroma-derived cultured cells from patients with neurofibromatosis 1. *J Dermatol* **29**, 713–717.

Kraft, A., Weindel, K., Ochs, A., Marth, C., Zmija, J., Schumacher, P., Unger, C., Marme, D. and Gastl, G. (1999). Vascular endothelial growth factor in the sera and effusions of patients with malignant and nonmalignant disease. *Cancer* **85**, 178–187.

Krieg, M., Haas, R., Brauch, H., Acker, T., Flamme, I. and Plate, K.H. (2000). Up-regulation of hypoxia-inducible factors HIF-1alpha and HIF-2alpha under normoxic conditions in renal carcinoma cells by von Hippel-Lindau tumor suppressor gene loss of function. *Oncogene* **19**, 5435–5443.

Kumar, R. and Yarmand-Bagheri, R. (2001). The role of HER2 in angiogenesis. *Semin Oncol* **28**, 27–32.

Laughner, E., Taghavi, P., Chiles, K., Mahon, P.C. and Semenza, G.L. (2001). HER2 (neu) signaling increases the rate of hypoxia-inducible factor 1alpha (HIF-1alpha) synthesis: novel mechanism for HIF-1-mediated vascular endothelial growth factor expression. *Mol Cell Biol* **21**, 3995–4004.

Leung, D.W., Cachianes, G., Kuang, W.J., Goeddel, D.V. and Ferrara, N. (1989). Vascular endothelial growth factor is a secreted angiogenic mitogen. *Science* **246**, 1306–1309.

Linder, S., Blasjo, M., von Rosen, A., Parrado, C., Falkmer, U.G. and Falkmer, S. (2001). Pattern of distribution and prognostic value of angiogenesis in pancreatic duct carcinoma: a semiquantitative immunohistochemical study of 45 patients. *Pancreas* **22**, 240–247.

Maeda, K., Chung, Y.S., Takatsuka, S., Ogawa, Y., Sawada, T., Yamashita, Y., Onoda, N., Kato, Y., Nitta, A., Arimoto, Y. and *et al.* (1995). Tumor angiogenesis as a predictor of recurrence in gastric carcinoma. *J Clin Oncol* **13**, 477–481.

Maehara, Y., Kabashima, A., Koga, T., Tokunaga, E., Takeuchi, H., Kakeji, Y. and Sugimachi, K. (2000). Vascular invasion and potential for tumor angiogenesis and metastasis in gastric carcinoma. *Surgery* **128**, 408–416.

Maisonpierre, P.C., Suri, C., Jones, P.F., Bartunkova, S., Wiegand, S.J., Radziejewski, C., Compton, D., McClain, J., Aldrich, T.H., Papadopoulos, N., Daly, T.J., Davis, S., Sato, T.N. and Yancopoulos, G.D. (1997). Angiopoietin-2, a natural antagonist for Tie2 that disrupts in vivo angiogenesis. *Science* **277**, 55–60.

Masui, T., Hosotani, R., Doi, R., Miyamoto, Y., Tsuji, S., Nakajima, S., Kobayashi, H., Koizumi, M., Toyoda, E., Tulachan, S.S. and Imamura, M. (2002). Expression of IL-6 receptor in pancreatic cancer: involvement in VEGF induction. *Anticancer Res* **22**, 4093–4100.

Matsushima, K., Baldwin, E.T. and Mukaida, N. (1992). Interleukin-8 and MCAF: novel leukocyte recruitment and activating cytokines. *Chem Immunol* **51**, 236–265.

Meert, A.P., Paesmans, M., Martin, B., Delmotte, P., Berghmans, T., Verdebout, J.M., Lafitte, J.J., Mascaux, C. and Sculier, J.P. (2002). The role of microvessel density on the survival of patients with lung cancer: a systematic review of the literature with meta-analysis. *Br J Cancer* **87**, 694–701.

Miyamoto, S., Teramoto, H., Gutkind, J.S. and Yamada, K.M. (1996). Integrins can collaborate with growth factors for phosphorylation of receptor tyrosine kinases and MAP kinase activation: roles of integrin aggregation and occupancy of receptors. *J Cell Biol* **135**, 1633–1642.

Monestiroli, S., Mancuso, P., Burlini, A., Pruneri, G., Dell'Agnola, C., Gobbi, A., Martinelli, G. and Bertolini, F. (2001). Kinetics and viability of circulating endothelial cells as surrogate angiogenesis marker in an animal model of human lymphoma. *Cancer Res* **61**, 4341–4344.

Moriyama, T., Kataoka, H., Hamasuna, R., Yokogami, K., Uehara, H., Kawano, H., Goya, T., Tsubouchi, H., Koono, M. and Wakisaka, S. (1998). Up-regulation of vascular endothelial growth factor induced by hepatocyte growth factor/scatter factor stimulation in human glioma cells. *Biochem Biophys Res Commun* **249**, 73–77.

Nagy, J.A., Masse, E.M., Herzberg, K.T., Meyers, M.S., Yeo, K.T., Yeo, T.K., Sioussat, T.M. and Dvorak, H.F. (1995). Pathogenesis of ascites tumor growth: vascular permeability factor, vascular hyperpermeability, and ascites fluid accumulation. *Cancer Res* **55**, 360–368.

Neuchrist, C., Erovic, B.M., Handisurya, A., Fischer, M.B., Steiner, G.E., Hollemann, D., Gedlicka, C., Saaristo, A. and Burian, M. (2003). Vascular endothelial growth factor C and vascular endothelial growth factor receptor 3 expression in squamous cell carcinomas of the head and neck. *Head Neck* **25**, 464–474.

Neufeld, G., Cohen, T., Gengrinovitch, S. and Poltorak, Z. (1999). Vascular endothelial growth factor (VEGF) and its receptors. *FASEB J* **13**, 9–22.

Nguyen, D.M. and Schrump, D.S. (2004). Growth factor receptors as targets for lung cancer therapy. *Semin Thorac Cardiovasc Surg* **16**, 3–12.

Oh, J.S., Kucab, J.E., Bushel, P.R., Martin, K., Bennett, L., Collins, J., DiAugustine, R.P., Barrett, J.C., Afshari, C.A. and Dunn, S.E. (2002). Insulin-like growth factor-1 inscribes a gene expression profile for angiogenic factors and cancer progression in breast epithelial cells. *Neoplasia* **4**, 204–217.

Paget, S. (1989). The distribution of secondary growths in cancer of the breast. *Cancer Metastasis Rev* **8**, 98–101.

Pardanaud, L., Altmann, C., Kitos, P., Dieterlen-Lievre, F. and Buck, C.A. (1987). Vasculogenesis in the early quail blastodisc as studied with a monoclonal antibody recognizing endothelial cells. *Development* **100**, 339–349.

Parikh, A.A., Fan, F., Liu, W.B., Ahmad, S.A., Stoeltzing, O., Reinmuth, N., Bielenberg, D., Bucana, C.D., Klagsbrun, M. and Ellis, L.M. (2004). Neuropilin-1 in human colon cancer: expression, regulation, and role in induction of angiogenesis. *Am J Pathol* **164**, 2139–2151.

Park, J.E., Keller, G.A. and Ferrara, N. (1993). The vascular endothelial growth factor (VEGF) isoforms: differential deposition into the subepithelial extracellular matrix and bioactivity of extracellular matrix-bound VEGF. *Mol Biol Cell* **4**, 1317–1326.

Partanen, J., Armstrong, E., Makela, T.P., Korhonen, J., Sandberg, M., Renkonen, R., Knuutila, S., Huebner, K. and Alitalo, K. (1992). A novel endothelial cell surface receptor tyrosine kinase with extracellular epidermal growth factor homology domains. *Mol Cell Biol* **12**, 1698–1707.

Partanen, T.A., Arola, J., Saaristo, A., Jussila, L., Ora, A., Miettinen, M., Stacker, S.A., Achen, M.G. and Alitalo, K. (2000). VEGF-C and VEGF-D expression in neuroendocrine cells and their receptor, VEGFR-3, in fenestrated blood vessels in human tissues. *FASEB J* **14**, 2087–2096.

Petit, A.M., Rak, J., Hung, M.C., Rockwell, P., Goldstein, N., Fendly, B. and Kerbel, R.S. (1997). Neutralizing antibodies against epidermal growth factor and ErbB-2/neu receptor tyrosine kinases down-regulate vascular endothelial growth factor production by tumor cells in vitro and in vivo: angiogenic implications for signal transduction therapy of solid tumors. *Am J Pathol* **151**, 1523–1530.

Plouet, J., Schilling, J. and Gospodarowicz, D. (1989). Isolation and characterization of a newly identified endothelial cell mitogen produced by AtT-20 cells. *EMBO J* **8**, 3801–3806.

Rajesh, L., Joshi, K., Bhalla, V., Dey, P., Radotra, B.D. and Nijhawan, R. (2004). Correlation between VEGF expression and angiogenesis in breast carcinoma. *Anal Quant Cytol Histol* **26**, 105–108.

Reinmuth, N., Fan, F., Liu, W., Parikh, A.A., Stoeltzing, O., Jung, Y.D., Bucana, C.D., Radinsky, R., Gallick, G.E. and Ellis, L.M. (2002). Impact of insulin-like growth factor receptor-I function on angiogenesis, growth, and metastasis of colon cancer. *Lab Invest* **82**, 1377–1389.

Reinmuth, N., Liu, W., Jung, Y.D., Ahmad, S.A., Shaheen, R.M., Fan, F., Bucana, C.D., McMahon, G., Gallick, G.E. and Ellis, L.M. (2001). Induction of VEGF in perivascular cells defines a potential paracrine mechanism for endothelial cell survival. *FASEB J* **15**, 1239–1241.

Reinmuth, N., Parikh, A.A., Ahmad, S.A., Liu, W., Stoeltzing, O., Fan, F., Takeda, A., Akagi, M. and Ellis, L.M. (2003). Biology of angiogenesis in tumors of the gastrointestinal tract. *Microsc Res Tech* **60**, 199–207.

Sato, N., Mizumoto, K., Beppu, K., Maehara, N., Kusumoto, M., Nabae, T., Morisaki, T., Katano, M. and Tanaka, M. (2000). Establishment of a new human pancreatic cancer cell line, NOR-P1, with high angiogenic activity and metastatic potential. *Cancer Lett* **155**, 153–161.

Schackert, G., Price, J.E., Bucana, C.D. and Fidler, I.J. (1989). Unique patterns of brain metastasis produced by different human carcinomas in athymic nude mice. *Int J Cancer* **44**, 892–897.

Senger, D.R., Claffey, K.P., Benes, J.E., Perruzzi, C.A., Sergiou, A.P. and Detmar, M. (1997). Angiogenesis promoted by vascular endothelial growth factor: regulation through alpha1beta1 and alpha2beta1 integrins. *Proc Natl Acad Sci USA* **94**, 13612–13617.

Senger, D.R., Galli, S.J., Dvorak, A.M., Perruzzi, C.A., Harvey, V.S. and Dvorak, H.F. (1983). Tumor cells secrete a vascular permeability factor that promotes accumulation of ascites fluid. *Science* **219**, 983–985.

Senger, D.R., Perruzzi, C.A., Feder, J. and Dvorak, H.F. (1986). A highly conserved vascular permeability factor secreted by a variety of human and rodent tumor cell lines. *Cancer Res* **46**, 5629–5632.

Senger, D.R., Van de Water, L., Brown, L.F., Nagy, J.A., Yeo, K.T., Yeo, T.K., Berse, B., Jackman, R.W., Dvorak, A.M. and Dvorak, H.F. (1993). Vascular permeability factor (VPF, VEGF) in tumor biology. *Cancer Metastasis Rev* **12**, 303–324.

Sengupta, S., Gherardi, E., Sellers, L.A., Wood, J.M., Sasisekharan, R. and Fan, T.P. (2003a). Hepatocyte growth factor/scatter factor can induce angiogenesis independently of vascular endothelial growth factor. *Arterioscler Thromb Vasc Biol* **23**, 69–75.

Sengupta, S., Sellers, L.A., Li, R.C., Gherardi, E., Zhao, G., Watson, N., Sasisekharan, R. and Fan, T.P. (2003b). Targeting of mitogen-activated protein kinases and phosphatidy-linositol 3 kinase inhibits hepatocyte growth factor/scatter factor-induced angiogenesis. *Circulation* **107**, 2955–2961.

Shaheen, R.M., Tseng, W.W., Davis, D.W., Liu, W., Reinmuth, N., Vellagas, R., Wieczorek, A.A., Ogura, Y., McConkey, D.J., Drazan, K.E., Bucana, C.D., McMahon, G. and Ellis, L.M. (2001). Tyrosine kinase inhibition of multiple angiogenic growth factor receptors improves survival in mice bearing colon cancer liver metastases by inhibition of endothelial cell survival mechanisms. *Cancer Res* **61**, 1464–1468.

Shi, Q., Abbruzzese, J.L., Huang, S., Fidler, I.J., Xiong, Q. and Xie, K. (1999). Constitutive and inducible interleukin 8 expression by hypoxia and acidosis renders human pancreatic cancer cells more tumorigenic and metastatic. *Clin Cancer Res* **5**, 3711–3721.

Shibata, A., Nagaya, T., Imai, T., Funahashi, H., Nakao, A. and Seo, H. (2002). Inhibition of NF-kappaB activity decreases the VEGF mRNA expression in MDA-MB-231 breast cancer cells. *Breast Cancer Res Treat* **73**, 237–243.

Smith, L.E., Shen, W., Perruzzi, C., Soker, S., Kinose, F., Xu, X., Robinson, G., Driver, S., Bischoff, J., Zhang, B., Schaeffer, J.M. and Senger, D.R. (1999). Regulation of vascular endothelial growth factor-dependent retinal neovascularization by insulin-like growth factor-1 receptor. *Nat Med* **5**, 1390–1395.

Soker, S., Miao, H.Q., Nomi, M., Takashima, S. and Klagsbrun, M. (2002). VEGF165 mediates formation of complexes containing VEGFR-2 and neuropilin-1 that enhance VEGF165-receptor binding. *J Cell Biochem* **85**, 357–368.

Soldi, R., Mitola, S., Strasly, M., Defilippi, P., Tarone, G. and Bussolino, F. (1999). Role of alphavbeta3 integrin in the activation of vascular endothelial growth factor receptor-2. *EMBO J* **18**, 882–892.

Staton, C.A., Stribbling, S.M., Tazzyman, S., Hughes, R., Brown, N.J. and Lewis, C.E. (2004). Current methods for assaying angiogenesis in vitro and in vivo. *Int J Exp Pathol* **85**, 233–248.

Stefanou, D., Batistatou, A., Arkoumani, E., Ntzani, E. and Agnantis, N.J. (2004). Expression of vascular endothelial growth factor (VEGF) and association with microvessel density in small-cell and non-small-cell lung carcinomas. *Histol Histopathol* **19**, 37–42.

Stoeltzing, O., Ahmad, S.A., Liu, W., McCarty, M.F., Parikh, A.A., Fan, F., Reinmuth, N., Bucana, C.D. and Ellis, L.M. (2002). Angiopoietin-1 inhibits tumour growth and ascites formation in a murine model of peritoneal carcinomatosis. *Br J Cancer* **87**, 1182–1187.

Stoeltzing, O., Ahmad, S.A., Liu, W., McCarty, M.F., Wey, J.S., Parikh, A.A., Fan, F., Reinmuth, N., Kawaguchi, M., Bucana, C.D. and Ellis, L.M. (2003a). Angiopoietin-1 inhibits vascular permeability, angiogenesis, and growth of hepatic colon cancer tumors. *Cancer Res* **63**, 3370–3377.

Stoeltzing, O., Liu, W., Reinmuth, N., Fan, F., Parikh, A.A., Bucana, C.D., Evans, D.B., Semenza, G.L. and Ellis, L.M. (2003b). Regulation of hypoxia-inducible factor-1alpha, vascular endothelial growth factor, and angiogenesis by an insulin-like growth factor-I receptor autocrine loop in human pancreatic cancer. *Am J Pathol* **163**, 1001–1011.

Sugino, T., Kusakabe, T., Hoshi, N., Yamaguchi, T., Kawaguchi, T., Goodison, S., Sekimata, M., Homma, Y. and Suzuki, T. (2002). An invasion-independent pathway of blood-borne metastasis: a new murine mammary tumor model. *Am J Pathol* **160**, 1973–1980.

Suri, C., Jones, P.F., Patan, S., Bartunkova, S., Maisonpierre, P.C., Davis, S., Sato, T.N. and Yancopoulos, G.D. (1996). Requisite role of angiopoietin-1, a ligand for the TIE2 receptor, during embryonic angiogenesis. *Cell* **87**, 1171–1180.

Takahashi, Y., Cleary, K.R., Mai, M., Kitadai, Y., Bucana, C.D. and Ellis, L.M. (1996). Significance of vessel count and vascular endothelial growth factor and its receptor (KDR) in intestinal-type gastric cancer. *Clin Cancer Res* **2**, 1679–1684.

Takahashi, Y., Kitadai, Y., Bucana, C.D., Cleary, K.R. and Ellis, L.M. (1995). Expression of vascular endothelial growth factor and its receptor, KDR, correlates with vascularity, metastasis, and proliferation of human colon cancer. *Cancer Res* **55**, 3964–3968.

Takebayashi, Y., Aklyama, S., Yamada, K., Akiba, S. and Aikou, T. (1996). Angiogenesis as an unfavorable prognostic factor in human colorectal carcinoma. *Cancer* **78**, 226–231.

Terayama, N., Terada, T. and Nakanuma, Y. (1996a). Histologic growth patterns of metastatic carcinomas of the liver. *Japan J Clin Oncol* **26**, 24–29.

Terayama, N., Terada, T. and Nakanuma, Y. (1996b). An immunohistochemical study of tumour vessels in metastatic liver cancers and the surrounding liver tissue. *Histopathology* **29**, 37–43.

Uehara, H., Kim, S.J., Karashima, T., Shepherd, D.L., Fan, D., Tsan, R., Killion, J.J., Logothetis, C., Mathew, P. and Fidler, I.J. (2003). Effects of blocking platelet-derived growth factor-receptor signaling in a mouse model of experimental prostate cancer bone metastases. *J Natl Cancer Inst* **95**, 458–470.

Ushijima, C., Tsukamoto, S., Yamazaki, K., Yoshino, I., Sugio, K. and Sugimachi, K. (2001). High vascularity in the peripheral region of non-small cell lung cancer tissue is associated with tumor progression. *Lung Cancer* **34**, 233–241.

Vermeulen, P.B., Van den Eynden, G.G., Huget, P., Goovaerts, G., Weyler, J., Lardon, F., Van Marck, E., Hubens, G. and Dirix, L.Y. (1999). Prospective study of intratumoral microvessel density, p53 expression and survival in colorectal cancer. *Br J Cancer* **79**, 316–322.

Walton, H.L., Corjay, M.H., Mohamed, S.N., Mousa, S.A., Santomenna, L.D. and Reilly, T.M. (2000). Hypoxia induces differential expression of the integrin receptors alpha(vbeta3) and alpha(vbeta5) in cultured human endothelial cells. *J Cell Biochem* **78**, 674–680.

Wang, G.L., Jiang, B.H., Rue, E.A. and Semenza, G.L. (1995). Hypoxia-inducible factor 1 is a basic-helix–loop–helix-PAS heterodimer regulated by cellular O2 tension. *Proc Natl Acad Sci USA* **92**, 5510–5514.

Warren, R.S., Yuan, H., Matli, M.R., Ferrara, N. and Donner, D.B. (1996). Induction of vascular endothelial growth factor by insulin-like growth factor 1 in colorectal carcinoma. *J Biol Chem* **271**, 29483–29488.

Wei, L.H., Kuo, M.L., Chen, C.A., Cheng, W.F., Cheng, S.P., Hsieh, F.J. and Hsieh, C.Y. (2001). Interleukin-6 in cervical cancer: the relationship with vascular endothelial growth factor. *Gynecol Oncol* **82**, 49–56.

Wei, L.H., Kuo, M.L., Chen, C.A., Chou, C.H., Lai, K.B., Lee, C.N. and Hsieh, C.Y. (2003). Interleukin-6 promotes cervical tumor growth by VEGF-dependent angiogenesis via a STAT3 pathway. *Oncogene* **22**, 1517–1527.

Weidner, N., Semple, J.P., Welch, W.R. and Folkman, J. (1991). Tumor angiogenesis and metastasis – correlation in invasive breast carcinoma. *N Engl J Med* **324**, 1–8.

Xiangming, C., Hokita, S., Natsugoe, S., Tanabe, G., Baba, M., Takao, S., Kuroshima, K. and Aikou, T. (1998). Angiogenesis as an unfavorable factor related to lymph node metastasis in early gastric cancer. *Ann Surg Oncol* **5**, 585–589.

Xu, L., Yoneda, J., Herrera, C., Wood, J., Killion, J.J. and Fidler, I.J. (2000). Inhibition of malignant ascites and growth of human ovarian carcinoma by oral administration of a potent inhibitor of the vascular endothelial growth factor receptor tyrosine kinases. *Int J Oncol* **16**, 445–454.

Yancopoulos, G.D., Davis, S., Gale, N.W., Rudge, J.S., Wiegand, S.J. and Holash, J. (2000). Vascular-specific growth factors and blood vessel formation. *Nature* **407**, 242–248.

Yang, W., Klos, K., Yang, Y., Smith, T.L., Shi, D. and Yu, D. (2002). ErbB2 overexpression correlates with increased expression of vascular endothelial growth factors A, C, and D in human breast carcinoma. *Cancer* **94**, 2855–2861.

Yano, S., Nokihara, H., Yamamoto, A., Goto, H., Ogawa, H., Kanematsu, T., Miki, T., Uehara, H., Saijo, Y., Nukiwa, T. and Sone, S. (2003). Multifunctional interleukin-1beta promotes metastasis of human lung cancer cells in SCID mice via enhanced expression of adhesion-, invasion- and angiogenesis-related molecules. *Cancer Sci* **94**, 244–252.

Yen, L., You, X.L., Al Moustafa, A.E., Batist, G., Hynes, N.E., Mader, S., Meloche, S. and Alaoui-Jamali, M.A. (2000). Heregulin selectively upregulates vascular endothelial growth factor secretion in cancer cells and stimulates angiogenesis. *Oncogene* **19**, 3460–3469.

Yuan, A., Yu, C.J., Chen, W.J., Lin, F.Y., Kuo, S.H., Luh, K.T. and Yang, P.C. (2000). Correlation of total VEGF mRNA and protein expression with histologic type, tumor angiogenesis, patient survival and timing of relapse in non-small-cell lung cancer. *Int J Cancer* **89**, 475–483.

Yuan, A., Yu, C.J., Luh, K.T., Kuo, S.H., Lee, Y.C. and Yang, P.C. (2002). Aberrant p53 expression correlates with expression of vascular endothelial growth factor mRNA and interleukin-8 mRNA and neoangiogenesis in non-small-cell lung cancer. *J Clin Oncol* **20**, 900–910.

Zebrowski, B.K., Yano, S., Liu, W., Shaheen, R.M., Hicklin, D.J., Putnam, J.B., Jr. and Ellis, L.M. (1999). Vascular endothelial growth factor levels and induction of permeability in malignant pleural effusions. *Clin Cancer Res* **5**, 3364–3368.

Zhang, H., Wu, J., Meng, L. and Shou, C.C. (2002). Expression of vascular endothelial growth factor and its receptors KDR and Flt-1 in gastric cancer cells. *World J Gastroenterol* **8**, 994–998.

Zhong, H., De Marzo, A.M., Laughner, E., Lim, M., Hilton, D.A., Zagzag, D., Buechler, P., Isaacs, W.B., Semenza, G.L. and Simons, J.W. (1999). Overexpression of hypoxia-inducible factor 1alpha in common human cancers and their metastases. *Cancer Res* **59**, 5830–5835.

4

Development of Agents that Selectively Disrupt Tumor Vasculature: A Historical Perspective

David J. Chaplin and Sally A. Hill

4.1 Introduction

Most cancer research is aimed at developing strategies to kill, or stop the proliferation of, tumor cells directly. For successful control of cancer, every cancer cell capable of indefinite proliferation must be reached by the therapeutic agent and either be eradicated or prevented from dividing. Even in very small tumor deposits of $1\,cm^3$ this may require contact with up to 10^9 cells. The difficulty of achieving this has led to the search for other approaches that can indirectly target tumor cells via influencing the function of associated host cells such as cells involved in the immune response and vascular endothelial cells.

The survival and growth of solid tumors depends on the development and function of a blood vessel network. This vascular network can be acquired, in part, by incorporation of host vessels. However, many of the vessels within the tumor result from active angiogenesis triggered by the release of specific growth factors, such as VEGF, by the tumor cells themselves or by incorporated host cells such as macrophages. It is therefore not surprising that blood vessel development has become a major target for new approaches to cancer therapy. The predominant focus over the last 25 years has been the development of strategies to prevent blood vessel growth within tumors, so-called antiangiogenic therapies. This approach was originally advocated and pioneered by Professor Judah Folkman and has led, most recently, to the approval of the first rationally developed anti-

Vascular-targeted Therapies in Oncology Edited by Dietmar W. Siemann
© 2006 John Wiley & Sons, Ltd.

angiogenic therapeutic, Avastin (bevacizumab). In contrast, relatively little effort has been made in the development of agents that compromise the function of the abnormal neovasculature already present in the tumor at the time of detection and treatment, so-called vascular disrupting agents (VDAs). This approach was originally advocated by the late Professor Juliana Denekamp (Figure 4.1).

VDAs differ from antiangiogenic agents (for a review see Siemann *et al.*, 2005) in that, rather than preventing new blood vessel formation, they are designed to cause a rapid and selective vascular shutdown in tumors, which occurs over a period of minutes to hours. Moreover, such agents are expected to be used in intermittent doses, to synergize with conventional treatments, rather than chronically over months or years, as is required for the antiangiogenic therapies. VDAs divide into two main classes, the ligand-based approaches, which utilize antibodies and peptides to deliver toxins, procoagulant and pro-apoptotic effectors to tumor endothelium, and the small molecules, which do not specifically localize to tumor endothelium but exploit the known differences between tumor and normal endothelial cells to induce selective vascular dysfunction.

The VDA approach has several advantages, including the following.

- Each vessel provides the nutrition for, and facilitates removal of waste products of metabolism from, many thousands of tumor cells.

- Since a vessel is much like any channel involved in transportation, it only has to be damaged at one point to block both upstream and downstream function.

- It is not necessary to kill endothelial cells; a change of shape or function could also be effective.

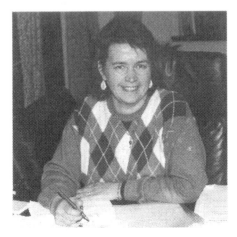

Figure 4.1 Juliana Denekamp (1943–2001), who first advocated the rational development of agents that selectively target and/or disrupt newly formed blood vessels in tumors

- The endothelial cell is adjacent to the blood stream, therefore delivery problems of any therapeutic are minimized.

- A surrogate marker of biological activity, i.e. blood flow, is readily measurable in the clinic.

As mentioned previously, in contrast to the focus on antiangiogenic approaches to therapy, there has until recently been relatively little effort afforded to VDA development. In this chapter we will focus on the historical background to the development of these agents, with a particular focus on the small-molecule-based VDAs.

4.2 Early history

Whilst the rational development of VDAs has only had a relatively short history, as will be documented in subsequent sections, there was evidence from early studies that vasculature was a key element in tumor viability and was involved in the therapeutic response to some agents.

William Henry Woglom (1879–1953)

The pivotal role of tumor vasculature and the effects of its selective destruction were first highlighted by Woglom, a scientist at Columbia University, over 80 years ago (Woglom, 1923). It had been reported in the mid-1800s that solid tumors in the clinic could occasionally be eradicated when their circulation was interrupted, either by torsion of the vascular pedicle or by thrombosis of a major feeding vessel (Walshe, 1844). A critical review of these findings and other evidence concerning tumor regression led Woglom to raise the question of whether 'the receding tumor may not differ from the growing one only in the extent to which its blood vessels have been obliterated by thrombosis'. Based on this and other findings, he suggested that damage to the capillary system might be the best way to inhibit tumor growth. He states that 'the problem of treatment would be to find some agent capable of thrombosing the vessels of a tumor and no others. The only reason for regarding such a discovery as anything but utterly chimerical is that the blood vessels of many tumors are more subject to thrombosis than are those of normal tissues'. He goes on to state that one of the problems with what we would now call an optimal VDA agent would be that 'even though all the vessels of a tumor could be thrombosed, there would often remain single cells or small groups of cells invading the surrounding tissue and supported, not by the blood vessels of the neoplasm from which they escaped, but by the fluids imbibed from the normal tissues about them', the latter predicting the so called 'viable rim' that characteristically remains following treatment with VDAs.

Bacterial products

Many early cancer therapies undoubtedly elicited part of their therapeutic effects via selective vascular damage. Early studies by Coley had shown that tumor regression was often observed following spontaneous or induced bacterial infection (Coley, 1893, 1894). This work stimulated many early investigators to evaluate further the effects of bacterial products administered to tumor-bearing mice. Work with a variety of bacterial extracts was shown to elicit rapid hemorrhagic necrosis, a now established hallmark of vascular damage in experimental tumors (Boyland and Boyland, 1937; Andervont, 1940). It is now believed that the antitumor effects of such toxins were mediated through the production of cytokines such as tumor necrosis factor alpha (TNFα) (Old, 1985). TNFα has been shown subsequently to mediate a significant part of its anti-tumor effects through damage to tumor vasculature (Pober, 1987; Kallinowski et al., 1989).

Lead colloids and arsenicals

Several metals are known to damage blood vessels; these include lead, arsenic and cadmium (Bekemeier and Hirschelmann, 1989). However, relatively little is known about their selectivity for tumor vasculature.

In the 1920s, Mottram attributed the anti-tumor effects of lead colloids, in part, to thrombosis of blood vessels (Mottram, 1928). In the 1950s, Leiter and colleagues at the National Cancer Institute evaluated approximately 100 organic arsenic compounds for their ability to induce rapid histological damage in sarcoma 37 tumors grown in mice (Leiter et al., 1952). We now know that the appearance of necrosis within a few hours of treatment is a hallmark of vascular damage. The studies by Leiter et al. showed that many of the compounds he tested could induce such changes, indicative of vascular disruption, with the trivalent arsenicals being the most active. However, they noted that activity was only observed at doses close to the maximum tolerated dose (MTD).

It is interesting to note that arsenic trioxide, an inorganic trivalent arsenical, which has been developed primarily as a cytotoxic agent for use in the treatment of promyelocytic leukemia, has been shown to induce blood flow reductions when used in experimental solid tumors (Lew et al., 1999; Griffin et al., 2003). However, no rational development of these agents has yet taken place to hone their vascular disrupting properties.

Colchicine

Studies with colchicine, reported in the mid-1930s by Boyland and Boyland, demonstrated that colchicine and a bacterial filtrate, when injected into mice, induced hemorrhage within tumors (Boyland and Boyland, 1937). Further evaluation of the vascular effects of colchicine was undertaken by Ludford (Ludford, 1945, 1948). These studies clearly demonstrated that colchicine preferentially damaged newly formed capillaries in tumors, with the consequence of inducing hemorrhage and extensive necrosis. Activity was noted in many different experimental tumor systems, but significant effects were only achieved at doses approaching the maximum tolerated dose. The activity of colchicines in the treatment of patients with advanced carcinomas was also evaluated (Seed *et al.*, 1940). Four patients in the study were treated at toxic doses; indeed, two patients died of colchicine poisoning. In the other two patients there was histological evidence of 'rapid degeneration' in the tumors within a few days. These findings, indicating rapid necrosis and regrowth from the periphery, are, based on our current knowledge, characteristic of the induction of vascular damage within the tumor. Because of the narrow therapeutic window associated with the use of colchicine to achieve anti-tumor activity, along with the fact that other cytotoxic agents were emerging as potent anti-cancer drugs, little further investigation was carried out in this area for over 40 years. In the 1950s, data obtained using another tubulin depolymerizing agent, podophyllotoxin, had indicated similar effects to colchicine in that it could rapidly induce hemorrhagic necrosis (Leiter *et al.*, 1950).

4.3 Formulation of the VDA concept

Despite all the interesting findings highlighted above, it was not until the early 1980s that the concept of rationally developing VDAs was put forward. In 1982 Juliana Denekamp first proposed that the very much higher proliferation rate of endothelial cells in tumors compared to normal tissues might enable them to be selectively targeted. Up until this time most investigators had considered the relatively poorly formed and inadequate vascular network in tumors to be a problem which limited the effectiveness of conventional therapies. Many tumor cells would be hypoxic and thus radiation resistant and many cells would be located distant from vessels and lack an optimal supply of nutrients to facilitate proliferation, thus limiting the delivery and effectiveness of cell cycle specific chemotherapy. In a series of papers Denekamp advocated that tumor vasculature, rather than being a problem, represented an opportunity for therapeutic approaches and should be considered the 'Achilles' heel' of solid tumors (Denekamp, 1982, 1984, 1986).

It was suggested that monoclonal antibodies, which targeted antigenic differences between tumor and normal endothelium, could be used to localize radioactive isotopes, cytotoxins and/or clotting factors to tumor endothelium (Denekamp, 1986). It was a few years later that some elegant work by Burrows and Thorpe provided the proof of concept for these theories (Burrows and Thorpe, 1993). These initial studies of Burrows and Thorpe involved using interferon-γ-transfected tumors, which were targeted using a ricin conjugated antibody against the MHC Class II antigen. Since IFN γ up-regulates MHC Class II on the tumor-associated endothelial cells, it was an ideal model to prove the feasibility of such antibody-directed approaches. These workers subsequently used the model to show the effectiveness of using the antibody to selectively deliver a truncated form of tissue factor, thus triggering thrombosis in tumor-associated vasculature (Huang *et al.*, 1997).

4.4   Effects of vascular occlusion on tumor cell survival

The initial study investigating the effects of induced ischemia within tumors was performed by Denekamp and colleagues in 1983 (Denekamp *et al.*, 1983). The ischemia was achieved by applying D-shaped metal clamps across the base of subcutaneously implanted tumors. Marked tumor regression, delayed growth and long-term tumor control were seen, with the magnitude of the response being proportional to the duration of clamping. Vessel occlusion for at least 15 hours was necessary to achieve local cure of the tumor. One potential issue with this study that was not addressed was the actual kinetics of tumor cell death and the potential effects of cooling likely to have occurred in the tissue during the clamping period. A subsequent study by Chaplin and Horsman investigated these issues in different tumor models (Chaplin and Horsman, 1994). The rate of tumor cell death following blood flow cessation in three different tumor models is shown in Figure 4.2. It can be seen that a two-hour period of ischemia reduced survival by over 99 per cent when the tumor temperature was maintained at 37 °C; similar results were obtained for other tumor types. The rate of cell death was much reduced if the tumors were allowed to cool during the ischemic insult. It was also shown in this study that a six-hour period of ischemia induced in C3H mammary tumors maintained at 37 °C could result in the local control of three of the seven tumors treated. Similar kinetics of tumor cell death was also reported for the CaNT tumor following ischemic insult under conditions where the tumor temperature was maintained (Parkins *et al.*, 1994). These authors attributed the decreased rate of cell death in tumors allowed to cool to a reduced metabolic process and showed a slower acidification of extracellular pH in these tumors.

4.5   Rational development of VDA therapeutics

Ligand-directed VDAs

As mentioned previously, the advantages of targeting the endothelium include a reduction in both delivery problems and in the number of cells that need to be targeted. These factors make the tumor vasculature a potentially ideal target for ligand-based approaches, where antibodies or peptides that recognize tumor-associated vasculature are linked to an effector molecule that can induce apoptosis, coagulation etc. Several groups are working on these approaches. For such

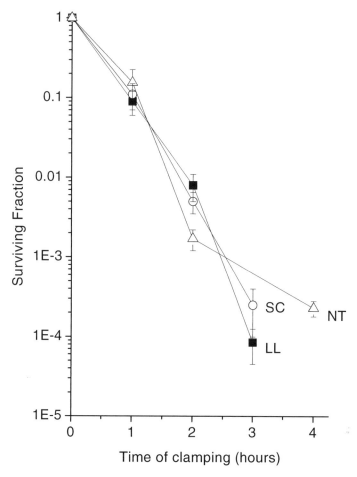

Figure 4.2   The kinetics of tumor cell death following vascular occlusion, when tumor temperature is maintained at 37 °C. The effects in three different murine tumours are shown, Lewis Lung Carcinoma (LL), Carcinoma NT (NT) and the SCCVII (SC)

strategies there is a need to identify antibodies and peptides that target unique determinants that are expressed on the tumor endothelium. Some determinants that have already been identified and/or used as targets for ligand-directed VDA approaches include endoglin (Burrows *et al.*, 1995; Seon, 2002), VEGF receptors (Brekken and Thorpe, 2001; Veenendaal *et al.*, 2002), αv integrins (Brooks *et al.*, 1994; Arap *et al.*, 1998), fibronectin ED-B domain (Nilsson *et al.*, 2001) and prostate specific membrane antigen (PSMA) (Chang *et al.*, 1999). Recent results in experimental tumor systems, with both VEGF linked to the toxin gelonin, which targets VEGF receptor expression, and with an antibody fragment specific for the oncofetal ED-B domain of fibronectin fused to the extracellular domain of tissue factor, have demonstrated selective vascular destruction

(Nilsson *et al.*, 2001; Veenendaal *et al.*, 2002). Also of interest is the recent finding that phosphatidyl serine is selectively found on the outside surface of endothelial cell membranes in solid tumors. An antibody to PS has now been developed and shown, even as a naked antibody, to induce evidence of vascular shutdown in experimental tumors (Thorpe AACR 2004). This concept is further explored in Chapter 10.

4.6   Development of small-molecule VDAs

Despite the early work with colchicines and podophyllotoxin in the 1930s through 1950s, which seemed to indicate that these low-molecular-weight drugs mediated their antitumor effects, at least in part, through vascular disruption, very little was done to develop small-molecule VDAs until the late 1980s. Since there were no clear molecular targets that could be used to screen for such drugs *in vitro*, early leads came from identifying drugs that elicited the classic hallmarks of vascular disruption and subsequent ischemic cell death:

*   rapid necrosis

*   hemorrhage

*   thrombosis.

Flavonoids

One of the first agents to be clearly identified as a VDA was flavone acetic acid (FAA) Evidence that this drug could elicit rapid hemorrhagic necrosis in experimental solid tumors was obtained by several investigators (Smith *et al.*, 1987; Bibby *et al.*, 1989; Hill *et al.*, 1992). Other studies confirmed that the drug elicited a rapid reduction in tumor blood flow (Evelhoch *et al.*, 1988; Bibby *et al.*, 1989; Hill *et al.*, 1989). The mechanism of action of the drug was attributed, in part, to its ability to induce the production of the cytokine tumor necrosis factor alpha (TNFα) in tumor cells and the tumor-associated host cells. Interestingly, the identification of the vascular action of FAA came after the compound had entered clinical trials. The lack of response seen in the trials when administered as a single agent (Kerr *et al.*, 1987; Weiss *et al.*, 1988; Kerr *et al.*, 1989) led to the discontinuation of the clinical program. The lack of effect of FAA was attributed at the time to its inability to induce significant TNF production in cells of human, rather than rodent, origin. This led to a search for other structurally related agents which could overcome this issue. The current lead compound is 5, 6-dimethylxanthenone 4-acetic acid (DMXAA, AS1404). This compound has shown activity in a number of experimental tumor models and has progressed through phase I clinical trials (Laws *et al.*, 1995; Jameson *et al.*,

2003). Evidence of blood flow reduction in these phase I trials has resulted in the movement of DMXAA, in combination with cytotoxic therapy, into phase II trials. Interestingly, the mechanism of action of this compound has not been clearly elucidated, but there is some evidence that it involves the induction of localized TNFα release from activated macrophages within the tumor and apoptosis of endothelial cells within the tumor vessels (Ching *et al.*, 1999, 2002). The utility of flavones and xanthenones as VDAs is discussed in detail in Chapter 9.

N-cadherin antagonists

The endothelial cell adhesion molecules neural and vascular endothelial cadherin play essential roles in the formation of stable and fully functional blood vessels (Blaschuk and Rowlands, 2000) (see also Chapter 11). If the integrity of the endothelial cell lining can be compromised, then blood flow in these vessels would be reduced. A cyclic peptide has been developed that targets N-cadherin. This molecule, called ADH-1 or Exherin, has been shown to selectively induce necrosis and hemorrhage within experimental tumors. ADH-1 works by mimicking the N-cadherin active site, thereby preventing cadherins from binding together, leading to leakage and rupture of the established tumor blood vessels. This compound has now moved into clinical trials.

Tubulin depolymerizing agents

As discussed above, early studies had indicated that colchicine and podophyllotoxin, two established tubulin depolymerizing agents, could induce rapid hemorrhagic necrosis in experimental tumors. The drawback was that these effects were only observed at, or close to, the MTD. Despite these early hints of vascular disrupting activity, efforts to discover other tubulin depolymerizing agents focused only on their ability to inhibit cell proliferation *in vitro*. These studies led to the discovery and development of many compounds including the vinca alkaloids.

In the early 1990s our group at the Gray Laboratory decided to take an active interest in the vascular disrupting properties of tubulin depolymerizing agents. First, we established that selective vascular shutdown in tumors could be obtained using high doses of both vincristine and vinblastine (Hill *et al.*, 1993). This work took place at the same time that we were developing a technique that facilitated rapid assessment of vascular function in tumors. This technique involved intravenous injection of the fluorochrome Hoechst 33342 (Chaplin *et al.*, 1987; Smith *et al.*, 1988). With this technique in hand we decided to screen tubulin-depolymerizing agents available from commercial and academic sources for their ability to decrease tumor blood flow at doses down to one-tenth of the MTD. Most agents lost their vascular effects at doses just below the MTD. However, two groups of novel compounds displayed quite potent vascular effects, notably the dolastatins and combretastatins (Chaplin *et al.*, 1996). The most exciting early data surrounded the water-soluble phosphate prodrug of combretastatin A4 (CA4P). This compound was shown to shut down blood flow in tumors at doses below one-tenth of the MTD in mice (Dark *et al.*, 1997). Moreover, this blood flow shutdown was shown to be selective for the tumor tissue. CA4P represented the first small-molecular-weight agent that could induce selective vascular disruption in tumors over a wide dose range. This discovery led to an intense search for other agents with similar properties. Over the past eight years several other tubulin-depolymerizing agents have been identified that possess similar properties, several of which have progressed into clinical trial (Table 4.1). Since CA4P has now become one of the most widely studied VDAs, we will focus the remainder of the chapter on this molecule.

Table 4.1 Small-molecule VDAs currently in late preclinical or clinical evaluation

Compound	Mechanism	Current development status	Notes
CA4P (OXi2021)	Tubulin-depolymerizing agent	Phase II clinical trials ongoing	Nine clinical trials including two in ophthalmology
ZD6126	Tubulin-depolymerizing agent	Phases I clinical trials completed	Futher preclinical evaluation ongoing
DMXAA(AS1404)	TNF induction	Phase II clinical trials ongoing	Combination study with carbo/taxol
AVE8062	Tubulin-depolymerizing agent	Phase I clinical trials ongoing	
NPI 2358	Tubulin-depolymerizing agent	Preclinical	IND filing 2005
MN 029	Tubulin-depolymerizing agent	Phase I clinical trials ongoing	
OXi4503	Tubulin-depolymerizing agent	Phase I clinical trials ongoing	
ADH-1 (Exherin)	N-cadherin antagonist	Phase I clinical trials ongoing	

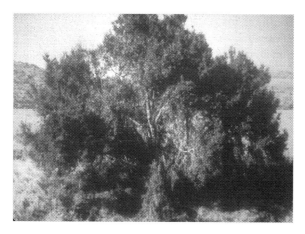

Figure 4.3 *Combretum caffrum*, from the bark of which combretastatin A4 was originally isolated by Pettit and co-workers at Arizona State University

4.7 Combretastatin A4 phosphate

Discovery and isolation

Combretastatin A4 was originally isolated from the bark of *Combretum caffrum* by Pettit and colleagues in the early 1980s. *Combretum caffrum* is a deciduous tree (growing to 15 m high) found principally in South Africa and Zimbabwe (Figure 4.3). The willow-like tree ('bushwillow') is a common sight overhanging stream beds. It has been reported that the powdered root bark has been used by the Zulu of South Africa as a charm to harm an enemy.

Tubulin binding activity

CA4P is a water-soluble pro-drug, which is activated when it is dephosphorylated into CA4. CA4P does not bind to tubulin, but CA4 is a known tubulin-binding agent and has been demonstrated to bind at or near the colchicine-binding site of β-tubulin ($k_d = 0.40 \pm 0.06\,\mu M$) (Lin *et al.*, 1988; Woods *et al.*, 1995). CA4 competitively inhibits the binding of colchicine to tubulin (K_i of $0.14\,\mu M$) and, like colchicine, inhibits the polymerization of tubulin (IC_{50} $2.4 + 1.4\,\mu M$). CA4 binds rapidly to tubulin, in contrast to colchicine, which binds in a relatively slow and temperature-dependent manner. However, CA4 dissociates from tubulin over 100 times faster than colchicine, with a half-life of 3.6 relative to 405 min at 37 °C (Lin *et al.*, 1989). Notably, the *trans*-isomer of CA4 does not significantly compete with colchicine in binding tubulin, nor does it interfere with tubulin assembly ($IC \geq 50\,\mu M$).

Mechanism responsible for vascular disruption

At the time that its vascular activity was discovered, little was known about the molecule that could clearly explain why it induced vascular shutdown. Studies have shown that combretastatin A-4 phosphate can induce selective cytotoxic/antiproliferative effects against dividing, compared to quiescent, endothelial cells in culture (Dark *et al.*, 1997). However, the rapidity of vascular shutdown (~10 min) observed in an isolated rat tumor model suggests that more immediate changes are responsible for the drug effects seen (Dark *et al.*, 1997; Tozer *et al.*, 1999). Work has shown that combretastatin A-4 phosphate and related compounds can have dramatic effects on the three-dimensional shape of newly formed endothelial cells, but less effect on quiescent endothelial cells (Watts *et al.*, 1997; Galbraith *et al.*, 2001). It is believed that the reason newly formed endothelial cells are more sensitive than more mature cells is that the latter have a more highly developed actin cytoskeleton, which maintains the cell shape despite depolymerization of the tubulin cytoskeleton (Chaplin and Dougherty, 1999). Clearly, rapid changes in endothelial cell shape *in vivo* would dramatically alter capillary blood flow, expose basement membrane and as a result induce hemorrhage and coagulation. The sensitivity of the immature tumor vasculature to CA4P probably relates to not only differences between newly formed and mature endothelial cells, but also to characteristics of the tumor microcirculation such as high vascular permeability, high interstitial fluid pressure, pro-coagulant status, vessel tortuosity and heterogeneous blood flow distribution (Tozer *et al.*, 2002).

Selectivity for abnormal neovasculature

Little work has been done to evaluate the selectivity of CA4P for the neovasculature specifically associated with abnormal disease processes such as cancer and ocular disorders such as age-related macular degeneration (AMD) and diabetic retinopathy, compared with new vessels formed during normal processes such as wound healing and embryo development. However, a study by Griggs and colleagues did look at the effect of CA4P in 12-day-old mouse pups where abnormal retinal neovascularization had been induced following exposure to a high-oxygen environment (Griggs *et al.*, 2002). After five days of CA4P treatment they evaluated the effect on both the abnormal neovascularization associated with the retinopathy and the continued neovascularization associated with the normal retinal development in these young mice. They concluded that 'CA4P permitted the development of normal retinal vasculature while inhibiting aberrant neovascularization'. This raises the question as to the reason for such selectivity. It has been reported that the abnormal neovascularization associated with cancer and certain eye diseases is associated with a shift in the balance between angiopoietins (Ang) 1 and 2 in favor of angiopoietin 2 (Otani *et al.*,

1999; Tait and Jones, 2004). Ang-1 is known to act as a maturation factor promoting the recruitment of pericytes and smooth muscle cells to the developing vessel, whereas Ang-2 destabilizes the vessel structure. It is interesting to speculate that a lack of pericytes and other support cells may make the endothelial cells more likely to undergo a change in shape in response to tubulin-depolymerizing agents. Indeed some ongoing work in transfected tumors indicates that overexpression of Ang-1 reduces the effectiveness of CA4P.

Reason for enhanced vascular effects with CA4P versus colchicine

It appears that almost all of the tubulin-depolymerizing agents that have been tested can disrupt vascular function in tumors when administered at doses close to the MTD. Based on the mechanisms described above, one would expect them all to do this. So the question is often asked as to why CA4P can shut down vasculature in tumors at much lower doses than colchicine. It is our belief, based on the data available, that the shift from anti-mitotic activity to vascular disrupting activity *in vivo*, seen as we move from colchicine to CA4P, is due to the reversibility of the tubulin binding, coupled with an increased rate of clearance. This would result in a reduced duration of tubulin depolymerization. Such an effect, while still allowing rapid morphological changes in endothelial cells, would greatly reduce the dose-limiting antiproliferative effects associated with prolonged periods of tubulin depolymerization.

What have we learned from the clinic

The clinical experience with CA4P has recently been reviewed (Young and Chaplin, 2004). CA4P underwent three phase I clinical trials. The dose-limiting toxicities seen in phase I, which resulted in an MTD of $68 \, \text{mg m}^{-2}$ being established, were ataxia, tumor pain and reversible myocardial effects. Tumor blood flow reductions were observed at clinically achievable doses of $33 \, \text{mg m}^{-2}$ and above. Currently nine further trials are ongoing, including two in ophthalmology. For more detailed reviews of clinical trials of CA4P and other VDAs see Chapters 17 and 18.

Dissociating vasoconstrictive effects from vascular disruption

There has been considerable focus on potential cardiovascular side effects of CA4P based around its known mechanism of action. In the reported phase I studies three cases of reversible myocardial effects were reported and these contributed to the establishment of the current MTD. In these patients hypertension was evident prior to the myocardial effects occurring. It is of interest that tubulin depolymerizing agents as a class can, in addition to their direct effects on endothelial cell morphology, induce arteriolar vasoconstriction even in endothelial cell denuded vessels (Platts *et al.*, 1999). Also, it has been established that concomitant use of vasodilators with CA4P can eliminate vasoconstriction in rats without altering the blood flow shutdown effects in the tumor, further indicating the independence of the two effects (Honess *et al.*, 2002). If, as we believe, the vasoconstrictive actions of CA4P contribute to the dose-limiting toxicities, including cardiovascular ones, there is a possibility that the prophylactic use of vasodilators may not only alter its toxicity profile, but also enable higher dose levels to be attained. This approach requires evaluation in a clinical setting.

4.8   The viable rim

It has become evident from the use of VDAs in a cancer setting that they have little or no effect on tumor growth and response when used alone. As mentioned earlier, this effect was predicted by Woglom as early as 1923 and is due to the fact that there will be tumor cells present, particularly at the outside edge or rim of the tumor, which derive their nutrients etc from blood vessels in the proximal normal tissue. Since such tumor cells are supported by a well formed and functional blood supply, not only should they be readily accessible to systemically administered agents, but because of relatively good nutrient and oxygen supplies, they should also be the cells most sensitive to conventional therapies, which by their design, target rapidly proliferating, well oxygenated cell populations. The use of VDAs in conjunction with chemotherapy, radiation and antibody-based therapeutics, which directly target tumor cells, has provided significantly enhanced tumor responses and this is covered in detail in subsequent chapters. Clearly the regrowth of this 'viable rim' of tumor cells into the central regions, necrosed following VDA treatment, is also dependent on revascularization, so potentially anti-angiogenic approaches could be used to enhance tumor response. Recent data by Siemann and colleagues (Siemann and Shi, 2004) have shown that combining a VDA with antiangiogenic therapy significantly augments tumor response in preclinical models, compared with either treatment alone.

4.9   Conclusions

Although the importance of tumor vasculature as a potential therapeutic target for drug development was first alluded to over 80 years ago, it is only over the last 10–15 years that a concerted effort has been made to develop such therapeutics. The concept and rationale for targeting the already formed neovasculature in tumors was put forward by the late Professor Julie Denekamp. Her enthusiasm and persistence in initiating this field of research has been rewarded with several compounds now in clinical trial and many more due to enter the clinical evaluation phase. It is of interest that the most widely studied group of compounds is the tubulin-depolymerizing drugs, and their development stems from early evidence that colchicine induced hemorrhagic necrosis in tumors. The lead compound CA4P has demonstrated the ability to disrupt tumor vascular function in clinical trials, thus establishing proof of concept.

As with all drug development the path has not been entirely smooth. Reversible myocardial events in a few patients raised the question of selectivity for abnormal neovasculature associated with disease processes as opposed to newly formed vessels that could occur normally following injury or ischemic events. Recent data indicates that vasoconstrictive properties of CA4P could also be responsible for the myocardial effects seen. If so, evidence that the control of drug-induced hypertension in rats does not alter the tumor-vascular-disrupting properties of the drug could be very important. Several ligand-based VDA approaches have demonstrated impressive effects in animal models and several are expected to enter clinical trials shortly. Conceptually, the ability to target unique antigenic determinants expressed on tumor endothelium is very appealing. It has become clear that even the most ideal VDA would not be curative, because of our knowledge that a small but significant number of tumor cells reside adjacent to normal tissue vessels. However, the combination of VDAs with many conventional and emerging therapeutic strategies, including anti-angiogenics, has produced impressive results in preclinical models (Chapters 7–9).

Although originally developed for use in oncology it has become evident that VDAs may have application in other diseases that are characterized by abnormal neovascularization, in particular certain ocular disorders such as wet AMD and myopic macular degeneration (MMD). Positive results in preclinical models have led to the initiation of two clinical trials evaluating the use of CA4P in both AMD and MMD (see also Chapter 18).

References

Andervont, H.B. (1940). Effect of colchicine and bacterial products on transplantable and spontaneous tumors in mice. *J Natl Cancer Inst* **1**, 361–366.

Arap, W., Pasqualini, R. *et al.* (1998). Cancer treatment by targeted drug delivery to tumor vasculature in a mouse model. *Science* **279** (5349), 377–380.

Bekemeier, H. and Hirschelmann, R. (1989). Reactivity of resistance blood vessels ex vivo after administration of toxic chemicals to laboratory animals: arteriolotoxicity. *Toxicol Lett* **49** (1), 49–54.

Bibby, M.C., Double, J.A. *et al.* (1989). Reduction of tumor blood flow by flavone acetic acid: a possible component of therapy. *J Natl Cancer Inst* **81** (3), 216–220.

Blaschuk, O.W. and Rowlands, T.M. (2000). Cadherins as modulators of angiogenesis and the structural integrity of blood vessels. *Cancer Metastasis Rev* **19** (1/2), 1–5.

Boyland, E. and Boyland, M.E. (1937). Studies in tissue metabolism. IX. The action of colchicine and *B. typhosus* extract. *Biochem J* 31, 454–460.

Brekken, R.A. and Thorpe, P.E. (2001). Vascular endothelial growth factor and vascular targeting of solid tumors. *Anticancer Res* 21 (6B), 4221–4229.

Brooks, P.C., Clark, R.A. *et al.* (1994). Requirement of vascular integrin alpha v beta 3 for angiogenesis. *Science* 264 (5158), 569–571.

Burrows, F.J., Derbyshire, E.J. *et al.* (1995). Up-regulation of endoglin on vascular endothelial cells in human solid tumors: implications for diagnosis and therapy. *Clin Cancer Res* 1 (12), 1623–1634.

Burrows, F.J. and Thorpe, P.E. (1993). Eradication of large solid tumors in mice with an immunotoxin directed against tumor vasculature. *Proc Natl Acad Sci USA* 90 (19), 8996–9000.

Chang, S.S., O'Keefe, D.S. *et al.* (1999). Prostate-specific membrane antigen is produced in tumor-associated neovasculature. *Clin Cancer Res* 5 (10), 2674–2681.

Chaplin, D.J. and Dougherty, G.J. (1999). Tumour vasculature as a target for cancer therapy. *Br J Cancer* 80 (Suppl. 1), 57–64.

Chaplin, D.J. and Horsman, M.R. (1994). The influence of tumour temperature on ischemia-induced cell death: potential implications for the evaluation of vascular mediated therapies. *Radiother Oncol* 30 (1), 59–65.

Chaplin, D.J., Olive, P.L. *et al.* (1987). Intermittent blood flow in a murine tumor: radiobiological effects. *Cancer Res* 47 (2), 597–601.

Chaplin, D.J., Pettit, G.R. *et al.* (1996). Antivascular approaches to solid tumour therapy: evaluation of tubulin binding agents. *Br J Cancer* 27 (Suppl.), S86–S88.

Ching, L.M., Cao, Z. *et al.* (2002). Induction of endothelial cell apoptosis by the antivascular agent 5,6-dimethylxanthenone-4-acetic acid. *Br J Cancer* 86 (12), 1937–1942.

Ching, L.M., Goldsmith, D. *et al.* (1999). Induction of intratumoral tumor necrosis factor (TNF) synthesis and hemorrhagic necrosis by 5,6-dimethylxanthenone-4-acetic acid (DMXAA) in TNF knockout mice. *Cancer Res* 59 (14), 3304–3307.

Coley, W.B. (1893). The treatment of malignant tumors by repeated inoculations of erysipelas, with a report of 10 original cases. *Am J Med Sci* 105, 488–511.

Coley, W.B. (1894). Treatment of inoperable malignant tumors with the toxins of erysipelas and the Bacillus prodigiosus. *Am J Med Sci* 108, 50–66.

Dark, G.G., Hill, S.A. *et al.* (1997). Combretastatin A-4, an agent that displays potent and selective toxicity toward tumor vasculature. *Cancer Res* 57 (10), 1829–1834.

Denekamp, J. (1982). Endothelial cell proliferation as a novel approach to targeting tumour therapy. *Br J Cancer* 45 (1), 136–139.

Denekamp, J. (1984). Vascular endothelium as the vulnerable element in tumours. *Acta Radiologica Oncol* 23 (4), 217–225.

Denekamp, J. (1986). Endothelial cell attack as a novel approach to cancer therapy. *Cancer Topics* 6, 6–8.

Denekamp, J., Hill, S.A. *et al.* (1983). Vascular occlusion and tumour cell death. *Eur J Cancer Clin Oncol* 19 (2), 271–275.

Evelhoch, J.L., Bissery, M.C. *et al.* (1988). Flavone acetic acid (NSC 347512)-induced modulation of murine tumor physiology monitored by in vivo nuclear magnetic resonance spectroscopy. *Cancer Res* 48 (17), 4749–4755.

Galbraith, S.M., Chaplin, D.J. *et al.* (2001). Effects of combretastatin A4 phosphate on endothelial cell morphology in vitro and relationship to tumour vascular targeting activity in vivo. *Anticancer Res* 21 (1A), 93–102.

Griffin, R.J., Monzen, H. *et al.* (2003). Arsenic trioxide induces selective tumour vascular damage via oxidative stress and increases thermosensitivity of tumours. *Int J Hypertherm* 19 (6), 575–589.

Griggs, J., Skepper, J.N. *et al.* (2002). Inhibition of proliferative retinopathy by the anti-vascular agent combretastatin-A4. *Am J Pathol* **160** (3), 1097–1103.

Hill, S.A., Lonergan, S.J. *et al.* (1993). Vinca alkaloids: anti-vascular effects in a murine tumour. *Eur J Cancer* **9** (4), 1320–1324.

Hill, S.A., Williams, K.B. *et al.* (1989). Vascular collapse after flavone acetic acid: a possible mechanism of its anti-tumour action. *Eur J Cancer Clin Oncol* **25**, 1419–1424.

Hill, S.A., Williams, K.B. *et al.* (1992). A comparison of vascular-mediated tumor cell death by the necrotizing agents GR63178 and flavone acetic acid. *Int J Radiat Oncol Biol Phys* **22** (3), 437–441.

Honess, D.J., Hylands, F., Chaplin, D.J. and Tozer, G.M. (2002). Comparison of strategies to overcome the hypertensive effect of combretastatin-A-4-phosphate in a rat model. *Br J Cancer* **86** (Suppl. 1), S118.

Huang, X., Molema, G. *et al.* (1997). Tumor infarction in mice by antibody-directed targeting of tissue factor to tumor vasculature. *Science* **275** (5299), 547–550.

Jameson, M.B., Thompson, P.I. *et al.* (2003). Clinical aspects of a phase I trial of 5,6-dimethylxanthenone-4-acetic acid (DMXAA), a novel antivascular agent. *Br J Cancer* **88** (12), 1844–1850.

Kallinowski, F., Schaefer, C. *et al.* (1989). In vivo targets of recombinant human tumour necrosis factor-alpha: blood flow, oxygen consumption and growth of isotransplanted rat tumours. *Br J Cancer* **60** (4), 555–560.

Kerr, D.J., Kaye, S.B. *et al.* (1987). Phase I and pharmacokinetic study of flavone acetic acid. *Cancer Res* **47** (24 Pt 1), 6776–6781.

Kerr, D.J., Maughan, T. *et al.* (1989). Phase II trials of flavone acetic acid in advanced malignant melanoma and colorectal carcinoma. *Br J Cancer* **60** (1), 104–106.

Laws, A.L., Matthew, A.M. *et al.* (1995). Preclinical in vitro and in vivo activity of 5,6-dimethylxanthenone-4-acetic acid. *Br J Cancer* **71** (6), 1204–1209.

Leiter, J., Downing, V. *et al.* (1950). Damage induced in sarcoma 37 with podophyllin, podophyllotoxin alpha-peltatin, beta-peltatin, and quercetin. *J Natl Cancer Inst* **10** (6), 1273–1293.

Leiter, J., Downing, V. *et al.* (1952). Damage induced in sarcoma 37 with chemical agents. II. Trivalent and pentavalent arsenicals. *J Natl Cancer Inst* **13** (2), 365–378.

Lew, Y.S., Brown, S.L. *et al.* (1999). Arsenic trioxide causes selective necrosis in solid murine tumors by vascular shutdown. *Cancer Res* **59** (24), 6033–6037.

Lin, C.M., Ho, H.H. *et al.* (1989). Antimitotic natural products combretastatin A-4 and combretastatin A-2: studies on the mechanism of their inhibition of the binding of colchicine to tubulin. *Biochemistry* **28** (17), 6984–6991.

Lin, C.M., Singh, S.B. *et al.* (1988). Interactions of tubulin with potent natural and synthetic analogs of the antimitotic agent combretastatin: a structure–activity study. *Mol Pharmacol* **34** (2), 200–208.

Ludford, R.J. (1945). Colchicine in the experimental chemotherapy of cancer. *J Natl Cancer Inst* **6**, 89–101.

Ludford, R.J. (1948). Factors determining the action of colchicine on tumour growth. *Br J Cancer* **2**, 75–86.

Mottram, J.C. (1928). Observations on the combined action of colloidal lead and radiation on tumours. *Br Med J* **1**, 928.

Nilsson, F., Kosmehl, H. *et al.* (2001). Targeted delivery of tissue factor to the ED-B domain of fibronectin, a marker of angiogenesis, mediates the infarction of solid tumors in mice. *Cancer Res* **61** (2), 711–716.

Old, L.J. (1985). Tumour necrosis factor (TNF). *Science* **230**, 630–633.

Otani, A., Takagi, H. *et al.* (1999). Expressions of angiopoietins and Tie2 in human choroidal neovascular membranes. *Invest Ophthalmol Vis Sci* **40** (9), 1912–1920.

Parkins, C.S., Hill, S.A. *et al.* (1994). Ischaemia induced cell death in tumors: importance of temperature and pH. *Int J Radiat Oncol Biol Phys* **29** (3), 499–503.

Platts, S.H., Falcone, J.C. *et al.* (1999). Alteration of microtubule polymerization modulates arteriolar vasomotor tone. *Am J Physiol* **277** (1 Pt 2), H100–H106.

Pober, J.S. (1987). Effects of tumour necrosis factor and related cytokines on vascular endothelial cells. *Ciba Found Symp* **131**, 170–184.

Seed, L., Slaughter, D.P. *et al.* (1940). Effect of colchicine on human carcinoma. *Surgery* **7**, 696–709.

Seon, B.K. (2002). Expression of endoglin (CD105) in tumor blood vessels. *Int J Cancer. J Int Cancer* **99** (2), 310–311; discussion 312.

Siemann, D.W., Bibby, M.C., Dark, G.G., Dicker, A.P., Eskens, F.A.L.M., Horsman, M.R., Marme, D. and LoRusso, P.M. (2005) Differentiation and definition of vascular-targeting therapies. *Clin Cancer Res* **11**, 416–420.

Siemann, D.W. and Shi, W. (2004). Efficacy of combined antiangiogenic and vascular disrupting agents in the treatment of solid tumors. *Int J Radiat Oncol Biol Phys* **60**, 1233–1240.

Smith, G.P., Calveley, S.B. *et al.* (1987). Flavone acetic acid (NSC 347512) induces haemorrhagic necrosis of mouse colon 26 and 38 tumours. *Eur J Cancer Clin Oncol* **23** (8), 1209–1211.

Smith, K.A., Hill S.A., Begg, A.C. and Denekamp, J. (1988). Validation of the fluorescent dye Hoechst 33342 as a vascular space marker in tumours. *Br J Cancer* **57**, 247–253.

Tait, C.R. and Jones, P.F. (2004). Angiopoietins in tumours: the angiogenic switch. *J Pathol* **204** (1), 1–10.

Tozer, G.M., Kanthou, C. *et al.* (2002). The biology of the combretastatins as vascular targeting agents. *Int J Exp Pathol* **83**, 21–38.

Tozer, G.M., Prise, V.E. *et al.* (1999). Combretastatin A-4 phosphate as a tumor vascular-targeting agent: early effects in tumors and normal tissues. *Cancer Res* **59** (7), 1626–1634.

Veenendaal, L.M., Jin, H. *et al.* (2002). In vitro and in vivo studies of a VEGF121/rGelonin chimeric fusion toxin targeting the neovasculature of solid tumors. *Proc Natl Acad Sci USA* **99** (12), 7866–7871.

Walshe, W.W. (1844). *The Anatomy, Physiology, Pathology and Treatment of Cancer*. Ticknor and Company, Boston.

Watts, M.E., Woodcock, M. *et al.* (1997). Effects of novel and conventional anti-cancer agents on human endothelial permeability: influence of tumour secreted factors. *Anticancer Res* **17** (1A), 71–75.

Weiss, R.B., Greene, R.F. *et al.* (1988). Phase I and clinical pharmacology study of intravenous flavone acetic acid (NSC 347512). *Cancer Res* **48** (20), 5878–5882.

Woglom, W.H. (1923). A critique of tumour resistance. *J Cancer Res* **7**, 283–311.

Woods, J.A., Hadfield, J.A. *et al.* (1995). The interaction with tubulin of a series of stilbenes based on combretastatin A-4. *Br J Cancer* **71** (4), 705–711.

Young, S.L. and Chaplin, D.J. (2004). Combretastatin A4 phosphate: background and current clinical status. *Exp Opin Invest Drugs* **13** (9), 1171–1182.

5

Morphologic Manifestations of Vascular-disrupting Agents in Preclinical Models

Mumtaz V. Rojiani and **Amyn M. Rojiani**

Abstract

An important aspect of tumor growth is the continued 'physiologic' functioning of intratumoral blood vessels, effectively delivering oxygen and nutrients. Vascular disrupting agents (VDA) target this component of tumor vasculature, bringing about a rapid and catastrophic shutdown and consequent tumor necrosis. Using three animal tumor models and different VDAs we detail the morphologic and morphometric evolution of VDA induced tumor injury. While there are quantitative and chronologic differences, qualitative morphologic alterations are strikingly similar between the tumor models and VDAs investigated. Functional vascular shutdown is identified by fluorescent microscopy within the first hour following parenteral delivery of the drug. As the tumor undergoes frank necrosis, intratumoral vessels are irreversibly damaged. The pattern of injury is typical of vascular compromise, with necrosis interspersed with areas of red cell extravasation. In each of the models, surviving tumor persists as a peripheral, viable rim of neoplastic elements that has a clear and significant potential for regrowth. The morphologic changes manifest by use of these agents, provide important clues to understanding the mechanisms that operate in the induction of this antitumor activity.

Keywords

Histopathology, preclinical models, KHT sarcoma, Kaposi's sarcoma, vascular disrupting agents, combretastatin, ZD6126, treatment effect

5.1   Introduction

The establishment and continued growth of tumors is predicated upon the development and ongoing maintenance of an adequate network of blood vessels. The initial process of neovascularization, also referred to as angiogenesis, is essential to all solid tumors (Dennekamp, 1984; Folkman and Shing, 1992; Denekamp, 1993; Folkman, 1995; Hahnfeldt *et al.*, 1999). This phenomenon is critical in the early growth of the neoplasm and its continued expansion, be it infiltration or metastasis. A second and arguably equally important aspect of this tumor growth is the maturation, development of a tubular component and continued patency of these vessels in order that they may effectively carry out the 'physiologic' function of blood vessels, *viz.* the adequate perfusion of cells to deliver oxygen and nutrients. It is recognized that a variety of agents target this latter component of tumor vasculature, bringing about a rapid and catastrophic shutdown of these vessels and consequent hemorrhagic tumor necrosis (Bicknell and Harris, 1992; Dark *et al.*, 1997). Included in this group of compounds are tubulin-binding agents (Baguley *et al.*, 1991; Hill, Sampson and Chaplin, 1995), most notably combretastatin A4 disodium phosphate (CA4DP) and OXI4503, as well as the phosphate prodrug of N-acetycolchinol (ZD6126) and the flavone derivative 5,6-dimethyl-xanthenone-4 acetic acid (DMXAA). These drugs, often referred to as vascular-disrupting agents (VDAs), have demonstrated potent antivascular and antitumor efficacy in a wide variety of preclinical tumor models at well tolerated doses (Rewcastle *et al.*, 1991; Ching, Joseph and Baguley, 1992; Laws *et al.*, 1995; Dark *et al.*, 1997; Li, Rojiani and Siemann, 1998; Horsman *et al.*, 1998; Grosios *et al.*, 1999; Tozer *et al.*, 1999; Hori *et al.*, 1999; Nelkin and Ball, 2001; Blakey *et al.*, 2002; Siemann and Rojiani, 2002; Rojiani *et al.*, 2002; Siemann *et al.*, 2002).

5.2   Animal models

The morphologic changes manifest by the use of these agents provide important clues to understanding the mechanisms that operate in the induction of this antitumor activity. We have used the human Kaposi's sarcoma (KSY-1) and renal cell carcinoma Caki-1 xenograft models as well as the rodent KHT sarcoma model with the VDAs CA4DP, OXI4503, DMXAA and ZD6126 and will rely on these models to illustrate the changes. Human tumor xenografts were generated by injecting tumor cells into the flank of 6–8-week-old athymic NCR nu/nu mice (Frederick Laboratories, Frederick, MD). KHT sarcomas were initiated by injecting tumor cells into the calf muscle of 6–8-week-old C3H/HeJ mice (Jackson Laboratories, Bar Harbor, ME). Details of these models have been described elsewhere (Rojiani *et al.*, 2002, Shi and Siemann, 2002, Siemann and Rojiani, 2002).

The KSY-1 cell line as previously characterized (Lunardi-Iskander *et al.*, 1995) was used. This cell line was derived from mononuclear cells from pleural effusion of an AIDS patient with KS, following selective removal of lymphocytes, monocytes/macrophages and fibroblasts. Histologic sections of untreated KS xenografts reveal a solid, vasoformative neoplasm with intervening fibrovascular septae along with scattered inflammatory cells (Figure 5.1(a)). Occasional areas of necrosis may be seen within the tumor (arrow).

The neoplastic cells are large and epithelioid or spindle shaped, with vesicular nuclei and modest pleomorphism. The tumor is a highly vascular, actively proliferating neoplasm with brisk mitotic activity. Areas of the tumor have slit-like spaces characteristic of endothelial-derived tumors with scattered red blood cells, while in other areas tumor cells appear to be forming abortive lumina (Figure 5.1(b)). The tumors are focally immunoreactive for CD31 and only minimally positive or negative for CD34 and FVIIIra

Electron microscopy (Figure 5.1(c)) show the tumor cells to be large, oval to spindle shaped with round to irregular nuclei and prominent nucleoli. Although well defined vascular lumina containing red blood cells are present (bottom left),

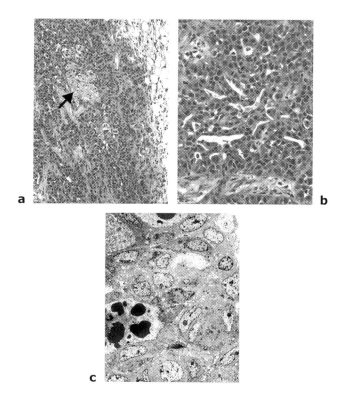

Figure 5.1 (a),(b) H&E stained, untreated KSY xenograft. (a) Original magnification 40×. (b) Original magnification 200×. (c) Untreated KS xenograft, electron micrograph, original magnification 12 000×. (Reproduced with permission from Rojiani A.M., *et al.* (2002). Activity of the vascular targeting agent combretastatin A-4 disodium phosphate in a xenograft model of AIDS-associated Kaposi's sarcoma. *Acta Oncologica*, Taylor and Francis)

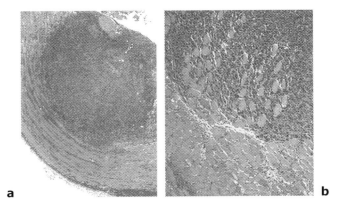

Figure 5.2   H&E stained sections from untreated KHT sarcoma. (a) The rodent KHT sarcoma grows as a well defined tumor mass, compressing adjacent soft tissue including skeletal muscle. Original magnification 40×. (b) On closer examination, however, tumor cells can be seen infiltrating soft tissue in the immediate vicinity, particularly skeletal muscle, resulting in host muscle fibers isolated within the body of the tumor. Original magnification 200×

there are multiple areas where the tumor cells have microvilli that appear to be projecting into an abortive lumen (top right). Endothelial cells with tubuloreticulated rod-shaped bodies suggestive of Weibel-Palade bodies are rarely seen (not illustrated). Junctions were present between cells, although they differed in appearance from typical desmosomes.

Caki-1 tumor cells represent the clear cell renal carcinoma cell line (Shi and Siemann, 2002). These tumors grow within the flanks of nude mice as well – circumscribed, almost spherical nodules, with formation of a pseudocapsule-like edge from compressed adjacent host tissue. The cells are large, round to oval, with a distinctly epithelial appearance. Normal vessels appear rounded and in some areas compressed.

The KHT sarcoma model (Thomson and Rauth, 1974; Siemann, 1995; Siemann, Johansen and Horsman, 1998; Siemann and Rojiani, 2002) differs from the above models in some morphologic aspects. By virtue of its mesenchymal derivation, the inherent properties of this tumor promote a more infiltrative growth pattern. Although it forms a measurable tumor nodule, its margins are poorly defined and the tumor insinuates itself within the endomysium of adjacent skeletal muscle, often entrapping isolated myofibers within the body of the tumor as is characteristic of many sarcomas (Figures 5.2(a) and (b)).

5.3   Morphologic and morphometric analysis

The tumor was dissected from the flank and adjacent connective tissue removed. Following fixation in 10 per cent neutral buffered formalin it was inked around its entire surface to define borders and then serially divided at 1 mm intervals. Alternate slices were submitted for routine histology processing. Sections were dehydrated through a series of graded alcohols, processed in xylene and embedded in paraffin. Four micrometer sections obtained from these paraffin blocks were stained with hematoxylin and eosin (H&E) stain. Each H&E stained tumor section was divided into multiple grids and individual grids were then assessed. Images were captured with a frame-grabber using a CCD camera attached to a Nikon ES600 microscope. Sections were then morphometrically assessed with the Image Pro Plus image analysis system (Media Cybernetics, Silver Spring, MD). With the aid of an 'irregular area of interest' tool, areas of necrosis were outlined and measured on each grid. Multiple grids for each tumor were combined and compared with the total area of the tumor, results being expressed as percent necrosis.

Hoechst-33342 (bisBenzimide, Sigma) solution made up in 0.9 per cent sterile saline was administered at 40 mg/kg intravenously (volume 5 ml kg^{-1}) at various times after treatment with CA4DP (Smith *et al.*, 1988). One minute after Hoechst-33342 injection the mice were killed and the tumors resected and immediately immersed in liquid nitrogen for subsequent frozen sectioning. For each tumor sample, 10 μm cryostat sections were cut at three different levels between one pole and the equatorial plane. The sections were air dried and then studied under UV illumination using a fluorescent microscope. Blood vessel outlines were identified by the surrounding halo of fluorescent H33342-labeled cells. Vessel counts were performed using a Chalkley point array for random sample analysis (Curtis, 1960).

Methods for immunohistochemistry were standard protocols with antigen retrieval methods and optimized antibody dilutions. Images for morphologic evaluation and illustration were captured on a SPOT Insight digital camera.

5.4 Effects of treatment

An important observation to be recognized in the context of VDA is that the morphologic changes characterizing this group of agents remain fairly consistent. While there are differences in the chronologic progression of treatment effects as well as variations in potency and efficacy, the overall morphology is strikingly similar. The histologic features described hereunder are therefore derived from studies utilizing various vascular disrupting agents (VDAs), including combretastatin CA4DP, its analog OXI4503 or ZD6126.

Following treatment with ZD6126 (150 mg kg^{-1}) or CA4DP (100 mg kg^{-1}), or OXI4503 (25 mg kg^{-1}), when tumors are removed, fixed and examined, prior to processing for histology, there are visible areas of hemorrhagic necrosis in tumors that are clearly smaller than untreated controls. These changes are seen within the boundaries of the tumor without tinctorial or structural changes in the surrounding tissue (Figure 5.3(a)). Similarly, with ZD6126 or

OXI4503, large, advanced tumors are more likely to show significant changes in size as we have previously reported (Figure 5.3(b)) (Siemann and Rojiani, 2005).

Fluorescent microscopy using the Hoechst-33342 dye identifies vascular changes in tumors within the first hour following parenteral delivery of the drug with CA4DP in the KSY tumor (Rojiani *et al.*, 2002) with a more extensive shut-down by 2 h (Figures 5.4(a) and (b)). Similarly, a significant reduction in functioning blood vessels was detected in KHT sarcoma as early as 30 minutes after ZD6126 although structural evidence of vascular injury was not seen at that early time point (Siemann and Rojiani, 2002).

This rapid and extensive shutdown in vascular function observed in the KSY model is similar to previously reported reductions in blood perfusion associated

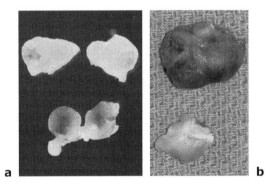

Figure 5.3   (a) Sections through KSY-1 xenografts treated with 100 mg kg^{-1} CA4DP, examined after 24 h. There is a visible reduction in tumor volume with discoloration secondary to the appearance of hemorrhagic necrosis. (b) External examination of large, bulky tumor treated with 150 mg kg^{-1} ZD6126, showing a marked decrease in overall tumor volume

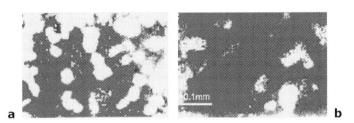

Figure 5.4   KSY xenograft, 1 min after injection of 40 mg of Hoechst-33342. Original magnification 32×. (a) Blood vessel outlines were identified by the surrounding halo of fluorescent Hoechst 33342-labeled cells in untreated animals. (b) Marked reduction in perivascular Hoechst-33342 stain reflecting significant shutdown of vasculature within the tumor in animals treated with CA4DP, 100 mg kg^{-1}, 2 h before sacrifice. (Modified and reproduced with permission from Rojiani *et al.* (2002). Activity of the vascular targeting agent combretastatin A-4 disodium phosphate in a xenograft model of AIDS-associated Kaposi's sarcoma. *Acta Oncologica*, Taylor and Francis)

with the vascular targeting agent CA4DP in other tumor models (Dark *et al.*, 1997; Horsman *et al.*, 1998; Grosios *et al.*, 1999; Chaplin, Pettit and Hill, 1999; Tozer *et al.*, 1999; Evelhoch *et al.*, 2001; Robinson *et al.*, 2001).

As recently reported (Sheng *et al.*, 2004), 12–24 h following administration of the drug there is a decrease in CD31-(PECAM-1-) labeled endothelial cells within the tumor. This decrease in vessel density progresses over the 24–48 h window and coincides with the appearance of damaged vessels in areas of incipient necrosis within the tumor.

As the tumor undergoes frank necrosis, intratumoral vessels are irreversibly compromised. Within this same time frame, blood vessels of various calibers and architecture, in the immediate vicinity of the tumor nodule, remain oblivious to this injurious effect (Figures 5.5(a)–(d)).

Necrosis within the tumor is a desirable early effect with administration of vascular-disrupting agents. In its earliest stages, the pattern of injury is one of vascular compromise with necrosis interspersed with areas of red cell extravasation. Geographic patterns of tissue loss, reminiscent of ischemic injury in

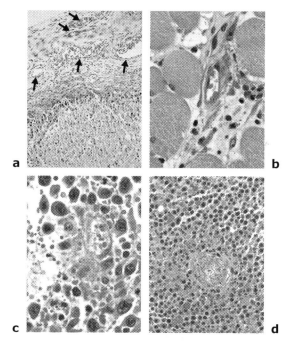

Figure 5.5 (a),(b) Vascular changes 24 h following treatment with VDA, H&E stained sections. (top) Blood vessels within the adjacent peritumoral soft tissue are preserved and undamaged following treatment with CA4DP (100 mg kg^{-1}). (a) Original magnification 100×; or OXI4503 (25 mg kg^{-1}). (b) Original magnification 400×. (c) (below) Early vessel damage with necrosis of the vessel wall within the tumor. OXI4503 (25 mg kg^{-1}) – original magnification 400×. (d) Almost complete obliteration of the structure of this thrombosed vessel with extensively necrotic surrounding tumor. Original magnification 200×

other models, are seen with lower doses of OXI 4503 (10 mg kg^{-1}). Necrosis becomes more widespread with higher doses (100 mg kg^{-1}), almost radiating outwards from the center until the vast majority of the tumor has undergone disintegration, from 80 to 95 per cent as measured by image analysis (Figures 5.6(a)–(c)).

The necrosis of tumor in focal areas is easily interpreted as being the result of shut-down of individual, dominant vessels with subsequent cell death in the distribution territory of that vessel. Over a period of time this necrosis extends to areas supplied by other intratumoral vessels, which eventually all undergo shut-down, leading to necrosis.

In all the models that we have examined, surviving tumor persists as a distinct edge, typically only a few cell layers thick, with no evidence of damage within adjacent peritumoral tissues of the host (Figures 5.7(a) and (b)). Following treat-

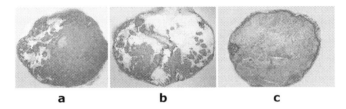

a   b   c

Figure 5.6 H&E stained, KSY xenograft, original magnification 20×. (a) Control, untreated KSY xenograft showing a solid tumor with focal tumor necrosis. (b) Treated animal, 24 h after parenteral administration of a single 10 mg kg^{-1} dose of OXI4503. Necrosis is focal and appears to progress from the center outwards. The pattern of tumor survival suggests limited involvement of some vessels and hence persistence of viable tumor in that vascular distribution. (c) Animals treated with 25 mg kg^{-1} of OXI4503 show most significant necrosis, with only about five per cent tumor persisting as a viable rim, perhaps nourished by normal, non-tumoral vessels at the periphery

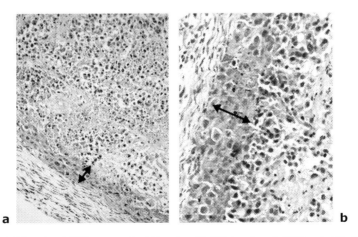

a   b

Figure 5.7 H&E stained KSY xenograft, 24 h after CA4DP treatment (100 mg kg^{-1}). (a) Original magnification 40×. (b) Original magnification 200×

ment with CA4DP (100 mg kg^{-1}) or ZD6126, large areas of necrosis, involving a major portion of the tumor, can be seen in this illustration. Only a small rim (3–5 cells wide) of viable tumor tissue is identifiable immediately below the normal host tissue (arrow). At higher magnification tissue breakdown and nuclear fragmentation is readily evident, along with a few layers of viable tumor.

This pattern of necrosis differs slightly in KHT sarcoma. As the tumor undergoes necrosis, a peripheral rim is evident and normal surrounding tissues including skeletal muscle fibers remain unaffected. Interestingly isolated skeletal muscle fibers entrapped within the bulk of the tumor undergo the same fate as tumor cells, i.e. ischemic necrosis, with loss of cross-striations and eventual breakdown of myofibers (Figures 5.8(a) and (b)).

Following ZD6126 treatment KHT tumors show extensive necrosis, extending in some areas up to the viable skeletal muscle edge. These muscle fibers however remain unaffected by the compound (Figure 5.8(a)).

Skeletal muscle fibers that have been surrounded by infiltrating tumor are compromised in the same manner as the tumor that undergoes necrosis following the vascular shut-down. Although a few viable tumor cells persist at the edge, entrapped muscle fibers are undergoing necrosis, with a glassy appearance, and loss of cross-striations and nuclei (arrow) (Figure 5.8(b)).

Although individual agents in different model systems may display some variance in the extent of necrosis induced, all of the agents bring about extensive tumor necrosis. In KSY and KHT tumors, CA4DP and ZD6126 often leave persistent viable rims between 10 and 15 per cent (Rojiani et al., 2002; Siemann and Rojiani, 2002), while in KSY OXI4503 is more effective than CA4DP, leaving a peripheral viable rim of only about five per cent (Figure 5.9(a) and (b)) (Holwell et al., 2002; Hill et al., 2002; Rojiani et al., 2004).

The necrosis seen in this context is similar to that seen in tissue death from ischemic injury. At higher magnification the cells adopt a discohesive and frag-

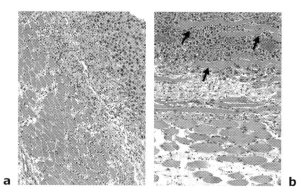

Figure 5.8 H&E stained KHT sarcoma, 24 h after ZD6126 treatment (150 mg kg^{-1}). (a) Original magnification 100×. (b) Original magnification 200×

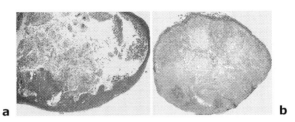

Figure 5.9 H&E stained, KSY xenograft. The extent of the persistent viable rim varies from model to model and from compound to compound, e.g. CA4DP (100 mg kg^{-1}) leaves a viable rim between 10 and 15 per cent or a few cells thick ((a), original magnification 40×) while OXI4503 at 25 mg kg^{-1} is more effective in the same model, leaving only about five per cent of the tumor ((b), original magnification 20×)

mented persona. Nuclei are condensed and round in the early stages and by 24 h this nuclear pyknosis gives way to complete disintegration. As indicated above, these changes progress from central areas of the tumor to the periphery, stopping short of the last few cell layers, which perhaps may derive their blood supply from normal vessels outside the boundaries of the neoplasm. There are frequent apoptotic bodies both in endothelial cells of intratumoral blood vessels and within neoplastic cells. Tumor cells are often enlarged or swollen, with a glassy, eosinophilic cytoplasm, reminiscent of early changes seen as a consequence of energy depletion in any ischemic process. The chromatin architecture is disrupted with many 'exploding' mitotic figures.

These changes suggest both an effect of VDAs on intratumoral blood vessels and a disruption of physiologic activities within the cells, perhaps reflecting arrested mitotic spindles and alterations in intracellular transport that are characteristics of most tubulin binding agents (Figure 5.10(a) and (b)). Tumor cells seen in Figure 5.10 at high magnification appear separated and discohesive. The cytoplasm of many cells is hyalinized and some nuclei are condensed and dark. Other cells display both cellular and nuclear fragmentation along with apoptotic bodies. Still others have both normal and abnormal nuclei. Not uncommonly, viable tumor cells at the periphery appear larger and reveal coarse, granular chromatin with many 'exploding' mitotic figures (arrow).

Despite the potent antivascular effects and large scale induction of central tumor necrosis observed following treatment with vascular targeting agents such as CA4DP and ZD6126, a narrow rim of viable tumor cells is typically observed at the tumor periphery near the surrounding normal tissues (Li, Rojiani and Siemann, 1998; Tozer *et al.*, 1999; Chaplin, Pettit and Hill, 1999; Siemann, Warrington and Horsman, 2000). In the days following single dose treatment, the previously described viable peripheral rim of the tumor proliferates to the extent that tumor regrowth occurs rapidly, thus defining limited growth delay. This has been widely reported for all vascular disrupting agents and at the current time remains the most significant limiting factor in the use of these agents in a therapeutic setting. Although the residual tumor cells can rapidly

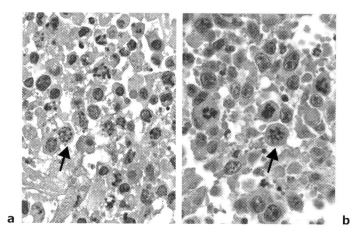

Figure 5.10 H&E stained sections, original magnification 400×, (a) KSY and (b) CAKI-1 xenografts, 24 h after treatment with OXI4503, 25 mg kg^{-1}

re-establish the tumor, its characteristic high proliferation rate and well oxygenated state make it susceptible to treatment with conventional anticancer therapies. An alternative strategy to eliminate the cells surviving the vascular targeting agent and hence to ultimately control the tumor is to combine this treatment with a therapy directly targeting these cells (Siemann, Warrington and Horsman, 2000). This approach has proven effective when combining CA4DP with conventional anticancer drugs (Chaplin, Pettit and Hill, 1999; Grosios *et al.*, 2000; Li, Rojiani and Siemann, 2002) and radiation (Li, Rojiani and Siemann, 1998; Murata *et al.*, 2001; Li, Rojiani and Siemann, 2002; Siemann and Rojiani, 2002).

In conclusion, the concept that attacking a tumor's supportive blood vessel network could offer a means of improving cancer cure rates has received a great deal of attention in recent years. One of the potentially most exploitable features of tumor blood vessels is that they are constantly growing in order to service the expanding tumor mass. Therefore, some part of each blood vessel network that supplies the tumor will be newly formed and immature, a feature not usually seen in normal adult tissues. Morphologic manifestations of vascular disrupting agents may be summarized as follows. Intratumoral vascular damage is readily evident, while normal blood vessels elsewhere in the body and even in the immediate vicinity of the tumor remain unaffected. Patterns of necrosis, both hemorrhagic and vascular shut-down induced, are similar, extending from central areas of the tumor to the periphery. Irrespective of differences in potency and efficacy of vascular disrupting agents, there persists a peripheral, viable rim of neoplastic elements that has a clear and significant potential for regrowth. Finally, although it is evident that morphologic patterns differ quantitatively and chronologically, their qualitative characteristics remain fairly consistent, from drug to drug and from animal model to animal model.

Acknowledgments

The studies described in this chapter were the result of significant interactions with Dietmar Siemann and his laboratory. The authors gratefully acknowledge this support and productive collaboration. The studies reported in this chapter were supported in part by a grant from the US National Cancer Institute (CA 84408).

References

Baguley, B.C., Holdaway, K.H., Thomsen, L.L. *et al.* (1991). Inhibition of growth of colon 38 adenocarcinoma by vinblastine and colchicine. Evidence for a vascular mechanism. *Eur J Cancer* 27, 482–487.

Bicknell, R. and Harris, A.L. (1992). Anticancer strategies involving the vasculature: vascular targeting and the inhibition of angiogenesis. *Semin Cancer Biol* 3, 399–407.

Blakey, D.C., Westwood, F.R., Walker, M., Hughes, G.D., Davis, P.D., Ashton, S.E. *et al.* (2002). Anti-tumor activity of the novel vascular targeting agent ZD6126 in a panel of tumor models. *Clin Cancer Res* 8 (6), 1974–1983.

Chaplin, D.J., Pettit, G.R. and Hill, S.A. (1999). Anti-vascular approaches to solid tumour therapy: evaluation of combretastatin A4 phosphate. *Anticancer Res* 19, 189–195.

Ching, L.M., Joseph, W.R. and Baguley, B.C. (1992). Antitumour responses to flavone-8-acetic acid and 5,6-dimethylxanthenone-4-acetic acid in immune deficient mice. *Br J Cancer* 66, 128–130.

Curtis, A.C.S. (1960). Area and volume measurements by random sampling methods. *Med Biol Illustration* 10, 261–266.

Dark, G.G., Hill, S.A., Prise, V.E. *et al.* (1997). Combretastatin A-4, an agent that displays potent and selective toxicity toward tumor vasculature. *Cancer Res* 57, 1829–1834.

Denekamp, J. (1984). Vasculature as a target for tumour therapy. *Prog Appl Microcirc* 4, 28–38.

Denekamp, J. (1993). Angiogenesis, neovascular proliferation and vascular pathophysiology as targets for cancer therapy. *Br J Radiol* 66, 181–196.

Evelhoch, J.L., He, Z., Polin, L., Corbett, T.H., Checkley, D.R., Blakey, D.C. *et al.* (2001). MRI evaluation of the effects of ZD6126 on tumor vasculature. *Proc Am Assoc Canc Res* 42, 107.

Folkman, J. (1995). Seminars in medicine of the Beth Israel Hospital, Boston. Clinical applications of research on angiogenesis. *N Engl J Med* 333, 1757–1763.

Folkman, J. and Shing, Y. (1992). Angiogenesis. *J Biol Chem* 267, 10931–10934.

Grosios, K., Holwell, S.E., McGown, A.T. *et al.* (1999). In vivo and in vitro evaluation of combretastatin A-4 and its sodium phosphate prodrug. *Br J Cancer* 81, 1318–1327.

Grosios, K., Loadman, P.M., Swaine, D.J. *et al.* (2000). Combination chemotherapy with combretastatin A-4 phosphate and 5- fluorouracil in an experimental murine colon adenocarcinoma. *Anticancer Res* 20, 229–233.

Hahnfeldt, P., Panigrahy, D., Folkman, J. and Hlatky, L. (1999). Tumor development under angiogenic signaling: a dynamical theory of tumor growth, treatment response, and post-vascular dormancy. *Cancer Res* 59 (19), 4770–4775.

Hill, S.A., Sampson, L.E. and Chaplin, D.J. (1995). Anti-vascular approaches to solid tumor therapy: evaluation of vinblastine and flavone acetic acid. *Int J Cancer* 63, 119–123.

Hill, S.A., Tozer, G.M., Pettit, G.R. and Chaplin, D.J. (2002). Preclinical evaluation of the antitumour activity of the novel vascular targeting agent Oxi 4503. *Anticancer Res* **22** (3), 1453–1458 [erratum: Anticancer Res. 2003;23:5369].

Holwell, S.E., Cooper, P.A., Thompson, M.J., Pettit, G.R., Lippert, L.W. III, Martin, S.W. and Bibby, M.C. (2002 Nov–Dec). Anti-tumor and anti-vascular effects of the novel tubulin-binding agent combretastatin A-1 phosphate. *Anticancer Res* **22** (6C), 3933–3940.

Hori, K., Saito, S., Nihei, Y. *et al.* (1999). Antitumor effects due to irreversible stoppage of tumor tissue blood flow: evaluation of a novel combretastatin A-4 derivative, AC7700. *Japan J Cancer Res* **90**, 1026–1038.

Horsman, M.R., Ehrnrooth, E., Ladekarl, M. *et al.* (1998). The effect of combretastatin A-4 disodium phosphate in a C3H mouse mammary carcinoma and a variety of murine spontaneous tumours. *Int J Radiat Oncol Biol Phys* **42**, 895–898.

Laws, A.L., Matthew, A.M., Double, J.A. and Bibby, M.C. (1995). Preclinical in vitro and in vivo activity of 5,6-dimethylxanthenone-4-acetic acid. *Br J Cancer* **71**, 1204–1209.

Li, L., Rojiani, A.M. and Siemann, D.W. (1998). Targeting the tumor vasculature with combretastatin A-4 disodium phosphate: effects on radiation therapy. *Int J Radiat Oncol Biol Phys* **42**, 899–903.

Li, L., Rojiani, A.M. and Siemann, D.W. (2002). Preclinical evaluations of therapies combining the vascular targeting agent combretastatin A-4 disodium phosphate and conventional anticancer therapies in the treatment of Kaposi's sarcoma. *Acta Oncologica* **41**, 91–97.

Lunardi-Iskandar, Y., Gill, P., Lam, V.H., Zeman, R.A., Michaels, F., Mann, D.L., Reitz, M.S. Jr., Kaplan, M., Berneman, Z.N., Carter, D. *et al.* (1995). Isolation and characterization of an immortal neoplastic cell line (KSY-1) from AIDS-associated Kaposi's sarcoma. *J Natl Cancer Inst* **87** (13), 974–981.

Murata, R., Siemann, D.W., Overgaard, J. and Horsman, M.R. (2001). Interaction between combretastatin A4 disodium phosphate and radiation in murine tumours. *Radiother Oncol* **60** (2), 155–161.

Nelkin, B.D. and Ball, D.W. (2001). Combretastatin A-4 and doxorubicin combination treatment is effective in a preclinical model of human medullary thyroid carcinoma. *Oncol Rep* **8**, 157–160.

Rewcastle, G.W., Atwell, G.J., Li, Z.A. *et al.* (1991). Potential antitumor agents. 61. Structure–activity relationships for in vivo colon 38 activity among disubstituted 9-oxo-9H-xanthene-4-acetic acids. *J Med Chem* **34**, 217–222.

Robinson, S.P., McIntyre, D.J., Howe, F.A., Griffiths, J.R., Blakey, D.C. and Waterton, J.C. (2001). Assessment of the novel tumor vascular targeting agent ZD6126 by non-invasive multi-gradient echo MRI. *Proc Am Assoc Cancer Res* **42**, 415.

Rojiani, A.M., Li, L., Rise, L. and Siemann, D.W. (2002). Activity of the vascular targeting agent combretastatin A-4 disodium phosphate in a xenograft model of AIDS-associated Kaposi's sarcoma. *Acta Oncologica* **41**, 98–105.

Rojiani, A.M., Rojiani, M.V. and Siemann, D.W. (2004). OXI 4503-second generation vascular targeting agent: histopathologic changes and preclinical efficacy. *Proc Am Assoc Cancer Res* **947**, 4103.

Sheng, Y., Hua, J., Pinney, K.G. *et al.* (2004). Combretastatin family member OXI4503 induces tumor vascular collapse through the induction of endothelial apoptosis. *Int J Cancer* **111** (4), 604–610.

Shi, W. and Siemann, D.W. (2002). Inhibition of renal cell carcinoma angiogenesis and growth by antisense oligonucleotides targeting vascular endothelial growth factor. *Br J Cancer* **87** (1), 119–126.

Siemann, D.W. (1995). Chemosensitization of CCNU in KHT murine tumor cells in vivo and in vitro by the agent RB 6145 and its isomer PD 144872. *Radiothel Oncol* **34**, 47–53.

Siemann, D.W., Johansen, I.M. and Horsman, M.R. (1998). Radiobiological hypoxia in the KHT sarcoma: predictions using the Eppendorf histograph. *Int J Radiat Oncol Biol Phys* **40**, 1171–1176.

Siemann, D.W., Mercer, E., Lepler, S.E. *et al.* (2002). Vascular targeting agents enhance chemotherapeutic agent activities in solid tumor therapy. *Int J Cancer* **99**, 1–6.

Siemann, D.W. and Rojiani, A.M. (2002). Enhancement of radiation therapy by the novel vascular targeting agent ZD6126. *Int J Radiat Oncol Biol Phys* **53**, 164–171.

Siemann, D.W. and Rojiani, A.M. (2005). The vascular disrupting agent ZD6126 shows enhanced antitumor efficacy and radiation sensitization in large, advanced tumors. *Int J Radiat Oncol Biol Phys* **62** (3), 846–853.

Siemann, D.W., Warrington, K.H. and Horsman, M.R. (2000). Targeting tumor blood vessels: an adjuvant strategy for radiation therapy. *Radiother Oncol* **57**, 5–12.

Smith, K.A., Hill, S.A., Begg, A.C. and Denekamp, J. (1988). Validation of the fluorescent dye Hoechst 33342 as a vascular space marker in tumours. *Br J Cancer* **57**, 247–253.

Thomson, J.E. and Rauth, A.M. (1974 May). An in vitro assay to measure the viability of KHT tumor cells not previously exposed to culture conditions. *Radiat Res* **58** (2), 262–276.

Tozer, G.M., Prise, V.E., Wilson, J. *et al.* (1999). Combretastatin A-4 phosphate as a tumor vascular-targeting agent: early effects in tumors and normal tissues. *Cancer Res* **59**, 1626–1634.

6

Molecular Recognition of the Colchicine Binding Site as a Design Paradigm for the Discovery and Development of Vascular Disrupting Agents

Kevin G. Pinney

Abstract

Successful molecular architecture, which can be viewed as the judicious combination of target molecule design and selection, synthetic chemistry, and structure activity relationship studies, remains one of the cornerstones of a well-focused drug design and development program. Several drugs that are currently in human clinical development as vascular disrupting agents function biologically (in parent drug form) through a binding interaction with the protein tubulin. This work briefly reviews the tubulin/microtubule protein system as a target for drug intervention and then focuses in a more comprehensive manner on the specific area of small molecule drug discovery and development of vascular disrupting agents (VDAs). Examples of new pre-clinical drug candidates are presented along with a working model for new molecule design and biological screening protocols deemed paramount for the discovery of viable pre-clinical and clinical small molecule drug candidates functioning biologically as VDAs.

6.1 Introductory comments

Vascular disruption represents an exciting, challenging and relatively new therapeutic approach to cancer treatment as well as the treatment of certain other diseases characterized by rapid and/or aberrant neovascularization (Chaplin and

Vascular-targeted Therapies in Oncology Edited by Dietmar W. Siemann
© 2006 John Wiley & Sons, Ltd.

Hill, 2002; Chaplin *et al.*, 2003a, 2003b; Siemann, 2002; Thorpe *et al.*, 2003). This technique involves treating the disease with a vascular disrupting agent (VDA), which is capable of inducing rapid and selective vascular damage in the microenvironment of the disease indication (Chaplin and Dougherty, 1999; Thorpe *et al.*, 2003). For solid tumor cancers, this shutdown in blood flow renders the tumor deficient in both nutrients and oxygen, which ultimately leads to tumor hypoxia and necrosis (Chaplin *et al.*, 1996). It is the intent of this current work to focus primarily on the discovery and development of small-molecule VDAs for cancer chemotherapy.

6.2 Colchicine binding site on tubulin

As a biological target suitable for disease intervention, the colchicine binding site on tubulin enjoys a rich historical past coupled with promise for present and future discoveries of significant relevance. Colchicine (Figure 6.1) is a small molecule natural product that originates from the *Colchicum autumnale* (Autumn crocus). As one of the first antimitotic agents that proved useful in furthering the understanding of tubulin's role in cellular processes, colchicine promotes necrosis in tumors by attacking vasculature (Baguley *et al.*, 1991; Ludford, 1948). At one time colchicine was used to treat cancer, particularly head and neck tumors; however, it proved to be relatively toxic and is now used clinically only in low doses to treat gout (Hartung, 1961). It is of tremendous historical significance that both synthetic analogs and other natural products reminiscent of the molecular structure of colchicine have emerged as potent, clinically relevant agents for the treatment of cancer as well as certain other diseases. Colchicine itself is comprised of three fused ring systems, the first being a six-member aromatic ring (A-ring) functionalized with three contiguous methoxy groups (Figure 6.1, McGown and Fox, 1989). The second ring (B-ring)

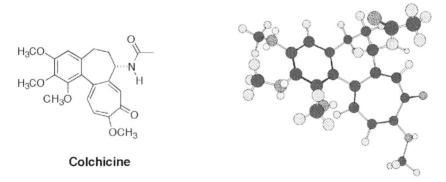

Colchicine

Figure 6.1 Molecular structure of colchicines along with the energy minimized (*mm2*) structure depicted in cylindrical bond format (energy minimization performed in the gas phase using CS Chem 3D Pro Version 5.0 by Cambridgesoft)

is seven membered, non-aromatic, and is functionalized with an amino acetate moiety. The third (C-ring) is an aromatic tropolone ring containing a single methoxy group. The planarity of the A and C rings is tempered by the conformationally flexible B-ring.

Accordingly, colchicine adopts a conformation in the gas phase that essentially orients the A and C rings with a twist towards each other, thus leaving the overall molecule in a puckered conformation (Figure 6.1). Void of the B-ring, the A and C rings approach a bi-aryl molecular structure with a dihedral angle of approximately 66°. The B-ring essentially serves to orient this bi-aryl ring system in a conformation that is ultimately appropriate for optimal binding to the protein tubulin. The X-ray crystallographic structure of colchicine has been determined (King et al., 1952). For molecules of relatively small size (such as colchicine) it is highly probable that solid state structures (from X-ray crystallographic analysis) and gas phase minimized structures bear a high degree of similarity to the conformation that the small molecule adopt in the liquid phase as well (Duax et al., 1985).

The colchicine binding site has been fertile ground for the development of both potent antimitotic agents and vascular disruption agents (VDAs) for the treatment of cancer. Antimitotic agents function biologically by disrupting the metaphase of the cell cycle at the point where chromosomes are poised to separate. Since cancer cells divide much more rapidly than healthy cells, this disruption of the cell cycle has been a viable way to treat cancer from a chemotherapy standpoint. A sampling of familiar antimitotic agents is illustrated in Figure 6.2.

Excellent reviews have addressed both the topic of antimitotic agents (Hamel, 1996; Jordon et al., 1998; Li and Sham, 2002) and the topic of vascular disruption for cancer chemotherapy (Gaya and Rustin, 2005; Jordan and Wilson, 2004; Siemann et al., 2005; Siemann, Chaplin and Horsman, 2004; Szala, 2004; Thorpe, 2004), and this chapter will make no attempt to duplicate these outstanding efforts. Instead, it seems instructive and prudent to journey through the complexities of drug discovery and development in the arena of small-molecule vascular disrupting agents for cancer chemotherapy as well as the treatment of other significant diseases, such as wet age-related macular degeneration. Attention will be tuned to both molecular design and synthesis and the establishment of appropriate biological screening protocols in the area of vascular disruption.

6.3 Brief overview of tubulin biology

Tubulin is a protein found in eukaryotic cells that is comprised of both α and β subunits that share a heterodimeric interface. These subunits are known as tubulin monomers. Both subunits bind one molecule of GTP, and upon hydrolysis of the GTP on the β subunit to GDP a slight conformational flux takes place, which results in assembly (also known as polymerization) of the

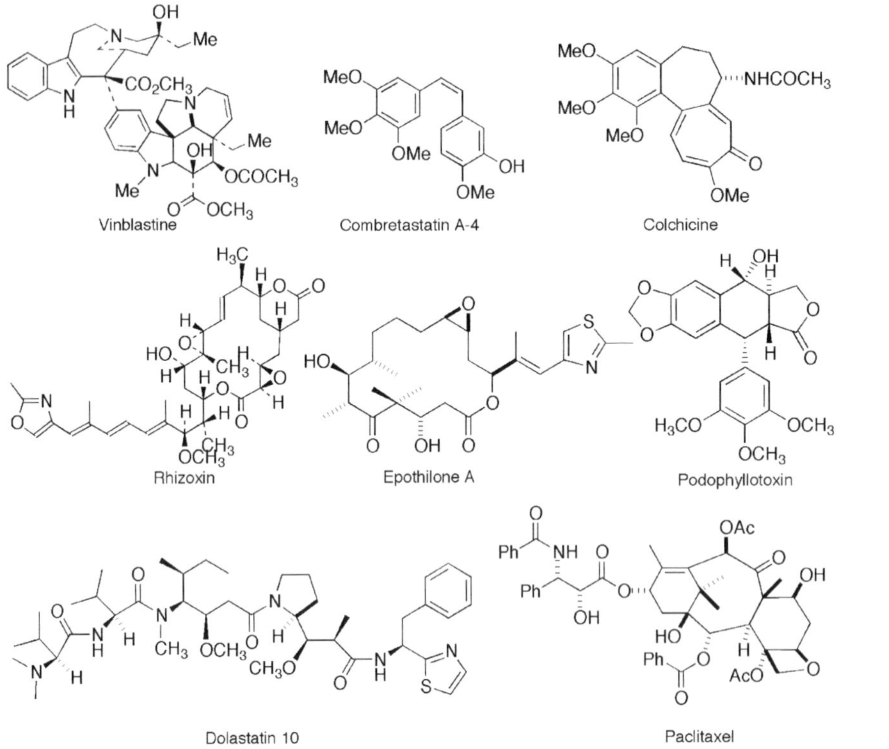

Figure 6.2   Representiative anti-cancer agents that interact with the tubulin-microtubule protein system (vinblastine, Owellen *et al.*, 1976; combretastatin A-4, Lin *et al.*, 1989; Chaplin, Pettit and Hill, 1999; Jordon *et al.*, 1998; colchicine, Boyland and Boyland, 1937; Ludford, 1948; rhizoxin, Nakada *et al.*, 1993; epothilone A, Nicolaou *et al.*, 1997; podophyllotoxin, Desbene and Giorgi-Renault, 2002; dolastatin 10, Pettit *et al.*, 1987c, 1998b; paclitaxel, Kingston, Samaranayake and Ivey, 1990)

tubulin monomers into microtubules (Downing, 2000). The microtubules have a cross-sectional diameter of approximately 20–24 nm, and as such are really perhaps one of nature's finest examples of self-assembly. A more than 50 year search for structural information on the tubulin-mictrotubule system concluded with the brilliant discovery by Nogales and Downing of the tertiary structure of a cross-sectional portion of the microtubule stabilized by paclitaxel (Nogales, Wolf and Downing, 1998). This was accomplished by electron crystallography and the structure was further refined to a resolution of 3.5 Å (Lowe *et al.*, 2001).

The process of tubulin assembly into microtubules occurs when an α/β subunit joins with another subunit causing one of the two bound guanosine triphosphates (GTPs) to hydrolyze to guanosine diphosphate (GDP) and inorganic phosphate (P_i) (Nogales, 2000). The tubulin heterodimer contains a plus end (α tubulin), which grows most rapidly, and a minus end (β tubulin). The minus end is usually oriented toward a centrosome, the center from which microtubules originate. Microtubules are in a constant dynamic instability because the second GTP at the plus end may become hydrolyzed to GDP before another tubulin subunit can join. The resulting GDP-subunit rapidly dissociates from the microtubule. Therefore, there is a regulation of growth or shrinkage depending on the rate of hydrolysis and availability of GTP-tubulin subunits (Nogales, 2000). This regulation causes cells to be able to vary their shape and form or dissolve the mitotic spindle (Nogales, 2000).

One classical approach to cancer treatment involves the use of small molecules as potent inhibitors of tubulin assembly into microtubules. Known as antimitotic agents, these compounds are effective at interfering with tubulin-mictrotubule dynamics and traditionally bind at one of three possible small-molecule binding domains (Figure 6.3; Wehbe, 2005; Hadimani, 2004; Pinney et al., 2000b).

Two of these domains (the colchicine binding site and the vinca alkaloid binding site) are located on the monomeric tubulin subunits, while the third domain (taxoid binding site) is located on the polymerized microtubule itself. The compounds that bind to monomeric tubulin are known to inhibit the formation of the microtubule and are often referred to as tubulin destabilizing agents. Alternatively, compounds that bind at the taxoid binding site are known as microtubule stabilizing agents. In either case, by interfering with the dynamics of the tubulin-microtubule system, cellular division is compromised.

The design of new molecules for optimal binding interaction at the colchicine binding site on tubulin remains a formidable challenge, primarily due to the fact that the colchicine binding site is not fully characterized to date. In fact, until very recently there was no structure available by X-ray crystallography or electron crystallography of tubulin with a small-molecule inhibitor located in the colchicine binding site; however, the recent description of a tubulinr colchicine complex stabilized with a stathmin-like domain offers the possibility for

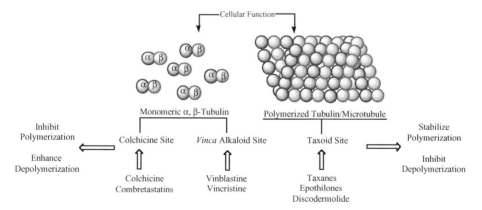

Figure 6.3 Tubulin and microtubule dynamics as influenced by selected small-molecule binding agents (from Wehbe, 2005 and Hall, 2005, with permission)

further characterization of tubulin at the molecular level (Ravelli *et al.*, 2004). Structural information has resulted primarily from chemical and photoaffinity labeling studies (Bai *et al.*, 1996; Chavan *et al.*, 1993; Floyd, Barnes and Williams, 1989; Hahn, Hastie and Sundberg, 1992; Olszewski *et al.*, 1994; Pinney *et al.*, 2000b; Safa, Hamel and Felsted, 1987; Sawada *et al.*, 1991, 1993a, 1993b; Staretz and Hastie, 1993; Williams *et al.*, 1985; Wolff *et al.*, 1991). Among the most noteworthy of these affinity labeling agents are those based on paclitaxel (Rao, Horwitz and Ringel, 1992) and colchicine (Bai *et al.*, 1996; Floyd, Barnes and Williams, 1989; Hahn, Hastie and Sundberg, 1992; Olszewski *et al.*, 1994; Staretz and Hastie, 1993; Wolff *et al.*, 1991). In addition, a diazoketone derivative of combretastatin A-4 (CA-4) has been prepared (Olszewski *et al.*, 1994). In each case, these affinity probes have provided useful information, but unequivocal identification of individual amino acid residues on tubulin responsible for binding at the colchicine site has remained elusive to date. Information of this nature is paramount for the design of new more potent inhibitors of tubulin polymerization and hence improved, more effective anti-tumor agents.

A working model for small-molecule binding at the colchicine site on tubulin has been proposed by Hamel and co-workers based on an electrophilic molecular probe of colchicine, which suggests a crucial 9 Å distance between Cys-239 and Cys-354 for effective binding of colchicine itself (Bai *et al.*, 1996).

6.4   Small-molecule inhibitors of tubulin assembly

One of the most productive approaches to drug development for cancer chemotherapy has traditionally centered on compounds that interact with the tubulin-microtubule protein system at one of the three known small-molecule binding sites (colchicine site, vinca alkaloid site and taxoid site). Vascular disruption agents (VDAs) that, in non-prodrug form, interact at the colchicine binding site are perhaps the most clinically advanced compounds in this emerging area of cancer treatment and, accordingly, this current work will focus in this area.

Interest in small-molecule (i.e. compounds with molecular weights in the range of approximately 300–800 g mol^{-1}) inhibitors of tubulin assembly at the colchicine binding site can be traced to the original discovery of colchicine. While colchicine clearly played a key role in helping to further elucidate the biological mechanism of action of tubulin as a therapeutic target, it is also important to keep in mind that this potent drug does interact directly with tumor vasculature, resulting in tissue death (Boyland and Boyland, 1937). The toxicity of colchicine has ultimately limited its use in humans; however, this drug has inspired the design and synthesis of a myriad of new analogs that inhibit tubulin assembly through a direct binding event at the colchicine binding site on tubulin.

Another group of naturally occurring compounds with pronounced biological activity is referred to as the combretastatins. These compounds are part of the Combretaceae plant family of natural products, originally discovered by Professor George R. Pettit (Arizona State University), and consist of a group of approximately 20 compounds that are isolated from the bush willow tree in South Africa known as *Combretum caffrum* (Pinney *et al.*, 2005a). Certain of these compounds are characterized by their remarkable biological activity as inhibitors of tubulin polymerization, potent *in vitro* cytotoxicity against human cancer cell lines and demonstrated *in vivo* efficacy as anti-angiogenesis agents and vascular disrupting agents (in suitable prodrug form; Bibby, 2002; Pinney *et al.*, 2005a). Among natural products of therapeutic interest, the combretastatins are striking, not only for their pronounced biological activity, but also for their elegance and remarkable simplicity in terms of molecular structure. The combretastatins demonstrate exceptional antimitotic, antivascular and, to a certain extent, antiangiogenic activity in biological systems (Cirla and Mann, 2003). A brief time-line depicting the history of the combretastatins from discovery through present clinical development is illustrated in Figure 6.4 (Jelinek, 2004). Guided and inspired by the folk lore attributed to the shaman of that region, Professor Pettit initiated a collecting trip to South Africa in 1979 following up on an original National Cancer Institute (NCI) collecting trip to Zimbabwe in 1973 (Pettit, Cragg and Singh, 1987a; Pinney *et al.*, 2005a). Intrigued by the further knowledge that the Zulu tribes of that region were known to dip their spears in boiled extracts from the *Combretum caffrum* trees to enhance the virulence of their weaponry during battle, the Pettit group focused their initial search in the bark of the tree (Pettit, Cragg and Singh, 1987a; Pinney *et al.*, 2005a).

Isolation of the first constituent of *Combretum caffrum*, (−)-combretastatin (Figure 6.5), was performed in 1982 by Pettit and co-workers (Pettit *et al.*, 1982). By 1987, the absolute stereochemistry, attributed to the single stereogenic center in the molecule, was determined to be the *R*-configuration (Pettit, Cragg and Singh, 1987a). The combretastatins are currently divided into four major groups based on their structural characteristics. These include the A-series (*cis*-stilbenoids), B-series (diaryl-ethylenes), C-series (quinone) and D-series (carbocyclic in nature). Representative members of each of these groups are depicted in Figure 6.5. Combretastatin A-4 (CA-4) and combretastatin A-1 (CA-1) have proven to be the most clinically important members of the combretastatin group of compounds. Both of these compounds are potent inhibitors of tubulin assembly ($IC_{50} = 1$–$2\,\mu M$; Pettit *et al.*, 1987c, 1995a). This activity is correlated with the *cis* configuration along with other structural features. Due to the poor solubility of CA-1 and CA-4, sodium phosphate prodrugs, CA-1P and CA-4P, were developed in the mid-1990s (Pettit and Lippert, 2000; Pettit *et al.*, 1995b). The prodrugs are cleaved to their active forms by phosphatase enzymes, which are taken up into cells. In preclinical studies, combretastatins have been shown to leave blood vessels associated with normal tissue

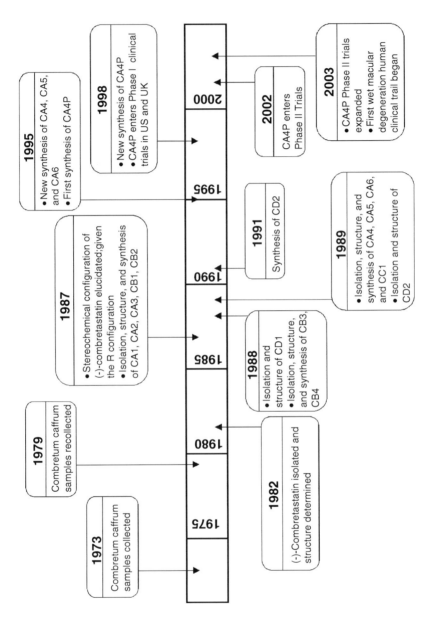

Figure 6.4 Timeline of discovery and development of combretastatin natural products (from Jelinek, 2004, with permission)

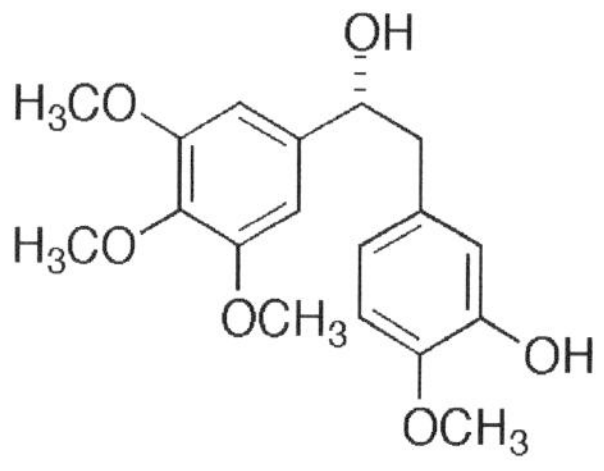

(-)-Combretastatin

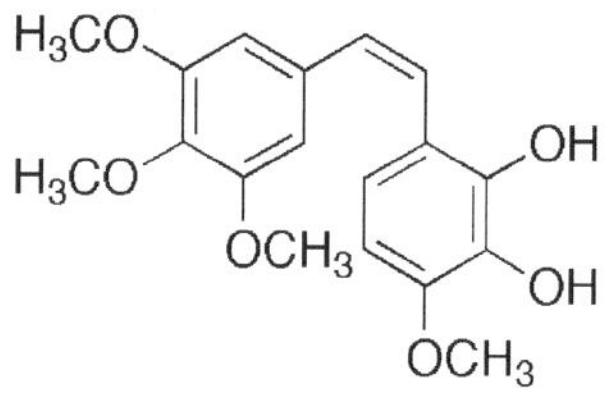

CA-1 (Oxi4503)

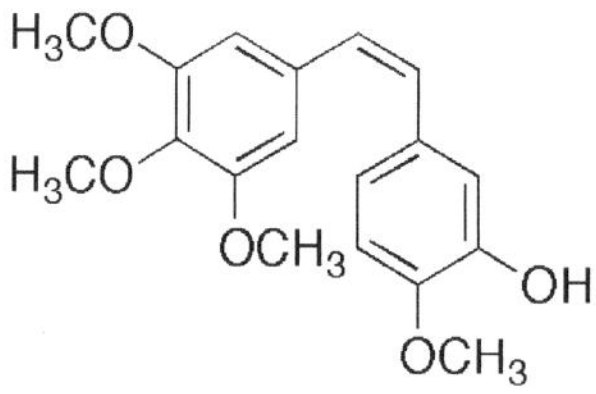

CA-4

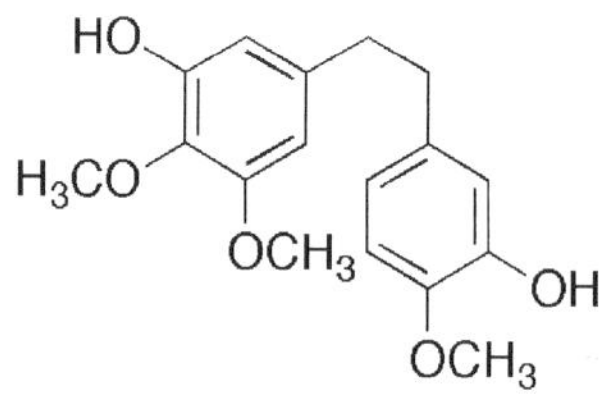

CB-2

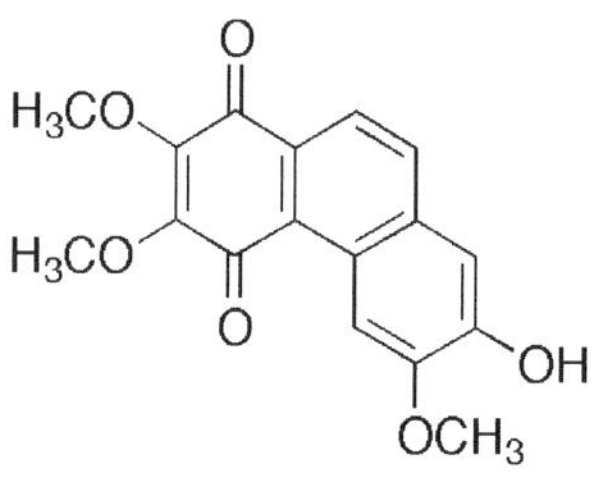

CC-1

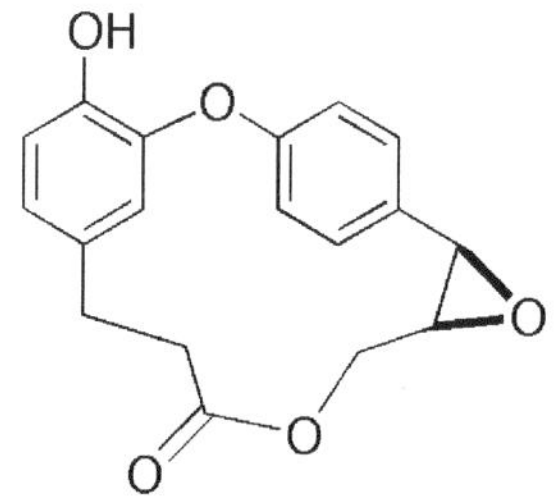

CD-1

Figure 6.5 A representative sampling of the naturally occurring combretastatins ((−)-combreta-statin, Pettit *et al.*, 1982; Pettit, Cragg and Singh, 1987a; CA-1, Pettit *et al.*, 1987c; CA-4, Pettit *et al.*, 1995a; CB-2, Pettit and Singh, 1987; CC-1, Singh and Pettit, 1989; CD-1, Pettit, Singh and Niven, 1988)

unaffected (Chaplin and Dougherty, 1999; Chaplin and Hill, 2002; Siemann, 2002; Thorpe, Chaplin and Blakey, 2003). Also, combretastatins have over-come other problems seen in some cancer treatments, including difficulty of application on a routine basis, tumor specificity, morbidity and narrow windows of activity (short duration of drug activity; Chaplin *et al.*, 1996; Young and Chaplin, 2004).

The combretastatins have inspired the design of numerous synthetic analogs, some of which are stilbenoid in nature, while others bear completely distinct molecular core components with similar aryl–aryl intramolecular spaces. Figure 6.6 illustrates a small sampling of such compounds; however, it is important to

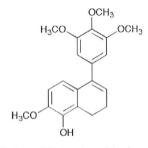

1,2-Disubstituted Imidazole Analog

3-Aroyl-2-aryl-indole-based Analog

3-Forymylindole Analog

2,3-Diaryl indole Analog

Indolyloxazoline Analog (A-289099)

Dihydronaphthalene-based Analog

Figure 6.6 A small sampling of synthetic analogs structurally inspired by the combretastatins (imidazole analog, Wang *et al.*, 2002; 3-aroyl-2-arylindoles, Hadimani *et al.*, 2002; Pinney, Wang and Del Pilar Mejia, 2001b; Flynn, Hamel and Jung, 2002b; formylindole, Gastpar *et al.*, 1998; 2,3-diarylindole, Flynn, Hamel and Jung, 2002b; indolyloxazoline analog, Li *et al.*, 2002; Tahir *et al.*, 2003; dihydronaphthalene analog, Pinney *et al.*, 2001a,b, 2003; Ghatak *et al.*, 2003; isoquinoline analog, Goldbrunner *et al.*, 1997; phenstatin, Pettit *et al.*, 1998b; benzofuran analogs, Flynn and Hamel, 2002a; Pinney *et al.*, 2004b; Flynn, Hamel and Jung, 2002b; sulfonamide analog, Medina *et al.*, 1999; Flygare *et al.*, 2000)

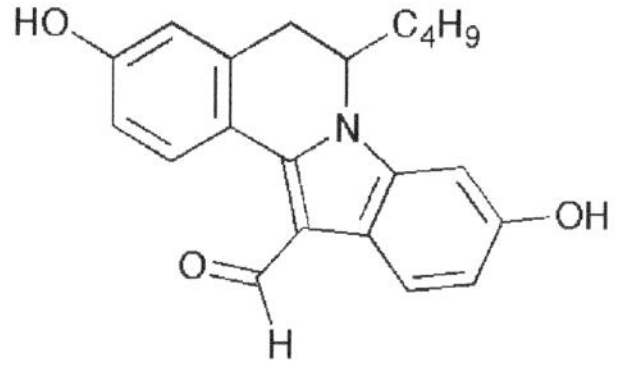

Isoquinoline Analog

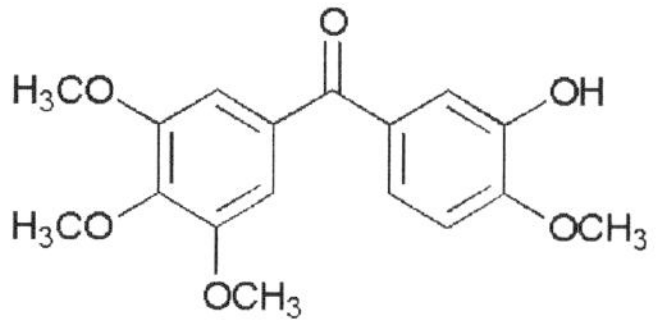

Phenstatin

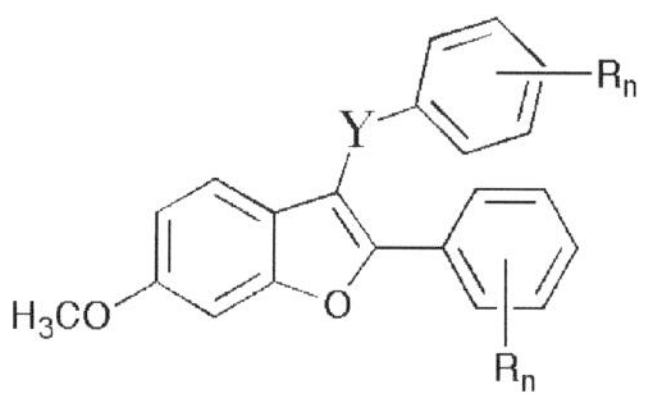

Y = carbonyl, covalent bond
R$_n$ = OCH$_3$, OH
Benzofuran Analogs

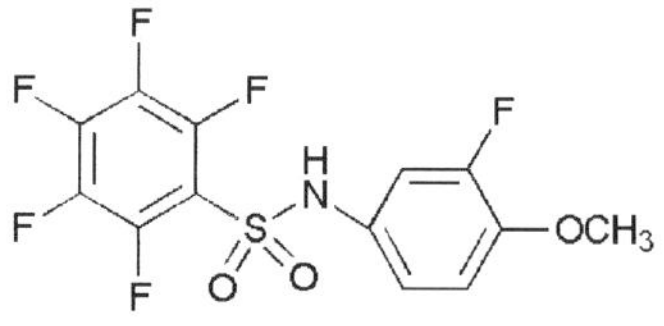

Sulfonamide Analog (T138067, T67)

Figure 6.6   *Continued*

note that the compounds depicted in this figure represent only a tiny fraction of the vast number of compounds based on the combretastatins that have appeared in the peer-reviewed literature (as publications, patent applications and patents issued) or become publicly known through presentations at scientific meetings (Chaplin *et al.*, 2003a, 2003b; Cushman *et al.*, 1991; Hamel, 1996; Li and Sham, 2002; Lin *et al.*, 1988; Pettit and Singh, 1996; Pinney *et al.*, 2000c).

6.5   Design paradigm for small-molecule vascular disrupting agents

Vascular disrupting agents (VDAs) hold great promise as improved chemotherapeutic agents for the treatment of solid tumor cancers. Distinct from antiangiogenesis compounds (which target the development of new blood vessels to tumors), VDAs are unique in their ability to selectively target and disrupt blood flow to both new microvessels and mature and established vessels, thereby effectively starving the tumor of necessary oxygen and nutrients needed for survival and growth. In prodrug form, the VDAs are largely inactive with the protein tubulin. However, once enzymatically cleaved to their parent free phenolic (or amino) derivatives, these compounds are potent inhibitors of tubulin assembly. Blood flow shut-down is most likely the result of morphological changes in the endothelial cells lining the microvessels of tumors induced by tubulin binding and subsequent inhibition of tubulin polymerization (Chaplin and Dougherty, 1999;

Galbraith *et al.*, 2001; Kanthou and Tozer, 2002; Tozer *et al.*, 2001). This blood flow shut-down essentially starves the tumor of important nutrients and oxygen and ultimately results in hypoxia and necrosis of the tumor. Morphology changes in the endothelial cells are induced by a direct binding interaction of the parent form of the VDA with tubulin and subsequent inhibition of tubulin assembly into microtubules. The selectivity of the VDAs for tumor vasculature most likely hinges on distinct differences in the cytoskeletal composition of endothelial cells in rapidly proliferating vasculature versus healthy cell vasculature, although this supposition is speculative at best and numerous current research efforts are focused on further elucidating this important mechanism of selectivity (Chaplin and Dougherty, 1999; Galbraith *et al.*, 2001; Kanthou and Tozer, 2002; Tozer *et al.*, 2001, 2002).

Currently, there are at least four compounds (which function biologically through a binding interaction with tubulin) that are in human clinical development as potential VDAs for cancer chemotherapy; however, none of these compounds have achieved approval by the Food and Drug Administration (FDA) to date and clinical trials, while promising, are on-going. Combretastatin A-4 phosphate (CA-4P), a prodrug of CA-4, is currently involved in seven on-going human clinical trials for cancer and one on-going clinical trials for myopic macular degeneration and one on-going clinical trial for myopic macular degeneration (Chaplin and Hill, 2002; Young and Chaplin, 2004; Oxigene Inc. website: www.oxigene.com). In addition, both ZD6126 (Blakey *et al.*, 2002; Micheletti *et al.*, 2003; Siemann and Rojiani, 2002b, 2002c) and AVE 8062A (Hori and Saito, 2003; Ohsumi *et al.*, 1998, 1999) are in human clinical development as small-molecule VDAs. The most recent entry into the clinic is Oxi 4503 (also known as CA-1P), which is a di-phosphate prodrug of the naturally occurring stilbenoid diphenol combretastatin family member CA-1 (Hill *et al.*, 2002; Holwell *et al.*, 2002; Hua *et al.*, 2003; Shnyder *et al.*, 2003). DMXAA (5,6-dimethylxanthenone-4-acetic acid) is another small-molecule VDA in human clinical development; however, its biological mechanism of action most likely involves the release of further vasoactive agents such as tumor necrosis factor, serotonin, other cytokines and nitric oxide from host cells rather than any interaction with tubulin (Baguley, 2003; Baguley and Wilson, 2002; Siemann, Chaplin and Horsman, 2004; Zhou *et al.*, 2002).

It is both instructive and timely to consider what might constitute a highly successful paradigm for the discovery and development of small-molecule VDAs. Through a long-standing basic research program focused on molecular recognition for the colchicine binding site on tubulin, we have discovered several new classes of compounds that in prodrug form are potent VDAs. Building on the success of this program, it continues to be our intention to develop new VDAs that will demonstrate improved molecular recognition for the colchicine binding site on β-tubulin, and will display a desirable *in vivo* therapeutic index, with the ultimate goal of discovering new compounds that hold the promise to be among the most interesting and clinically relevant VDAs known to date. It is important for the reader not to infer that the emphasis placed in this current work on VDAs developed in the Pinney group at Baylor University is suggestive that this represents the only effort or even the best research program in this regard. To the contrary, there are numerous excellent efforts underway around the world, both in academia and industry, to discover and develop new VDAs. The present focus is intended only to familiarize the reader with a successful discovery paradigm and development protocol that is in place for the preparation of new and biologically active VDAs.

Obviously, two key components must exist for the discovery and development of new, highly functional VDAs. First, suitable molecular targets must be chosen and workable synthetic routes devised for the preparation of these targets. Second, and of equal importance, there must be appropriate biochemical and biological assays in place (both *in vitro* and *in vivo*) to evaluate new molecular targets and aid in the selection of the most promising target molecules for further development.

A protocol that seems both effective and efficient involves the following aspects.

(i)   Design new ligands for binding to the colchicine binding site on tubulin through a strategy that is inspired and guided by nature's vast pharmacopoeia of natural products that are already known as colchicine site binding ligands.

(ii) Engineer additional degrees of rotational freedom and conformational flexibility into the new ligands at appropriate points, while conserving the approximate 5 Å aryl–aryl distance that seems paramount for effective inhibition of tubulin assembly through a binding event at the colchicine site.

(iii) Initially evaluate the new VDA candidates in terms of their ability to inhibit tubulin polymerization (assembly) in a pure protein assay. Although not always predictive, there remains a high correlation between compounds (in non-prodrug form) that inhibit tubulin assembly in the range of 1–5 µM and successful *in vivo* vascular targeting capability of their corresponding prodrug analogs.

(iv) Screen the new VDA candidates for their *in vitro* cytotoxicity against human cancer cell lines (either SRB total protein assay, or MTT assay).

(v)   Take all compounds that have reasonable numbers for inhibition of tubulin assembly in non-prodrug form into *in vivo* evaluation through both a blood flow shut-down assay and a tumor growth delay study in SCID mice. For the blood flow shut-down assay, it is important to evaluate efficacy at a minimum of two concentrations including a relatively high concentration ($100\,\mathrm{mg\,kg^{-1}}$) and a moderately low concentration ($10\,\mathrm{mg\,kg^{-1}}$).

We have synthesized approximately 100 new final target molecules and advanced intermediates as potential molecular probes for tubulin and potential inhibitors of tubulin assembly (Chen *et al.*, 2000; Pinney *et al.*, 1999, 2000c, 2000a, 2001b, 2001a, 2003, 2004b, 2004c). In several cases, new synthetic methodology was developed to facilitate the synthesis of certain target molecules that were not readily available through established methodologies. Each of these molecules was designed and chosen as a synthetic target based on our growing knowledge of molecular recognition for the colchicine binding site on β-tubulin. From this molecular library, approximately 20 compounds (refer to Figure 6.7 for representative examples) have recently emerged that demonstrate both strong *in vitro* cytotoxicity against selected human cancer cell lines and potent inhibition of tubulin assembly (cytotoxicity studies are carried out in collaboration with Professor George R. Pettit, Arizona State University; tubulin biochemical assays are done in collaboration with Dr. Ernest Hamel, National Cancer Institute and Dr. Mary Lynn Trawick, Baylor University). The indole-based analog **1** as well as the dihydronaphthalene ligand **2** are among the most potent inhibitors of tubulin assembly known to date, which function through a direct binding interaction to the colchicine site (Pinney *et al.*, 2003, 2004b, 2004c; Pinney, Wang and Hadimani, 2005b).

Structure–activity relationship (SAR) studies associated with this molecular library have guided our continued refinement of a working model for the structural and electronic features paramount for enhanced binding at the colchicine site on tubulin. The working model (in cartoon format) depicted in Figure 6.8 has been developed based primarily on the library of tubulin-specific molecules that we have prepared over the past several years. Although the model is highly subjective in nature, it does provide a reasonably accurate summary of the electronic and structural motifs which are nearly always present in molecules which demonstrate inhibition of tubulin polymerization at the level of 0.5–$4.0\,\mu\mathrm{M}$. These values are representative of the most potent inhibitors of tubulin assembly (interacting at the colchicine site) known to date ($\mathrm{IC}_{50} = 1$–$2\,\mu\mathrm{M}$ for CA-4, one of the most active tubulin inhibitors, Pettit *et al.*, 1987c, 1995a). This model complements and further expands the model proposed by Hamel and co-workers based on an electrophilic molecular probe of colchicines (Bai *et al.*, 1996). Not surprisingly, the seven molecules presented in Figure 6.7 all fit comfortably into this model along with numerous other analogs developed by us and others including several pseudo-peptidomimetic ligands, β-turn analogs and triple-bond derivatives (with one aryl ring replaced by the pi bond rich alkynyl moiety) that we have recently prepared (Pinney *et al.*, 2004b).

In order to further investigate the potential role that molecular recognition and pharmacokinetics may play in terms of enhanced VDA activity, we prepared a series of diphosphate and monophosphate prodrug congeners of our most

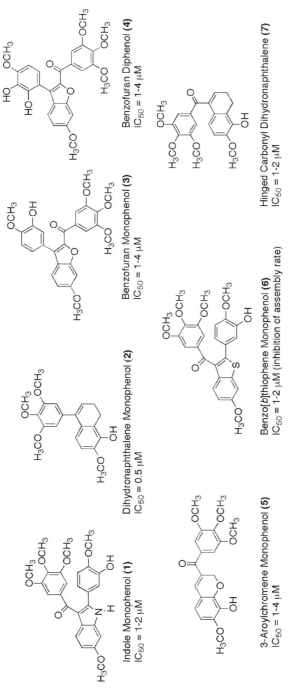

Figure 6.7 Representative synthetic ligands prepared by Pinney and co-workers that display molecular recognition for tubulin (IC_{50} for inhibition of tubulin assembly) (see references cited within the text as well as Pinney *et al.*, 2004b (for compounds **3** and **4**) and Pinney *et al.*, 2003 (for compound **7**))

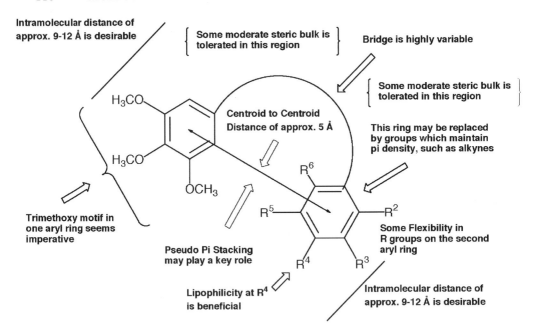

Figure 6.8 Salient SAR features paramount for molecular recognition of the colchicine binding site on tubulin (Pinney, 2005, unpublished)

potent tubulin binding ligands and evaluated them *in vivo* to determine both their efficacy in shutting down blood flow to tumors as well as the ability of several of these compounds to establish tumor growth delay in xenograft tumors in SCID mice (*in vivo* studies carried out in collaboration with Professor Klaus Edvardsen, University of Lund, Sweden). The indole monophosphate 8 (Oxi 8007) and the dihydronaphthalene monophosphate (DHN-P) **9** (Oxi 6197) (Figure 6.9) are exemplary in this regard (Pinney *et al.*, 2003, 2004c; Pinney, Wang and Hadimani, 2005b).

DHN-P **9** (Oxi 6197) effects a >90% shut-down of tumor blood flow within one hour of administration at a well tolerated dose of 25 mg kg^{-1} (Pinney *et al.*, 2003, 2004a). In addition, DHN-P **9** shows promising, dose-dependent tumor growth delay of the MDA-MB-231 breast carcinoma (Edvardsen and Pinney, 2005). In free phenol form, compound **2** is a potent inhibitor of tubulin assembly (IC$_{50}$ = 0.5 μM) (Hamel and Pinney, 2005). In addition, both DHN **2** and DHN-P **9** are strongly cytotoxic (*in vitro*) against human cancer cell lines. For example, DHN **2** has a GI$_{50}$ value of more than 3×10^{-10} against the MCF-7 cell line (Pettit and Pinney, 2005).

Oxi 8007 demonstrates significant preclinical activity as a VDA as well. This compound (as free phenol **1**) is a potent inhibitor of tubulin assembly with an IC$_{50}$ value in the range of 1–2 μM (Hamel and Pinney, 2005), and has pronounced activity in terms of *in vitro* cytotoxicity against selected human cancer cell lines (Pettit and Pinney, 2005; Pinney *et al.*, 2004a). In prodrug form,

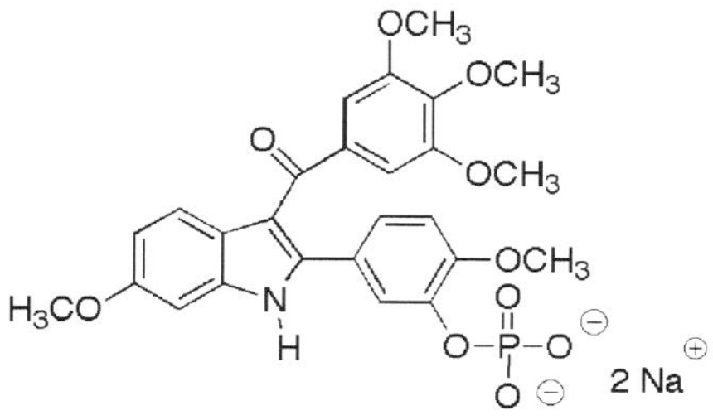

Indole Monophosphate Prodrug **(8)**
Oxi 8007

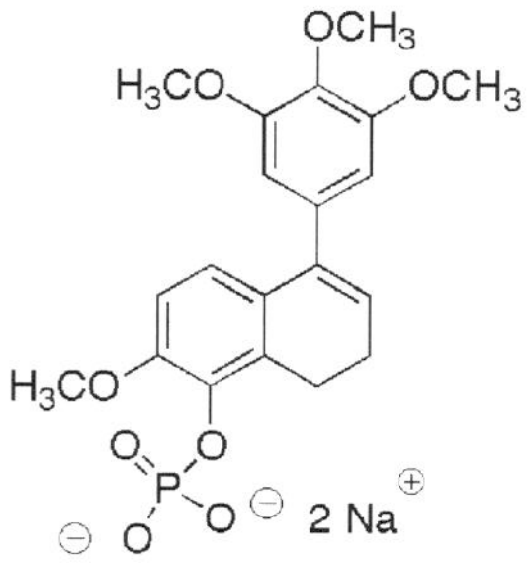

Dihydronaphthalene Monophosphate Prodrug (DHN-P) **(9)**
Oxi 6197

Figure 6.9 Monophosphate prodrug molecular structures of Oxi 8007 and Oxi 6197. (see references cited within the text)

Oxi 8007 shows nearly complete tumor blood flow shutdown (approximately 98 per cent) at a dose of $100\,mg\,kg^{-1}$ in the hemanagioendothelioma/SCID mouse tumor model after 24h (Edvardsen and Pinney, 2005; Pinney *et al.*, 2004a). In addition, Oxi 8007 shows significant tumor growth delay at doses of $100\,mg\,kg^{-1}$ and beyond in the MDA-MB-231 breast tumor model in SCID mice (Edvardsen and Pinney, 2005; Pinney *et al.*, 2004a). Furthermore, the maximum tolerated dose (MTD) in this tumor model is greater than $800\,mg\,kg^{-1}$ (Edvardsen and Pinney, 2005; Pinney *et al.*, 2004a).

It is instructive to note (as mentioned above) that the non-prodrug free phenol precursors to Oxi 8007 and Oxi 6197 (compounds **1** and **2** respectively (Figure 6.7)) are both potent inhibitors of tubulin assembly (IC_{50} = 1–2 μM for **1** and 0.5 μM for **2**). This data (albeit limited in scope) appears to establish a strong correlation between the demonstration of pronounced inhibition of tubulin assembly for the non-prodrug analogs and potent *in vivo* blood flow shut-down for the corresponding prodrug constructs. This correlation is mirrored with the combretastatins (CA-4/CA-4P and CA-1/CA-1P) as well. This correlation would be especially useful if it established a non-*in-vivo*-based assay that proved diagnostic in terms of predicting successful *in vivo* activity of corresponding prodrug VDAs in the SCID mouse animal model. It is important to attempt to establish such a model in order to be able to screen large numbers of compounds without incurring the necessary time delays and cost constraints of carrying out statistically relevant animal model studies. Fortunately, most if not all of the small-molecule VDAs that demonstrate noteworthy *in vivo* blood flow shut-down are also active inhibitors of tubulin assembly in their corresponding non-prodrug formulation. Unfortunately, this correlation is not always 100 per cent predictive. In our own hands, two molecules that show excellent inhibition of tubulin assembly as free phenols, chromene analog **5** (Pinney *et al.*, 2004a; Shirali, 2002) and benzo[*b*]thiophene **6** (Figure 6.7, Chen *et al.*, 2000; Edvardsen and Pinney, 2005; Flynn *et al.*, 2001a, 2001b; Pinney *et al.*, 1999, 2000a, 2001a), proved to be inactive (as their corresponding disodium phosphate prodrugs) in the *in vivo* blood flow shut-down assay at the higher dose of $100\,mg\,kg^{-1}$. Plausible reasons for this are not entirely clear, although one can speculate that issues of bioavailability and pharmacokinetics most likely contributed to the lack of measurable *in vivo* activity in terms of tumor blood flow shut-down. Therefore, while it seems prudent to rely heavily on tubulin activity in free drug formulation as a prognostic tool for *in vivo* success of the related prodrug analogs as VDAs, one must also be cautious of relying solely on this information. In other words, one must be prudent not to make the *a priori* presumption that this correlation is always valid, since a myriad of other factors come into play once compounds enter the *in vivo* environment.

The therapeutic window for VDA activity is also extremely important. It is our contention that drugs that are reversible (at a certain pharmacokinetic time-point) in terms of inhibition of tubulin assembly are much more prone to demonstrate wider therapeutic windows as compared with other tubulin binding drugs that are less reversible. A certain degree of conformational flexibility engineered into the otherwise fairly rigid structure paramount for enhanced binding at the colchicine site seems advantageous in regard to *in vivo* success (in terms of therapeutic window with blood flow shut-down). Accordingly, one can note that the indole analog **1** that features a conformationally flexible trimethoxy aroyl ring moiety (Hadimani *et al.*, 2002) appears (in preliminary *in vivo* dose studies) to have a fairly high therapeutic window of activity (Edvardsen and Pinney, 2005; Pinney *et al.*, 2004a). Not enough information is currently available in regard to the structure of the colchicine binding site on tubulin to make any significant or predictive comments about molecular flexibility and its potential link to reversibility of colchicine binding site activity; however, it is a parameter that is important to observe as more information regarding molecular recognition for the colchicine site is revealed with time.

6.6 Concluding remarks

Vascular disruption therapy has clearly found a lasting, and in fact growing, place of significance in terms of disease intervention for cancer and certain other diseases characterized by aberrant neovascularization (such as wet age-related macular degeneration). First-generation small-molecule based drugs (such as CA-4P, ZD6126 and AVE8062A) are well along in human clinical development. These compounds are highly effective at inducing rapid cessation of blood flow in the tumor microenvironment, resulting in hypoxia and necrosis in the core of the solid tumor. Interestingly, healthy tissue often still approaches the edges of the tumor and must be dealt with through adjunct therapy to avoid tumor re-growth after treatment has stopped. This healthy tissue, often referred to as the viable rim, can be treated through combination therapy. Accordingly, VDAs are most often used clinically in combination with traditional cytotoxic agents, radiation, immunoradiotherapy, monoclonal antibodies etc. in order to cause both blood flow shut-down (due to the VDA) along with destruction of the viable rim (through the combination choice of therapy, Chaplin, Pettit and Hill, 1999; Eikesdal *et al.*, 2000; Grosios *et al.*, 2000; Horsman *et al.*, 2000; Horsman and Murata, 2002; Landuyt *et al.*, 2001; Li, Rojiani and Siemann, 1998; Nelkin and Ball, 2001; Pedley *et al.*, 2001; Siemann *et al.*, 2002a; Wildiers *et al.*, 2004).

Second-generation small-molecule VDAs are also beginning to emerge. One approach to second-generation VDA discovery and development is to engineer bifunctionality, in terms of dual mechanisms of biological activity, into the same small molecule. The concept might take the form of using the selectivity of a VDA for the tumor microenvironment both as a treatment modality and also as a selective delivery mechanism for an entity with a separate and distinct mechanism of tumor destruction. CA-1P (Oxi 4503) is an example of one such second-generation drug (although in parent form it is also a natural product), which has recently (Spring 2005) entered the clinical arena in a phase I trial as an experimental drug (Hill *et al.*, 2002; Holwell *et al.*, 2002; Hua *et al.*, 2003; Pettit and Lippert, 2000; Sheng *et al.*, 2004). This compound appears to function first as a selective VDA, resulting in rapid blood flow shut-down to solid tumor cancers. However, once the vessels are damaged and leaky, the drug is selectively isolated in the tumor microenvironment, where it most likely undergoes a chemical redox reaction to convert from an *ortho*-phenol to an *ortho*-quinone moiety (Chaplin *et al.*, 2004). The *ortho*-quinone is then able to attack the viable rim cells through an alternate mechanism of action.

The field of vascular disruption therapies for specific disease intervention is dynamic and rapidly growing. At present, the well established first-generation small-molecule VDAs are making their way through phase I, Ib and II clinical trials with encouraging results, continuing to usher in cautious but persistent optimism for successful therapeutic treatment. The present merges with the future in regard to second- and third-generation VDA discovery and development, where even more targeted and aggressive therapies are both the present reality and on the envisioned close horizon.

Acknowledgments

The author is grateful for the important contributions of many talented graduate and undergraduate students as well as postdoctoral associates and summer high-school students that are reflected in some of the original research presented in this chapter. The assistance of Mr. Charlie Manzanares and Ms. Tracy Carter in the final stages of preparation of this manuscript is greatly appreciated. Funding for portions of this work was provided by Baylor University, The Welch Foundation (grant No. AA-1278) and Oxigene Inc., for which the author is most appreciative.

References

Baguley, B.C. (2003). Antivascular therapy of cancer: DMXAA. *Lancelot Oncol* **4**, 141–148.

Baguley, B.C., Holdaway, K.M., Thomsen, L.L., Zhuang, Li and Zwi, L.J. (1991). Inhibition of growth of colon 38 adenocarcinoma by vinblastine and colchicines: evidence for a vascular mechanism. *Eur J Cancer* **27**, 482–487.

Baguley, B.C. and Wilson, W.R. (2002). Potential of DMXAA combination therapy for solid tumors. *Exp Rev Anticancer Ther* **2**, 593–603.

Bai, R., Pei, X.F., Boye, O., Getahun, Z., Grover, S., Bekisz, J., Nguyen, N.Y., Brossi, A. and Hamel, E. (1996). Identification of cysteine 354 of beta-tubulin as part of the binding site for the a ring of colchicines. *J Biol Chem* **271**, 12639–12645.

Bibby, M.C. (2002). Combretastatin anticancer drugs. *Drugs Future* **27**, 475–480.

Blakey, D.C., Ashton, S.E., Westwood, F.R., Walker, M. and Ryan, A.J. (2002). ZD6126: a novel small molecule vascular targeting agent. *Int J Radiat Oncol Biol Phys* **54**, 1497–1502.

Boyland, E. and Boyland, M.E. (1937). Studies in tissue metabolism. IX. The action of col-chicine and *B typhosus* extract. *Biochem J* **31**, 454–460.

Chaplin, D.J. and Dougherty, G.J. (1999). Tumour vasculature as a target for cancer therapy. *Br J Cancer* **80**, 57–64.

Chaplin, D.J., Edvardsen, K., Pinney, K.G., Prezioso, J.A. and Wood, M. (2004). Preparation of quinone and catechol derivatives for the treatment of cancers and other vascular pro-liferative disorders. *PCT Int Application* WO 2004078126 A2.

Chaplin, D.J., Garner, C.M., Kane, R.R., Pinney, K.G, and Prezioso, J.A. (2003a). Preparation of stilbenes as vascular targeting agents (VTAs) for treatment of solid tumors and retinal neovascularization. *PCT Int Application* WO2003035008 A2.

Chaplin, D.J., Garner, C.M. III, Kane, R.R., Pinney, K.G. and Prezioso, J.A. (2003b). Functionalized stilbene derivatives as improved vascular targeting agents. *US Patent Application* 20030149003 A1.

Chaplin, D.J. and Hill, S.A. (2002). The development of combretastatin A4 phosphate as a vascular targeting agent. *Int J Radiat Oncol Biol Phys* **54**, 1491–1496.

Chaplin, D.J., Pettit, G.R. and Hill, S.A. (1999). Anti-vascular approaches to solid tumor therapy: evaluation of combretastatin A4 phosphate. *Anticancer Res* **19**, 189–196.

Chaplin, D.J., Pettit, G.R., Parkins, C.S. and Hill, S.A. (1996). Antivascular approaches to solid tumour therapy: evaluation of tubulin binding agents. *Br J Cancer* **27**, S86–S88.

Chavan, A.J., Richardson, S.K., Kim, H., Haley, B.E. and Watt, D.S. (1993). Forskolin photoaffinity probes for the evaluation of tubulin binding sites. *Bioconj Chem* **4**, 268–274.

Chen, Z., Mocharla, V.P., Farmer, J.M., Pettit, G.R., Hamel, E. and Pinney, K.G. (2000). Preparation of new anti-tubulin ligands through a dual-mode, addition–elimination reac-tion to a bromo-substituted α,β-unsaturated sulfoxide. *J Org Chem* **65**, 8811–8815.

Cirla, A. and Mann, J. (2003). Combretastatins: from natural products to drug discovery. *Nat Prod Rep* **20**, 558–564.

Cushman, M., Nagarathnam, D., Gopal, D., Chakraborti, A.K., Lin, C.M. and Hamel, E. (1991). Synthesis and evaluation of stilbene and dihydrostilbene derivatives as potential anticancer agents that inhibit tubulin polymerization. *J Med Chem* **34**, 2579–2588.

Desbene, S. and Giorgi-Renault, S. (2002). Drugs that inhibit tubulin polymerization: the particular case of podophyllotoxin and analogues. *Curr Medicinal Chem: Anti-Cancer Agents* **2**, 71–90.

Downing, K.H. (2000). Structural basis for the interaction of tubulin with proteins and drugs that affect microtubule dynamics. *Annu Rev Cell Biol* **16**, 89–111.

Duax, W.L., Griffin, J.F., Weeks, C.M. and Korach, K.S. (1985). Molecular conformation, receptor binding, and hormone action of natural and synthetic estrogens and antiestro-gens. *Environ Health Perspect* **61**, 111–121.

Edvardsen, K. and Pinney, K.G. (2005). Unpublished results, University of Lund, Sweden, and Baylor University, Waco, TX.

Eikesdal, H.P., Schem, B.C., Mella, O. and Dahl, O. (2000). The new tubulin-inhibitor com-bretastatin A-4 enhances thermal damage in the BT4An rat glioma. *Int J Radiat Oncol Biol Phys* **46**, 645–652.

Floyd, L.J., Barnes, L.D. and Williams, R.F. (1989) Photoaffinity labeling of tubulin with (2-nitro-4-azidophenyl)deacetylcolchicine: direct evidence for two colchicine binding sites. *Biochemistry* **28**, 8515–8525.

Flygare, J.A., Medina, J.C., Shan, B., Clark, D.L. and Rosen, T.J. (2000). Pentafluoroben-zenesulfonamides and analogs. *US Patent* 6121304.

Flynn, B.L., Flynn, G.P., Hamel, E. and Jung, M.K. (2001a). The synthesis and tubulin binding activity of thiophene-based analogues of combretastatin A-4. *Bioorg Med Chem Lett* **11**, 2341–2343.

Flynn, B.L. and Hamel, E. (2002a). Synthesis of indoles, benzofurans, and related compounds as potential tubulin binding agents. *PCT Int Application* WO2002060872 A1.

Flynn, B.L., Hamel, E. and Jung, M.K. (2002b). One-pot synthesis of benzo[b]furan and indole inhibitors of tubulin polymerization. *J Med Chem* **45**, 2670–2673.

Flynn, B.L., Verdier-Pinard, P. and Hamel, E. (2001b). A novel palladium-mediated coupling approach to 2,3-disubstituted benzo[b]thiophenes and its application to the synthesis of tubulin binding agents. *Org Lett* **3**, 651–654.

Galbraith, S.M., Chaplin, D.J., Lee, F., Stratford, M.R.L., Locke, R.J., Vojnovic, B. and Tozer, G.M. (2001). Effects of combretastatin A4 phosphate on endothelial cell morphology in vitro and relationship to tumor vascular targeting activity in vivo. *Anticancer Res* **21**, 93–102.

Gastpar, R., Goldbrunner, M., Marko, D. and Von Angerer, E. (1998). Methoxy-substituted 3-formyl-2-phenylindoles inhibit tubulin polymerization, *J Med Chem* **41**, 4965–4972.

Gaya, A.M. and Rustin, G.J.S. (2005). Vascular disrupting agents: a new class of drug in cancer therapy. *Clin Oncol* **17**, 277–290.

Ghatak, A., Dorsey, J.M., Garner, C.M. and Pinney, K.G. (2003). Synthesis of methoxy and hydroxy containing tetralones: versatile intermediates for the preparation of biologically relevant molecules. *Tetrahedron Lett* **44**, 4145–4148.

Goldbrunner, M., Loidl, G., Polossek, T., Mannschreck, A. and Von Angerer, E. (1997). Inhibition of tubulin polymerization by 5,6-dihydroindolo[2,1-α]isoquinoline derivatives. *J Med Chem* **40**, 3524–3533.

Grosios, K., Loadman, P.M., Swaine, D.J., Pettit, G.R. and Bibby, M.C. (2000). Combination chemotherapy with combretastatin A-4 phosphate and 5-fluorouracil in an experimental murine colon adenocarcinoma. *Anticancer Res* **20**, 229–233.

Hadimani, M., Kessler, R.J., Kautz, J.A., Ghatak, A., Shirali, A., O'Dell. H., Garner, C.M. and Pinney, K.G. (2002). 2-(3-tert-Butyldimethylsiloxy-4-methoxyphenyl)-6 methoxy-3-(3,4,5-trimethoxybenzoyl)indole. *Acta Cryst C: Crystal Struct Comm* **C58**, 330–332.

Hadimani, M.B. (December 2004). *Studies Toward the Discovery of New Classes of Privileged Molecules as Colchicine-Site Binding Ligands for Tubulin: Structure-Based Design, Synthesis, and Bioactivity of Small Ligands Targeted at Tumor Vasculature*, Ph.D. Dissertation, Baylor University.

Hahn, K.M., Hastie, S.B. and Sundberg, R.J. (1992). Synthesis and evaluation of 2-diazo-3,3,3-trifluopropanoyl derivatives of colchicine and podophyllotoxin as photoaffinity labels: reactivity, photochemistry, and tubulin binding. *Photochem Photobiol* **55**, 17–27.

Hall, J. (2005). Baylor University, (personal communication).

Hamel, E. (1996). Antimitotic natural products and their interactions with tubulin. *Med Res Rev* **16**, 207–231.

Hamel, E. and Pinney, K.G. 2005. Unpublished results, National Institutes of Health, National Cancer Institute – Frederick, MD, and Baylor University, Waco, TX.

Hartung, E.F. (1961). Colchicine and its analogs in gout: a brief review. *Arthritis Rheumatism* **4**, 18–26.

Hill, S.A., Tozer, G.M., Pettit, G.R. and Chaplin, D.J. (2002). Preclinical evaluation of the antitumour activity of the novel vascular targeting agent OXi 4503. *Anticancer Res* **22**, 1453–1458.

Holwell, S.E., Cooper, P.A., Grosios, K., Lippert, J.W. III, Pettit, G.R., Shnyder, S.D. and Bibby, M.C. (2002). Anti-tumor and anti-vascular effects of the novel tubulin-binding agent combretastatin A-1 phosphate. *Anticancer Res* **22**, 3933–3940.

Hori, K. and Saito, S. (2003). Microvascular mechanisms by which the combretastatin A-4 derivative AC7700 (AVE8062) induces tumour blood flow stasis. *Br J Cancer* **89**, 1334–1344.

Horsman, M.R. and Murata, R. (2002). Combination of vascular targeting agents with thermal or radiation therapy. *Int J Radiat Oncol Biol Phys* **54**, 1518–1523.

Horsman, M.R., Murata, R., Breidahl, T., Nielsen, F.U., Maxwell, R.J., Stodkiled-Jorgensen, H. and Overgaard, J. (2000). Combretastatins: novel vascular targeting drugs for improving anti-cancer therapy. Combretastatins and conventional therapy. *Adv Exp Med Biol* **476**, 311–323.

Hua, J., Sheng, Y., Pinney, K.G., Garner, C.M., Kane, R.R., Prezioso, J.A., Pettit, G.R., Chaplin, D.J. and Edvardsen, K. (2003). Oxi4503, a novel vascular targeting agent: effects on blood flow and antitumor activity in comparison to combretastatin A-4 phosphate. *Anticancer Res* **23**, 1433–1440.

Jelinek, C.J. (December 2004). *Discovery and Development of Dihydronaphthalene-Based Vascular Targeting Agents and Combretastatin-Related Analogs*, Thesis, Baylor University.

Jordan, M.A. and Wilson, L. (2004). Microtubules as a target for anticancer drugs. *Nature Rev* **4**, 253–265.

Jordon, A., Hadfield, J.A., Lawrence, N.J. and McGown, A.T. (1998). Tubulin as a target for anticancer drugs: agents which interact with the mitotic spindle. *Med Res Rev* **18**, 259–296.

Kanthou, C. and Tozer, G.M. (2002). The tumor vascular targeting agent combretastatin A-4-phosphate induces reorganization of the actin cytoskeleton and early membrane blebbing in human endothelial cells. *Blood* **99**, 2060–2069.

King, M.V., DeVries, J.L. and Pepinsky, R. (1952). X-ray diffraction determination of the chemical structure of colchicine. *Acta Crystallosr* **5**, 437–440.

Kingston, D.G.I., Samaranayake, G. and Ivey, C.A. (1990). The chemistry of taxol, a clinically useful anticancer agent. *J Nat Prod* **53**, 1–12.

Landuyt, W., Ahmed, B., Nuyts, S., Theys, J., Op de Beeck, M., Rijnders, A., Anne, J., Van Oosterom, A., Van Den Bogaert, W. and Lambin, P. (2001). In vivo antitumor effect of vascular targeting combined with either ionizing radiation or anti-angiogenesis treatment. *Int J Radiat Oncol Biol Phys* **49**, 443–450.

Li, L., Rojiani, A. and Siemann, D.W. (1998). Targeting the tumor vasculature with combretastatin A-4 disodium phosphate: effects on radiation therapy. *Int J Radiat Oncol Biol Phys* **42**, 899–903.

Li, Q. and Sham, H.L. (2002). Discovery and development of antimitotic agents that inhibit tubulin polymerization for the treatment of cancer. *Exp Opin Ther Pat* **12**, 1663–1702.

Li, Q., Woods, K.W., Claiborne, A., Gwaltney, S.L. II, Barr, K.J., Liu, G., Gehrke, L., Credo, R.B., Hui, Y.H., Lee, J., Warner, R.B., Kovar, P., Nukkala, M.A., Zielinski, N.A., Tahir, S.K., Fitzgerald, M., Kim, K.H., Marsh, K., Frost, D., Ng, S.C., Rosenberg, S. and Sham, H.L. (2002). Synthesis and biological evaluation of 2-indolyloxazolines as a new class of tubulin polymerization inhibitors. Discovery of A-289099 as an orally active antitumor agent. *Bioorg Med Chem Lett* **12**, 465–469.

Lin, C.M., Ho, H.H., Pettit, G.R. and Hamel, E. (1989). Antimitotic natural products combretastatin A-4 and combretastatin A-2: studies on the mechanism of their inhibition of the binding of colchicine to tubulin. *Biochemistry* **28**, 6984–6991.

Lin, C.M., Singh, S.B., Chu, P.S., Dempcy, R.O., Schmidt, J.M., Pettit, G.R. and Hamel, E. (1988). Interactions of tubulin with potent natural and synthetic analogs of the antimitotic agent combretastatin: a structure–activity study. *Mol Pharmacol* **34**, 200–208.

Lowe, J., Li, H., Downing, K.H., Nogales, E. (2001). Refined structure of αβ-tubulin at 3.5 Å resolution. *J Mol Biol* **313**, 1045–1057.

Ludford, R.J. (1948). Factors determining the action of colchicine on tumor growth. *Br J Cancer* **2**, 75–86.

McGown, A.T. and Fox, B.W. (1989). Structural and biochemical comparison of the antimitotic agents colchicine, combretastatin A4 and amphethinile. *Anti-Cancer Drug Des* **3**, 249–254.

Medina, J.C., Clark, D.L., Flygare, J.A., Rosen, T.J. and Shan, B. (1999). Pentafluorobenzenesulfonamides and analogs. *US Patent* 5880151.

Micheletti, G., Poli, M., Borsotti, P., Martinelli, M., Imberti, B., Taraboletti, G. and Giavazzi, R. (2003). Vascular-targeting activity of ZD6126, a novel tubulin-binding agent. *Cancer Res* **63**, 1534–1537.

Nakada, M., Kobayashi, S., Shibasaki, M., Iwasaki, S. and Ohno, M. (1993). The first total synthesis of the antitumor macrolide, rhizoxin. *Tetrahedron Lett* **34**, 1039–1042.

Nelkin, B.D. and Ball, D.W. (2001) Combretastatin A-4 and doxorubicin combination treatment is effective in a preclinical model of human medullary thyroid carcinoma. *Oncol Rep* **8**, 157–160.

Nicolaou, K.C., Winssinger, N., Pastor, J., Ninkovic, S., Sarabia, F., He, Y., Vourloumis, D., Yang, Z., Li, T., Giannakakou, P. and Hamel, E. (1997). Synthesis of epothilones A and B in solid and solution phase. *Nature* **387**, 268–272.

Nogales, E. (2000). Structural insights into microtubule function. *Annu Rev Biochem* **69**, 277–302.

Nogales, E., Wolf, S.G. and Downing, K.H. (1998). Structure of the α,β tubulin dimer by electron crystallography. *Nature* **391**, 199–203.

Ohsumi, K., Hatanaka, T., Nakagawa, R., Fukuda, Y., Morinaga, Y., Suga, Y., Nihei, Y., Ohishi, K., Akiyama, Y. and Tsuiji, T. (1999). Synthesis and antitumor activities of amino acid prodrugs of amino-combretastatins. *Anti-Cancer Drug Des* **14**, 539–548.

Ohsumi, K., Nakagawa, R., Fukuda, Y., Hatanaka, T., Morinaga, Y., Nihei, Y., Ohishi, K., Suga, Y., Akiyama, Y. and Tsuji, T. (1998). Novel combretastatin analogues effective against murine solid tumors: design and structure–activity relationships. *J Med Chem* **41**, 3022–3032.

Olszewski, J.D., Marshalla, M., Sabat, M. and Sundberg, R.J. (1994). Potential photoaffinity labels for tubulin. Synthesis and evaluation of diazocyclohexadienone and azide analogs of colchicine, combretastatin, and 3,4,5-trimethoxybiphenyl. *J Org Chem* **59**, 4285–4296.

Owellen, R.J., Hartke, C.A., Dickerson, R.M. and Hains, F.O. (1976). Inhibition of tubulin-microtubule polymerization by drugs of the vinca alkaloid class. *Cancer Res* **36**, 1499–1502.

Pedley, R.B., Hill, S.A., Boxer, G.M., Flynn, A.A., Boden, R., Watson, R., Dearling, J., Chaplin, D.J. and Begent, R.H.J. (2001). Eradication of colorectal xenografts by combined radioimmunotherapy and combretastatin A-4 3-O-phosphate. *Cancer Res* **61**, 4716–4722.

Pettit, G.R., Cragg, G.M., Herald, D.L., Schmidt, J.M. and Lohavanijaya, P. (1982). Isolation and structure of combretastatin. *Can J Chem* **60**, 1374–1376.

Pettit, G.R., Cragg, G.M. and Singh, S.B. (1987a). Antineoplastic agents, 122. Constituents of *Combretum caffrum*. *J Nat Prod* **50**, 386–391.

Pettit, G.R., Kamano, Y., Herald, C.L., Tuinman, A.A., Boettner, F.E., Kizu, H., Schmidt, J.M., Baczynskyj, L., Tomer, K.B. and Bontems, R.J. (1987b). The isolation and structure of a remarkable marine animal antineoplastic constituent: dolastatin 10. *J Am Chem Soc* **109**, 6883–6885.

Pettit, G.R. and Lippert, J.W. (2000). Antineoplastic agents 429. Syntheses of the combretastatin A-1 and combretastatin B-1 prodrugs. *Anti-Cancer Drug Des* **15**, 203–216.

Pettit, G.R. and Pinney, K.G. (2005). Unpublished results. Arizona State University, Tempe, AZ, and Baylor University, Waco, TX.

Pettit, G.R. and Singh, S.B. (1987). Isolation, structure, and synthesis of combretastatin A-2, A-3, and B-2. *Can J Chem* **65**, 2390–2396.

Pettit, G.R. and Singh, S.B. (1996). Isolation, structural elucidation and synthesis of novel antineoplastic substances denominated 'combretastatins'. *US Patent* 5569786.

Pettit, G.R., Singh, S.B., Boyd, M.R., Hamel, E., Pettit, R.K., Schmidt, J.M. and Hogan, F. (1995a). Antineoplastic agents. 291. Isolation and synthesis of combretastatins A-4, A-5, and A-6. *J Med Chem* **38**, 1666–1672.

Pettit, G.R., Singh, S.B. and Niven, M.L. (1988). Isolation and structure of combretastatin D-1: a cell growth inhibitory macrocyclic lactone from *Combretum caffrum*. *J Am Chem Soc* **110**, 8539–8540.

Pettit, G.R., Singh, S.B., Niven, M.L., Hamel, E. and Schmidt, J.M. (1987c). Isolation, structure, and synthesis of combretastatins A-1 and B-1, potent new inhibitors of microtubule assembly, derived from *Combretum caffrum*. *J Nat Prod* **50**, 119–131.

Pettit, G.R., Srirangam, J.K., Barkoczy, J., Williams, M.D., Boyd, M.R., Hamel, E., Pettit, R.K., Hogan, F., Bai, R., Chapuis, J.C., McAllister, S.C. and Schmidt, J.M. (1998a). Antineoplastic agents 365. Dolastatin 10 SAR probes. *Anticancer Drug Des* **13**, 243–277.

Pettit, G.R., Temple, C. Jr., Narayanan, V.L., Varma, R., Simpson, M.J., Boyd, M.R., Rener, G.A. and Bansal, N. (1995b). Antineoplastic agents 322. Synthesis of combretastatin A-4 prodrugs. *Anti-Cancer Drug Des* **10**, 299–309.

Pettit, G.R., Toki, B., Herald, D.L., Verdier-Pinard, P., Boyd, M.R., Hamel, E. and Pettit, R.K. (1998b). Antineoplastic agents. 379. Synthesis of phenstatin phosphate. *J Med Chem* **41**, 1688–1695.

Pinney, K.G., Bounds, A.D., Dingeman, K.M., Mocharla, V.P., Pettit, G.R., Bai, R. and Hamel, E. (1999). A new anti-tubulin agent containing the benzo[b]thiophene ring system. *Bioorg Med Chem Lett* **9**, 1081–1086.

Pinney, K.G., Edvardsen, K., Chaplin, D.J., Hadimani, M.B., Kessler, R.J., Jelinek, C. and Arthesary, P. (2004a). Molecular recognition of the colchicine binding site as a design paradigm for the discovery and development of new vascular targeting (disrupting) agents. *Second International Vascular Targeting Conference*, Miami Beach, FL, 2004.

Pinney, K.G., Jelinek, C.J., Edvardsen, K., Chaplin, D.J. and Pettit, G.R. (2005a). The discovery and development of the combretastatins. In *Antitumor Agents from Natural Products*, D. Kingston, D. Newman and G. Cragg (eds). CRC Press, Boca Raton, FL, Chapter 3, pp. 23–46.

Pinney, K.G., Mejia, P., Mocharla, V.P., Shirali, A. and Pettit, G.R. (2000a). Anti-mitotic agents which inhibit tubulin polymerization. *US Patent* 6162930.

Pinney, K.G., Mejia, M.P., Villalobos, V.M., Rosenquist, B.E., Pettit, G.R., Verdier-Pinard, P. and Hamel, E. (2000b). Synthesis and biological evaluation of aryl azide derivatives of combretastatin A-4 as molecular probes for tubulin. *Bioorg Med Chem* **8**, 2417–2425.

Pinney, K.G., Mocharla, V.P., Chen, Z., Garner, C.M., Ghatak, A. and Dorsey, J.M. (2003). Tubulin binding ligands and corresponding prodrug constructs. *US Patent* 6593374.

Pinney, K.G., Mocharla, V.P., Chen, Z., Garner, C.M., Ghatak, A., Hadimani, M., Kessler, J. and Dorsey, J.M. (2001a). Preparation of trimethoxyphenyl-containing tubulin binding ligands and corresponding prodrug constructs as inhibitors of tubulin polymerization and antimitotic agents. *PCT Int Application* WO2001068654.

Pinney, K.G., Mocharla, V.P., Chen, Z., Garner, C.M., Hadimani, M., Kessler, R., Dorsey, J.M., Edvardsen, K., Chaplin, D.J., Prezioso, J., Ghatak, A. and Ghatak, U. (2004b). Tubulin binding ligands and corresponding prodrug constructs. *US Patent Application* 2004044059 A1.

Pinney, K.G., Mocharla, V.P., Chen, Z., Garner, C.M., Hadimani, M., Kessler, R., Dorsey, J.M., Edvardsen, K., Chaplin, D.J., Prezioso, J., Ghatak, A. and Ghatak, U. (2004c). Tubulin binding ligands and corresponding prodrug constructs. *US Patent Application* 20040043969 A1.

Pinney, K.G., Pettit, G.R., Mocharla, V.P., Mejia, M.P. and Shirali, A. (2000c). Description of anti-mitotic agents which inhibit tubulin polymerization. *US Patent* 6350777.

Pinney, K.G., Wang, F. and Del Pilar Mejia, M. (2001b). Preparation of indole-containing and combretastatin-related anti-mitotic and anti-tubulin polymerization agents. *PCT Int Application* WO2001019794 A2.

Pinney, K.G., Wang, F. and Hadimani, M. (2005b). Indole-containing and combretastatin-related anti-mitotic and anti-tubulin polymerization agents. *US Patent* 6849656.

Rao, S., Horwitz, S.B. and Ringel, I. (1992). Direct photoaffinity labeling of tubulin with taxol. *J Natl Cancer Inst* **84**, 785–788.

Ravelli, R.B.G., Gigant, B., Curmi, P.A., Jourdain, I., Lachkar, S., Sobel, A., Knossow, M. (2004). Insight into tubulin regulation from a complex with colchicine and a stathmin-like domain. *Nature* **428**, 198–202.

Safa, A.R., Hamel, E., Felsted, R.L. (1987). Photoaffinity labeling of tubulin subunits with a photoactive analogue of vinblastine. *Biochemistry* **26**, 97–102.

Sawada, T., Hashimoto, Y., Li, Y., Kobayashi, H. and Iwasaki, S. (1991). Fluorescent and photoaffinity labeling derivatives of rhizoxin. *Biochem Biophys Res Comm* **178**, 558–562.

Sawada, T., Kato, Y., Kobayashi, H., Hashimoto, Y., Watanabe, T., Sugiyama, Y. and Iwasaki, S. (1993a). A fluorescent probe and a photoaffinity labeling reagent to study the binding site of maytansine and rhizoxin on tubulin. *Bioconj Chem* **4**, 284–289.

Sawada, T., Kobayashi, H., Hashimoto, Y. and Iwasaki, S. (1993b). Identification of the fragment photoaffinity-labeled with azidodansyl-rhizoxin as Met-363–Lys-379 on beta-tubulin. *Biochem Pharmacol* **45**, 1387–1394.

Sheng, Y., Hua, J., Pinney, K.G., Garner, C.M., Kane, R.R., Prezioso, J.A., Chaplin, D.J. and Edvardsen, K. (2004). Combretastatin family member OXI4503 induces tumor vascular collapse through the induction of endothelial apoptosis. *Int J Cancer* **111**, 604–610.

Shirali, A.R. (2002). *Inhibitors of Tubulin Assembly: Designed Ligands Featuring Benzo[b]thiophene, Dihydronaphthalene and Aroylchromene Molecular Core Structures*, Ph.D. Dissertation, Baylor University.

Shnyder, S.D., Cooper, P.A., Pettit, G.R., Lippert, J.W. III, and Bibby, M.C. (2003). Combretastatin A-1 phosphate potentiates the antitumour activity of cisplatin in a murine adeno-carcinoma model. *Anticancer Res* **23**, 1619–1623.

Siemann, D.W. (2002). Vascular targeting agents: an introduction. *Int J Radiat Oncol Biol Phys* **54**, 1472.

Siemann, D.W., Bibby, M.C., Dark, G.G., Dicker, A.P., Eskens, F.A.L.M., Horsman, M.R., Marme, D. and LoRusso, P.M. (2005). Differentiation and definition of vascular-targeted therapies. *Clin Cancer Res* **11**, 416–420.

Siemann, D.W., Chaplin, D.J. and Horsman, M.R. (2004). Vascular-targeting therapies for treatment of malignant disease. *Cancer* **100**, 2491–2499.

Siemann, D.W., Mercer, E., Lepler, S. and Rojiani, A.M. (2002a). Vascular targeting agents enhance chemotherapeutic agent activities in solid tumor therapy. *Int J Cancer* **99**, 1–6.

Siemann, D.W. and Rojiani, A.M. (2002b). Enhancement of radiation therapy by the novel vascular targeting agent ZD6126. *Int J Radiat Oncol Biol Phys* **53**, 164–171.

Siemann, D.W. and Rojiani, A.M. (2002c). Antitumor efficacy of conventional anticancer drugs is enhanced by the vascular targeting agent ZD6126. *Int J Radiat Oncol Biol Phys* **54**, 1512–1517.

Singh, S.B. and Pettit, G.R. (1989). Isolation, structure, and synthesis of combretastatin C-1. *J Org Chem* **54**, 4105–4114.

Staretz, M.E. and Hastie, S.B. (1993). Synthesis, photochemical reactions, and tubulin binding of novel photoaffinity labeling derivatives of colchicines. *J Org Chem* **58**, 1589–1592.

Szala, S. (2004). Two-domain vascular disruptive agents in cancer therapy. *Curr Cancer Drug Targets* **4**, 501–509.

Tahir, S.K., Nukkala, M.A., Mozny, N.A.Z., Credo, R.B., Warner, R.B., Li, Q., Woods, K.W., Claiborne, A., Gwaltney, S.L. II, Frost, D.J., Sham, H.L., Rosenberg, S.H. and Ng, S.C. (2003). Biological activity of A-289099: an orally active tubulin-binding indolyloxazoline derivative. *Mol Cancer Ther* **2**, 227–233.

Thorpe, P.E. (2004). Vascular targeting agents as cancer therapeutics. *Clin Cancer Res* **10**, 415–427.

Thorpe, P.E., Chaplin, D.J. and Blakey, D.C. (2003). The first international conference on vascular targeting: meeting overview. *Cancer Res* **63**, 1144–1147.

Tozer, G.M., Kanthou, C., Parkins, C.S. and Hill, S.A. (2002). The biology of the combretastatins as tumour vascular targeting agents. *Int J Exp Pathol* **83**, 21–38.

Tozer, G.M., Prise, V.E., Wilson, J., Cemazar, M., Shan, S., Dewhirst, M.W., Barber, P.R., Vojnovic, B. and Chaplin, D.J. (2001). Mechanisms associated with tumor vascular shutdown induced by combretastatin A-4 phosphate: intravital microscopy and measurement of vascular permeability. *Cancer Res* **61**, 6413–6422.

Wang, L., Woods, K.W., Li, Q., Barr, K.J., McCroskey, R.W., Hannick, S.M., Gherke, L., Credo, R.B., Hui, Y.H., Marsh, K., Warner, R., Lee, J.Y., Zielinski-Mozng, N., Frost, D., Rosenberg, S.H. and Sham, H.L. (2002). Potent, orally active heterocycle-based combretastatin A-4 analogues: synthesis, structure–activity relationship, pharmacokinetics, and in vivo antitumor activity evaluation. *J Med Chem* **45**, 1697–1711.

Wehbe, H. (2005). *Towards Enhanced Chemotherapy: Studies on Drug Design, Synergy, and Drug Target Expression and Resistance with the Combretastatins and Other Chemotherapeutics*, Ph.D. Dissertation, Baylor University.

Wildiers, H., Ahmed, B., Guetens, G., De Boeck, G., De Bruijn, E.A., Landuyt, W. and Van Oosterom, A.T. (2004). Combretastatin A-4 phosphate enhances CPT-11 activity independently of the administration sequence. *Eur J Cancer* **40**, 284–290.

Williams, R.F., Mumford, C.L., Williams, G.A., Floyd, L.J., Aivaliotis, M.J., Martinez, R.A., Robinson, A.K. and Barnes, L.D. (1985). A photoaffinity derivative of colchicine: 6′-(4′-azido-2′-nitrophenylamino)hexanoyldeacetylcolchicine. Photolabeling and location of the colchicine binding site on the alpha-subunit of tubulin. *J Biol Chem* **260**, 13 794–13 802.

Wolff, J., Knipling, L., Cahnman, H.J. and Palumbo, G. (1991). Direct photoaffinity labeling of tubulin with colchicines. *Proc Natl Acad Sci USA* **88**, 2820–2824.

Young, S. and Chaplin, D.J. (2004). Combretastatin A4 phosphate: background and current clinical status. *Exp Opin Invest Drugs* **13**, 1171–1182.

Zhou, S., Kestell, P., Baguley, B.C. and Paxton, J.W. (2002). 5,6-Dimethylxanthenone-4-acetic acid (DMXAA): a new biological response modifier for cancer therapy. *Investigational New Drugs* **20**, 281–295.

7

Combined Modality Approaches Using Vasculature-disrupting Agents

Wenyin Shi, Michael R. Horsman and Dietmar W. Siemann

Abstract

Extensive preclinical investigations have established the efficacy of vascular disrupting agents (VDAs), such as DMXAA, CA4DP, ZD6126 and OXi4503. However, a thin rim of viable tumor tissue typically survives VDA treatment due to its location at the periphery where it receives nutritional support from adjacent normal tissue blood vessels. In order to eradicate that part of the tumor which survives VDA exposure, additional therapy needs to be administered. This review will summarize the preclinical status and conceptual basis of combining VDAs in combination with conventional cytotoxic approaches such as chemotherapy and radiation.

Keywords

Vascular targeting, Vascular disrupting agent, Anti-angiogenesis, Combretastatin, ZD6126, DMXAA, OXi4503, Radiotherapy, Chemotherapy, Hyperthermia

7.1 Tumor vasculature

Impact on conventional antitumor therapies

Tumor vessels differ greatly from vessels in normal tissues (Vaupel, Kallinowski and Okunieff, 1989). They are primitive in nature and morphologically and functionally abnormal. The structural defects and ineffective perfusion capacity of tumor microvessels lead to chaotic and heterogeneous blood flow, which inevitably fails to meet the metabolic demands of the tumor tissue. As a result areas of nutrient deprivation, hypoxia, and acidosis are common features of

Vascular-targeted Therapies in Oncology   Edited by Dietmar W. Siemann
© 2006 John Wiley & Sons, Ltd.

solid neoplasia (Vaupel, Kallinowski and Okunieff, 1989). The impact of these abnormal microenvironments on tumor response to conventional anticancer treatments such as radiation therapy and chemotherapy has been well documented (Siemann, 1984; Sartorelli, 1988; Durand, 1991; Okunieff *et al.*, 1993; Brizel *et al.*, 1994; Nordsmark, Overgaard and Overgaard 1996; Brizel *et al.*, 1999; Knocke *et al.*, 1999; Walenta, Schweder and Mueller-Klieser, 2002).

Targeting the tumor vasculature

Two key approaches to targeting the tumor blood vessel network have been developed (Denekamp, 1993; Folkman, 1995). The first approach aims to inhibit the tumor-initiated angiogenic process (Folkman, 1995). The second seeks to preferentially destroy the existing tumor vasculature (Denekamp, 1990; Chaplin and Dougherty, 1999; Siemann and Shi, 2003). Though both selectively target tumor vasculature, distinctions between antiangiogenic and vascular-disrupting therapies should be made. The two approaches differ in their mode of action as well as in their therapeutic applications (Siemann *et al.*, 2005).

7.2 Vascular-disrupting strategies

Vascular-disrupting agents exert their selective action by exploiting differences between tumor and normal endothelium (Thorpe, 2004). Destruction of the endothelium results in secondary tumor cell death from lack of oxygen and nutrients due to the rapid and extensive vascular shutdown. Treatment with these agents ultimately leads to widespread central necrosis in solid tumors (Rojiani *et al.*, 2002). The efficacies of small-molecule VDAs, such as DMXAA, CA4DP, AVE8062A, ZD6126 and OXi4503, have now been established in a wide variety of preclinical tumor models, including transplanted and spontaneous rodent tumors, orthotopically transplanted tumors and human tumor xenografts (Rewcastle *et al.*, 1991; Ching, Joseph and Bapuley, 1992; Laws *et al.*, 1995; Dark *et al.*, 1997; Li Rojiani and Siemann, 1998; Horsman *et al.*, 1998; Hori *et al.*, 1999; Murata *et al.*, 2001b; Blakey *et al.*, 2002b; Hill *et al.*, 2002a; Kim *et al.*, 2003; Hua *et al.*, 2003). Yet, despite the potent antivascular effects and large-scale induction of central tumor necrosis following treatment with VDAs, a narrow rim of viable tumor cells is typically observed at the tumor periphery near the surrounding normal tissues (Chaplin, Pettit and Hill, 1999; Siemann and Rojiani, 2002a; Rojiani *et al.*, 2002; Thorpe, 2004). The most plausible explanation is that these areas of the tumor survive because they are supplied by normal vessels, which are not susceptible to damage by these agents (Siemann, Chaplin and Horsman, 2004). The residual pockets of tumor tissue can act as a source of tumor regrowth. Recent studies with a second-generation VDA (OXi4503) have shown that reductions in the viable rim are possible (Hua *et al.*, 2003; Hill *et al.*, 2002b). In general, it is not likely that VDA treatment alone will eradicate the tumor mass.

A reasonable approach to eliminate the tumor cells that survive VDA treatment is to combine these agents with cytotoxic anticancer therapies such as radiation or chemotherapy (Siemann and Shi, 2003; Siemann and Horsman, 2004). The rationale for such a strategy is that cells that make up this viable rim of tumor tissue are likely to be oxygenated and in a state of high proliferation. In addition, these tumor cells are also readily accessible to systemically administered agents since they are adjacent to normal tissue vasculature. All these factors should make the surviving tumor cells susceptible to radiotherapy and chemotherapy. Conversely, VDAs cause the destruction of large areas of the interior of tumors and show excellent activity against large bulky disease (Siemann and Shi, 2003), which is typically resistant to conventional anticancer therapies. Taken together, the application of VDAs in a combined modality setting should hold considerable promise.

7.3   VDAs and chemotherapy

Chemotherapeutic agents target the neoplastic cell population and have direct cytotoxic effect. VDAs are directed against the tumor endothelium. By combining VDAs and cytotoxic drugs, enhanced antitumor effects may be expected on the basis of these therapies having distinctive target cell populations and independent mechanisms of action and potential interactions. Several studies have reported on the use of VDAs combined with conventional chemotherapy in a variety of tumor model systems (Cliffe *et al.*, 1994; Pruijn *et al.*, 1997; Lash *et al.*, 1998; Chaplin, Pettit and Hill, 1999; Grosios *et al.*, 2000; Horsman *et al.*, 2000; Nelkin and Ball, 2001; Blakey *et al.*, 2002b; Siemann and Rojiani, 2002a; Li, Rojiani and Siemann, 2002; Siim *et al.*, 2003; Shnyder *et al.*, 2003; Hori *et al.*, 2003; Morinaga *et al.*, 2003) (Table 7.1). In general, marked enhancements in antitumor activities were observed when VDAs were combined with anticancer drugs. For example, Figure 7.1 demonstrates significant enhancement of antitumor effect of cisplatin with the use of a VDA (OXi4503). However, the timing and sequencing of agents are of significant consideration in such treatments. Typically, optimal enhancements were obtained by administrating the VDAs within a few hours after chemotherapy (Cliffe *et al.*, 1994; Pruijn *et al.*, 1997; Lash *et al.*, 1998; Chaplin, Pettit and Hill, 1999; Grosios *et al.*, 2000; Nelkin and Ball, 2001; Blakey *et al.*, 2002b; Siemann and Rojiani, 2002a; Li, Rojiani and Siemann, 2002). The rationale for such sequencing was to minimize the possible interference of distribution and uptake of the chemotherapeutic agents by the VDAs. Indeed, some evidence exists that combination therapy may be less effective when VDAs are administered immediately prior to the administration of the cancer chemotherapy agent (Pruijn *et al.*, 1997; Chaplin, Pettit and Hill, 1999; Siemann *et al.*, 2002). One possible explanation for the

Table 7.1 Combination therapy of VDAs with chemotherapy agents

VDAs	Chemotherapy agent	Tumor model	Reference
DMXAA	Tirapazamine	Mouse	(Cliffe *et al.*, 1994; Lash *et al.*, 1998)
	Melphalan	Mouse	(Pruijn *et al.*, 1997)
	Dinitrobenzamide mustard	Mouse	(Lash *et al.*, 1998)
	5-FU	Mouse	(Siim *et al.*, 2003)
	Etoposide	Mouse	(Siim *et al.*, 2003)
	Carboplatin	Mouse	(Siim *et al.*, 2003)
	Cyclophosphamide	Mouse	(Siim *et al.*, 2003)
	Doxorubicin	Mouse	(Siim *et al.*, 2003)
	Cisplatin	Mouse	(Siim *et al.*, 2003)
	Docetaxel	Mouse	(Siim *et al.*, 2003)
	Vincristine	Mouse	(Siim *et al.*, 2003)
	Paclitaxel	Mouse	(Siim *et al.*, 2003)
CA4DP	Doxorubicin	Human xenograft	(Nelkin and Ball, 2001)
	Cisplatin	Mouse	(Chaplin, Pettit and Hill, 1999; Horsman *et al.*, 2000; Siemann *et al.*, 2002; Shnyder *et al.*, 2003)
	5-FU	Mouse	(Grosios *et al.*, 2000)
	Vinblastine	Human xenograft	(Li, Rojiani and Siemann, 2002)
	Cyclophosphamide	Mouse	(Siemann *et al.*, 2002)
AVE8062A	Cisplatin	Mouse, human xenograft	(Morinaga *et al.*, 2003)
	Doxorubicin	Mouse	(Hori *et al.*, 2003)
	Mitomycin C	Mouse	(Hori *et al.*, 2003)
ZD6126	Cisplatin	Human xenograft, mouse	(Siemann and Rojiani, 2002a; Goto *et al.*, 2004; Blakey *et al.*, 2002b)

latter results is that when VDAs are given just before chemotherapy they cause parts of the tumor to undergo transient reductions in blood flow. If these reductions are sufficient to impair delivery of the subsequently administered chemotherapy agent, but insufficient to lead to tumor cell death due to ischemia, then a suboptimal antitumor effect could be the consequence.

Although most preclinical investigations have demonstrated improved tumor responses through the combination therapy, such a result will only be of benefit if the treatment does not lead to enhanced critical normal tissue reactions.

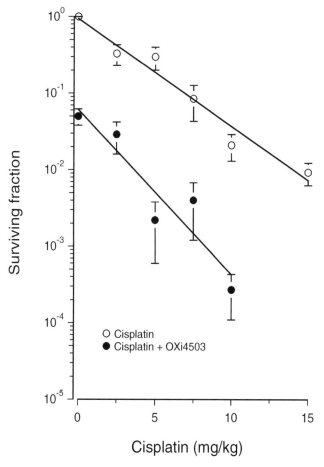

Figure 7.1 Tumor cell survival in KHT sarcomas treated with a 10 mg kg^{-1} dose of OXi4503 1 h after a range of doses of cisplatin. Results are the means ± 1 SE of four to nine tumors per treatment group

Because VDAs and conventional chemotherapy agents have distinctive target populations and mechanisms of action, it should be possible to achieve an increase in treatment efficacy with little or no increase in toxicity. In general, this has been observed in preclinical studies. Combinations of VDAs with anti-cancer drugs have shown improved antitumor effects without concomitant increases in host toxicity (Cliffe *et al.*, 1994; Pruijn *et al.*, 1997; Lash *et al.*, 1998; Chaplin, Pettit and Hill, 1999; Grosios *et al.*, 2000; Nelkin and Ball, 2001; Siemann and Rojiani, 2002a; Li, Rojiani and Sieimann, 2002; Siemann *et al.*, 2002) or chemotherapy-agent-specific side-effects (Siemann *et al.*, 2002; Siemann and Rojiani, 2002a). Current preclinical data therefore support the notion of combining VDAs with chemotherapy regimens to improve treatment outcomes.

7.4 VDAs and radiation therapy

Currently, approximately 60 per cent of all cancer patients receive radiotherapy as a component of their treatment (Feldmann, Molls and Vaupel, 1999). Indeed, substantial numbers of patients with common cancers achieve long-term tumor control largely by the use of radiation therapy. Broad estimations of the relative roles of the main treatment modalities suggest that local treatment, including surgery and/or radiation, could be expected to be successful in ~40 per cent of these cases (DeVita *et al.*, 1979; Souhami R and Tobias, 1986; Tubiana, 1992). Still, significant numbers of radiotherapy patients with definitive treatment ultimately fail. Major reasons for radiotherapy failures include intrinsic genetic resistance, tumor progression, unfavorable tumor microenvironments, especially tumor hypoxia, and metastatic spread of the primary disease (DeVita Hellman and Rosenberg, 1997). Tumor vasculature may be an important contributor underlying many of the treatment failures (Overgaard and Horsman, 1996).

Since VDAs cause the destruction of the poorly oxygenated and radiation refractory cores of tumors, the tumor response to radiation may be improved when combined with VDAs. Moreover, since the tumor cells surviving VDA treatment are located predominantly at the tumor periphery adjacent to normal tissues, the residual tumor tissue is likely to be well oxygenated (Wilson *et al.*, 1998; Li, Rojiani and Siemann, 1998; Siemann and Rojiani, 2002b). Given the frequent use of radiotherapy and its mechanisms of action and reasons for treatment failure, a substantial number of preclinical investigations evaluating the therapeutic efficacy of combining radiation with VDAs have been initiated. By and large these studies have shown that VDAs can be combined successfully with radiation to improve therapeutic efficacy (Wilson *et al.*, 1998; Li, Rojiani and Siemann, 1998; Horsman *et al.*, 2000; Murata, Overgaard and Horsman, 2001; Murata *et al.*, 2001a, 2001b; Landuyt *et al.*, 2001; Siemann and Rojiani, 2002b) (Table 7.2). Similar to the combination with chemotherapy agents, one critical issue in such combination therapy is the importance of sequence and timing between the VDA and radiation. As with chemotherapy, the greatest benefit was achieved when VDAs were administered post-radiotherapy (Li, Rojiani and Siemann, 1998; Wilson *et al.*, 1998; Siemann and Rojiani, 2002b; Siemann and Shi, 2003). Once again, administrating VDAs just prior to radiation typically fails to enhance the radiation response possibly due to transient induction of hypoxia. This postulation is consistent with the observation that the hypoxic cell cytotoxin tirapazamine (SR-4233, NSC-130181, Tirazone, SanofiSynthelabo/National Cancer Institute) could increase the efficacy of the combination treatment of radiation and DMXAA (Wilson *et al.*, 1998). On the basis of such findings, most investigators have chosen to administer VDAs post-radiation (Wilson *et al.*, 1998; Li, Rojiani and Siemann, 1998; Horsman *et al.*, 2000; Murata Overgaard and Horsman, 2001; Murata *et al.*, 2001a, 2001b; Landuyt *et al.*, 2001; Siemann and Rojiani, 2002b; Horsman and Murata, 2003; Siemann and Horsman, 2004). In general these studies demonstrated enhanced

Table 7.2 Combination therapy of VDAs with radiation therapy

VDA	Tumor model	Radiation	Reference
DMXAA	RIF-1 fibrosarcoma	Single dose; fractionated dose	(Wilson *et al.*, 1998)
	MDAH-Mca4 mammary carcinoma	Single dose; fractionated dose	(Wilson *et al.*, 1998)
	C3H mammary carcinoma	Single dose	(Murata *et al.*, 2001a)
	KHT sarcoma	Single dose	(Murata *et al.*, 2001a)
CA4DP	KHT sarcoma	Single dose	(Li, Rojiani and Siemann 1998; Murata *et al.*, 2001b)
	C3H mammary carcinoma	Single dose	(Murata *et al.*, 2001b)
	Rat rhabdomyosarcoma	Single dose	(Landuyt *et al.*, 2001)
	KSY-1 Kaposi's sarcoma	Single dose	(Li, Rojiani and Siemann, 2002)
ZD6126	KHT sarcoma	Fractionated dose	(Siemann and Rojiani, 2002b)

antitumor response in a variety of murine and human tumor xenograft models while utilizing response endpoints including tumor growth delay, surviving fraction and tumor control. Figure 7.2 is an example showing markedly enhanced antitumor effect of radiation with the use of a VDA (OXi4503) in a murine tumor model of KHT. These findings are of particular relevance in light of preclinical results that showed no enhancement of the radiation response of normal skin (Wilson *et al.*, 1998; Murata *et al.*, 2001a, 2001b), bladder or lung by VDAs (Horsman and Murata, 2002).

The aforementioned investigations all utilized single-dose radiation therapy; importantly, the limited number of preclinical studies which incorporated fractionated dose external beam radiation in combination with a VDA also reported enhanced tumor responses (Wilson *et al.*, 1998; Chaplin, Pettit and Hill, 1999; Siemann and Rojiani, 2002b). While the issue of sequence and timing has not been unequivocally resolved in the fractionated radiation protocols, both a schedule that administered a VDA after the final dose of week-long daily fractionated radiation treatments (Chaplin, Pettit and Hill, 1999; Siemann and Rojiani, 2002b) and one in which the VDA was given daily after the second dose of a twice a day schedule (Wilson *et al.*, 1998) resulted in improved tumor responses. These findings suggest that VDAs can be successfully incorporated into fractionated radiation protocols and that it may be feasible to administrate VDAs more frequently during the course of radiation therapy than initially anticipated.

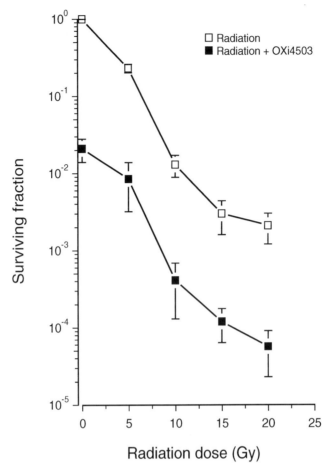

Figure 7.2 Tumor cell survival in KHT-sarcoma-bearing mice treated with a range of single doses of radiation administered 1 h after giving a 10 mg kg^{-1} dose of OXi4503. Data are the mean ± SE. Six to ten animals per treatment group

In addition to combining VDAs with photon radiation, a recent study also investigated the efficacy of adding ZD6126 to boron neutron capture therapy (Masunaga *et al.*, 2004). When this VDA was administered 15 min after boron compounds sodium borocaptate-^{10}B or I-p-boronophenylalanine-^{10}B, both the ^{10}B concentration and the resultant tumor cell kill were greatly increased. This study implies that VDAs may have utility in combination with other forms of radiotherapy, including high-LET radiotherapy and brachytherapy.

Moreover, novel approaches combining VDAs with radioimmunetherapy (RIT) demonstrated marked enhancement of antitumor efficacies in the human colorectal tumor xenograft model (Pedley *et al.*, 1996, 1999, 2001, 2002). Antibody distribution, modeling and immunohistochemistry studies showed radioimmunotherapy effectively treated the outer, well oxygenated tumor region only (Pedley *et al.*, 2002), while as discussed earlier VDAs are effective against the more hypoxic tumor center. These two spacial complementary approaches are found to be synergetic, which resulted in eradication of the tumors (Pedley *et al.*, 2002). Optimization of the combination therapy and clinical evaluation are warranted.

7.5   VDAs and antiangiogenic agents

Vascular disrupting and antiangiogenic therapies are two major vascular target-ing avenues that have evolved (Siemann *et al.*, 2005). Both the initiation of new blood formation and the integrity of the existing blood vessel network are critical to a tumor's survival, growth and spread. Therefore, a strategy aimed at compromising both aspects of a tumor's blood vessel network ought to result in an improved tumor response. Mechanistically, such a combination is likely to be complimenting rather than duplicative (Siemann and Shi, 2003). Antian-giogenic agents appear especially well suited to treat metastatic disease or early stage tumors (O'Reilly *et al.*, 1994; Yoon *et al.*, 1999; Lozonschi *et al.*, 1999), whereas VDAs may be particularly effective against large bulky tumors (Landuyt *et al.*, 2001). One rationale for combining such agents is that antiangiogenic agents may significantly slow down, or block the regrowth of the tumor from the rim that survived VDA treatment. Thus their combination should prove to be extremely efficacious. Indeed, data are beginning to emerge that such a com-bination may provide particularly beneficial antitumor effects (Wedge *et al.*, 2002; Blakey *et al.*, 2002a). Another reason for considering the combination of these approaches is that, based on their distinct mechanisms, antiangiogenic and vascular disrupting strategies are likely to have no overlapping toxicities. Con-sequently, their application in combination in both primary and secondary disease warrants further investigation and promises considerable merit.

7.6   Summary

The fact that a single tumor blood vessel can sustain thousands of tumor cells has been well established. The continuous growth and expansion of solid tumor masses as well as the metastatic spread of tumor cells are critically reliant on the tumor blood vessel network. Strategies that aim to target tumor blood vessels therefore have emerged as promising anticancer treatments. VDAs target the existing tumor vasculature. Recently, small-molecule VDAs such as CA4DP and ZD6126 have been shown to exert their anti-vascular effects at well toler-ated doses. Extensive preclinical studies have established the efficacy of this class of drugs in a variety of tumor models. However, a characteristic feature of this group of agents is that a thin rim of tumor tissue survives near the tumor periphery following VDA treatment. As a consequence, a number of strategies have evaluated the efficacy of combining VDAs with other anti-cancer therapies.

Preclinical investigations have demonstrated that VDAs can markedly enhance the response of tumors to radiation and chemotherapy. The results support the notion that such a combination allows the two treatments to act in a complementary fashion. Specifically, the VDA significantly reduces the central tumor burden, which typically tends to be resistant to conventional therapies, while radiation or chemotherapy destroys the rim of tumor cells surviving VDA treatment. It is also clear that there is benefit in combining VDAs with other agents that target the tumor vasculature such as, for example, antiangiogenic agents. Indeed such a combination could be considered as a single vascular-targeting regimen to be incorporated into a multi-modality anticancer treatment, which includes chemotherapy or radiotherapy.

Results from preclinical tumor response investigations have advanced VDAs into clinical trials. Evidence now suggests that the combination of therapies that target tumor vasculature in conjunction with conventional anticancer therapies offers the promise of providing significant improvement in treatment outcomes. The investigation of such combination in clinical trials appears warranted.

Acknowledgments

Work described in this article was supported in part by Grants RO1 CA84408 and RO1 CA89655 from the National Institutes of Health.

References

Blakey, D.C., Ashton, S.E., Westwood, F.R., Walker, M. and Ryan, A.J. (2002a). ZD6126: a novel small molecule vascular targeting agent. *Int J Radiat Oncol Biol Phys* **54**, 1497–1502.

Blakey, D.C., Westwood, F.R., Walker M, Hughes, G.D., Davis, P.D., Ashton, S.E. and Ryan, A.J. (2002b). Antitumor activity of the novel vascular targeting agent ZD6126 in a panel of tumor models. *Clin Cancer Res* **8**, 1974–1983.

Brizel, D.M., Dodge, R.K., Clough, R.W. and Dewhirst, M.W. (1999). Oxygenation of head and neck cancer: changes during radiotherapy and impact on treatment outcome. *Radiother Oncol* **53**, 113–117.

Brizel, D.M., Rosner, G.L., Harrelson, J., Prosnitz, L.R. and Dewhirst, M.W. (1994). Pretreatment oxygenation profiles of human soft tissue sarcomas. *Int J Radiat Oncol Biol Phys* **30**, 635–642.

Chaplin, D.J. and Dougherty, G.J. (1999). Tumor vasculature as a target for cancer therapy. *Br J Cancer* **80** (Suppl. 1), 57–64.

Chaplin, D.J., Pettit, G.R. and Hill, S.A. (1999). Anti-vascular approaches to solid tumor therapy: evaluation of combretastatin A4 phosphate. *Anticancer Res* **19**, 189–195.

Ching, L.M., Joseph, W.R. and Baguley, B.C. (1992). Stimulation of macrophage tumoricidal activity by 5,6-dimethyl-xanthenone-4-acetic acid, a potent analogue of the antitumour agent flavone-8-acetic acid. *Biochem Pharmacol* **44**, 192–195.

Cliffe, S., Taylor, M.L., Rutland, M., Baguley, B.C., Hill, R.P. and Wilson, W.R. (1994). Combining bioreductive drugs (SR 4233 or SN 23862) with the vasoactive agents flavone acetic acid or 5,6-dimethylxanthenone acetic acid. *Int J Radiat Oncol Biol Phys* **29**, 373–377.

Dark, G.G., Hill, S.A., Prise, V.E., Tozer, G.M., Pettit, G.R. and Chaplin, D.J. (1997). Combretastatin A-4, an agent that displays potent and selective toxicity toward tumor vasculature. *Cancer Res* **57**, 1829–1834.

Denekamp, J. (1990). Vascular attack as a therapeutic strategy for cancer. *Cancer Metastasis Rev* **9**, 267–282.

Denekamp, J. (1993). Review article: angiogenesis, neovascular proliferation and vascular pathophysiology as targets for cancer therapy. *Br J Radiol* **66**, 181–196.

DeVita, V.T., Goldin, A. and Oliverio, V.T. *et al.* (1979). The drug development and clinical trials programs of the division of cancer treatment. *Cancer Clin Trials* **2**, 195–216.

DeVita, V.T., Hellman, S. and Rosenberg, S. (1997). *Cancer: Principles and Practice of Oncology*. Lippincott-Raven, Philadelphia, PA.

Durand, R.E. (1991). Keynote address: the influence of microenvironmental factors on the activity of radiation and drugs. *Int J Radiat Oncol Biol Phys* **20**, 253–258.

Feldmann, H.J., Molls, M. and Vaupel, P. (1999). Blood flow and oxygenation status of human tumors. Clinical investigations. *Strahlenther Onkol* **175**, 1–9.

Folkman, J. (1995). Seminars in Medicine of the Beth Israel Hospital, Boston. Clinical applications of research on angiogenesis. *N Engl J Med* **333**, 1757–1763.

Goto, H., Yano, S., Matsumori, Y., Ogawa, H., Blakey, D.C. and Sone, S. (2004). Sensitization of tumor-associated endothelial cell apoptosis by the novel vascular-targeting agent ZD6126 in combination with cisplatin. *Clin Cancer Res* **10**, 7671–7676.

Grosios, K., Loadman, P.M., Swaine, D.J., Pettit, G.R. and Bibby, MC. (2000). Combination chemotherapy with combretastatin A-4 phosphate and 5-fluorouracil in an experimental murine colon adenocarcinoma. *Anticancer Res* **20**, 229–233.

Hill, S.A., Chaplin, D.J., Lewis, G. and Tozer, G.M. (2002a). Schedule dependence of combretastatin A4 phosphate in transplanted and spontaneous tumor models. *Int J Cancer* **102**, 70–74.

Hill, S.A., Toze, G.M., Pettit, G.R. and Chaplin, D.J. (2002b). Preclinical evaluation of the antitumour activity of the novel vascular targeting agent Oxi 4503. *Anticancer Res* **22**, 1453–1458.

Hori, K., Saito, S., Nihei, Y., Suzuki, M. and Sato, Y. (1999). Antitumor effects due to irreversible stoppage of tumor tissue blood flow: evaluation of a novel combretastatin A-4 derivative, AC7700. *Japan J Cancer Res* **90**, 1026–1038.

Hori, K., Saito, S., Sato, Y., Akita, H., Kawaguchi, T., Sugiyama, K. and Sato, H. (2003). Differential relationship between changes in tumor size and microcirculatory functions induced by therapy with an antivascular drug and with cytotoxic drugs. Implications for the evaluation of therapeutic efficacy of AC7700 (AVE8062). *Eur J Cancer* **39**, 1957–1966.

Horsman, M.R., Ehrnrooth, E., Ladekarl, M. and Overgaard, J. (1998). The effect of combretastatin A-4 disodium phosphate in a C3H mouse mammary carcinoma and a variety of murine spontaneous tumors. *Int J Radiat Oncol Biol Phys* **42**, 895–898.

Horsman, M.R. and Murata, R. (2002). Combination of vascular targeting agents with thermal or radiation therapy. *Int J Radiat Oncol Biol Phys* **54**, 1518–1523.

Horsman, M.R. and Murata, R. (2003). Vascular targeting effects of ZD6126 in a C3H mouse mammary carcinoma and the enhancement of radiation response. *Int J Radiat Oncol Biol Phys* **57**, 1047–1055.

Horsman, M.R., Murata, R., Breidahl, T., Nielsen, F.U., Maxwell, R.J., Stodkiled-Jorgensen, H. and Overgaard, J. (2000). Combretastatins novel vascular targeting drugs for improving anti-cancer therapy. Combretastatins and conventional therapy. *Adv Exp Med Biol* **476**, 311–323.

Hua, J., Sheng, Y., Pinney, K.G., Garner, C.M., Kane, R.R., Prezioso, J.A., Pettit, G.R., Chaplin, D.J. and Edvardsen, K. (2003). Oxi4503, a novel vascular targeting agent: effects on blood flow and antitumor activity in comparison to combretastatin A-4 phosphate. *Anticancer Res* 23, 1433–1440.

Kim, S., Min, S.Y., Lee, S.K. and Cho, W.J. (2003). Comparative molecular field analysis study of stilbene derivatives active against A549 lung carcinoma. *Chem Pharm Bull (Tokyo)* 51, 516–521.

Knocke, T.H., Weitmann, H.D., Feldmann, H.J., Selzer, E. and Potter, R. (1999). Intratumoral pO2-measurements as predictive assay in the treatment of carcinoma of the uterine cervix. *Radiother Oncol* 53, 99–104.

Landuyt, W., Ahmed, B., Nuyts, S., Theys, J., Op, d.B., Rijnders, A., Anne, J., van Oosterom, A., van den, B.W. and Lambin, P. (2001). In vivo antitumour effect of vascular targeting combined with either ionizing radiation or anti-angiogenesis treatment. *Int J Radiat Oncol Biol Phys* 49, 443–450.

Lash, C.J., Li, A.E., Rutland, M., Baguley, B.C., Zwi, L.J. and Wilson, W.R. (1998). Enhancement of the anti-tumor effects of the antivascular agent 5,6-dimethylxanthenone-4-acetic acid (DMXAA) by combination with 5-hydroxytryptamine and bioreductive drugs. *Br J Cancer* 78, 439–445.

Laws, A.L., Matthew, A.M., Double, J.A. and Bibby, M.C. (1995). Preclinical in vitro and in vivo activity of 5,6-dimethylxanthenone-4-acetic acid. *Br J Cancer* 71, 1204–1209.

Li, L., Rojiani, A.M. and Siemann, D.W. (1998). Targeting the tumor vasculature with combretastatin A-4 disodium phosphate: effects on radiation therapy. *Int J Radiat Oncol Biol Phys* 42, 899–903.

Li, L., Rojiani, A.M. and Siemann, D.W. (2002). Preclinical evaluations of therapies combining the vascular targeting agent combretastatin A-4 disodium phosphate and conventional anticancer therapies in the treatment of Kaposi's sarcoma. *Acta Oncol* 41, 91–97.

Lozonschi, L., Sunamura, M., Kobari, M., Egawa, S., Ding, L. and Matsuno, S. (1999). Controlling tumor angiogenesis and metastasis of C26 murine colon adenocarcinoma by a new matrix metalloproteinase inhibitor, KB-R7785, in two tumor models. *Cancer Res* 59, 1252–1258.

Masunaga, S., Sakurai, Y., Suzuki, M., Nagata, K., Maruhashi, A., Kinash, Y. and Ono, K. (2004). Combination of the vascular targeting agent ZD6126 with boron neutron capture therapy. *Int J Radiat Oncol Biol Phys* 60, 920–927.

Morinaga, Y., Suga, Y., Ehara, S., Harada, K., Nihei. Y. and Suzuki, M. (2003). Combination effect of AC-7700, a novel combretastatin A-4 derivative, and cisplatin against murine and human tumors in vivo. *Cancer Sci* 94, 200–204.

Murata, R., Overgaard, J. and Horsman, M.R. (2001). Combretastatin A-4 disodium phosphate: a vascular targeting agent that improves that improves the anti-tumor effects of hyperthermia, radiation, and mild thermoradiotherapy. *Int J Radiat Oncol Biol Phys* 51, 1018–1024.

Murata, R., Siemann, D.W., Overgaard, J. and Horsman, M.R. (2001a). Improved tumor response by combining radiation and the vascular-damaging drug 5,6-dimethylxanthenone-4-acetic acid. *Radiat Res* 156, 503–509.

Murata, R., Siemann, D.W., Overgaard, J. and Horsman, M.R. (2001b). Interaction between combretastatin A-4 disodium phosphate and radiation in murine tumors. *Radiother Oncol* 60, 155–161.

Nelkin, B.D. and Ball, D.W. (2001). Combretastatin A-4 and doxorubicin combination treatment is effective in a preclinical model of human medullary thyroid carcinoma. *Oncol Rep* 8, 157–160.

Nordsmark, M., Overgaard, M. and Overgaard, J. (1996). Pretreatment oxygenation predicts radiation response in advanced squamous cell carcinoma of the head and neck. *Radiother Oncol* **41**, 31–39.

Okunieff, P., Hoeckel, M., Dunphy, E.P., Schlenger, K., Knoop, C. and Vaupel, P. (1993). Oxygen tension distributions are sufficient to explain the local response of human breast tumors treated with radiation alone. *Int J Radiat Oncol Biol Phys* **26**, 631–636.

O'Reilly, M.S., Holmgren, L., Shing, Y., Chen, C., Rosenthal, R.A., Moses, M., Lane, W.S., Cao, Y., Sage, E.H. and Folkman, J. (1994). Angiostatin: a novel angiogenesis inhibitor that mediates the suppression of metastases by a Lewis lung carcinoma. *Cell* **79**, 315–328.

Overgaard, J. and Horsman, M.R. (1996). Modification of hypoxia-induced radioresistance in tumors by the use of oxygen and sensitizers. *Semin Radiat Oncol* **6**, 10–21.

Pedley, R.B., Boden, J.A., Boden, R., Boxer, G.M., Flynn, A.A., Keep, P.A. and Begent, R.H. (1996). Ablation of colorectal xenografts with combined radioimmunotherapy and tumor blood flow-modifying agents. *Cancer Res* **56**, 3293–3300.

Pedley, R.B., El Emir, E., Flynn, A.A., Boxer, G.M., Dearling, J., Raleigh, J.A., Hill, S.A., Stuart, S., Motha, R. and Begent, R.H. (2002). Synergy between vascular targeting agents and antibody-directed therapy. *Int J Radiat Oncol Biol Phys* **54**, 1524–1531.

Pedley, R.B., Hill, S.A., Boxer, G.M., Flynn, A.A., Boden, R., Watson, R., Dearling. J., Chaplin, D.J. and Begent, R.H. (2001). Eradication of colorectal xenografts by combined radioimmunotherapy and combretastatin a-4 3-O-phosphate. *Cancer Res* **61**, 4716–4722.

Pedley, R.B., Sharma, S.K., Boxer, G.M., Boden, R., Stribbling, S.M., Davies L., Springer, C.J. and Begent, R.H. (1999). Enhancement of antibody-directed enzyme prodrug therapy in colorectal xenografts by an antivascular agent. *Cancer Res* **59**, 3998–4003.

Pruijn, F.B., van Daalen, M., Holford, N.H. and Wilson, W.R. (1997). Mechanisms of enhancement of the antitumour activity of melphalan by the tumor-blood-flow inhibitor 5,6-dimethylxanthenone-4-acetic acid. *Cancer Chemother Pharmacol* **39**, 541–546.

Rewcastle, G.W., Atwell, G.J., Li, Z.A., Baguley, B.C. and Denny, W.A. (1991). Potential antitumour agents. 61. Structure–activity relationships for in vivo colon 38 activity among disubstituted 9-oxo-9H-xanthene-4-acetic acids. *J Med Chem* **34**, 217–222.

Rojiani, A.M., Li, L., Rise, L. and Siemann, D.W. (2002). Activity of the vascular targeting agent combretastatin A-4 disodium phosphate in a xenograft model of AIDS-associated Kaposi's sarcoma. *Acta Oncol* **41**, 98–105.

Sartorelli, A.C. (1988). Therapeutic attack of hypoxic cells of solid tumors: presidential address. *Cancer Res* **48**, 775–778.

Shnyder, S.D., Cooper, P.A., Pettit, G.R., Lippert, J.W., III. and Bibby, M.C. (2003). Combretastatin A-1 phosphate potentiates the antitumour activity of cisplatin in a murine adenocarcinoma model. *Anticancer Res* **23**, 1619–1623.

Siemann, D.W. (1984). Modification of chemotherapy by nitroimidazoles. *Int J Radiat Oncol Biol Phys* **10**, 1585–1594.

Siemann, D.W., Bibby, M.C., Dark, G.G., Dicker, A.P., Eskens, F.A., Horsman, M.R., Marme, D. and LoRusso, P.M. (2005). Differentiation and definition of vascular-targeted therapies. *Clin Cancer Res* **11**, 416–420.

Siemann, D.W., Chaplin, D.J. and Horsman, M.R. (2004). Vascular-targeting therapies for treatment of malignant disease. *Cancer* **100**, 2491–2499.

Siemann, D.W. and Horsman, M.R. (2004). Targeting the tumor vasculature: a strategy to improve radiation therapy. *Expert Rev Anticancer Ther* **4**, 321–327.

Siemann, D.W., Mercer, E., Lepler, S. and Rojiani, A.M. (2002). Vascular targeting agents enhance chemotherapeutic agent activities in solid tumor therapy. *Int J Cancer* **99**, 1–6.

Siemann, D.W. and Rojiani, A.M. (2002a). Antitumour efficacy of conventional anticancer drugs is enhanced by the vascular targeting agent ZD6126. *Int J Radiat Oncol Biol Phys* **54**, 1512–1517.

Siemann, D.W. and Rojiani, A.M. (2002b). Enhancement of radiation therapy by the novel vascular targeting agent ZD6126. *Int J Radiat Oncol Biol Phys* **53**, 164–171.

Siemann, D.W. and Shi, W. (2003). Targeting the tumor blood vessel network to enhance the efficacy of radiation therapy. *Semin Radiat Oncol* **13**, 53–61.

Siim, B.G., Lee, A.E., Shalal-Zwain, S., Pruijn, F.B., McKeage, M.J. and Wilson, W.R. (2003). Marked potentiation of the antitumour activity of chemotherapeutic drugs by the antivascular agent 5,6-dimethylxanthenone-4-acetic acid (DMXAA). *Cancer Chemother Pharmacol* **51**, 43–52.

Souhami, R. and Tobias, J. (1986). *Cancer and its Management*. Blackwell, Oxford.

Thorpe, P.E. (2004). Vascular targeting agents as cancer therapeutics. *Clin Cancer Res* **10**, 415–427.

Tubiana, M. (1992). The role of local treatment in the cure of cancer. *Eur J Cancer* **28A**: 2061–2069.

Vaupel, P., Kallinowski, P. and Okunieff, P. (1989). Blood flow, oxygen and nutrient supply, and metabolic microenvironment of human tumors: a review. *Cancer Res* **46**, 6449–6465.

Walenta, S., Schroeder, T. and Mueller-Klieser, W. (2002). Metabolic mapping with bioluminescence: basic and clinical relevance. *Biomol Eng* **18**, 249–262.

Wedge, S.R., Kendrew, J., Ogilvie, D.J. *et al.* (2002). Combination of the VEGF receptor tyrosine kinase inhibitor ZD6474 and vascular-targeting agent ZD6126 produces an enhanced anti-tumor response. *Proc Am Assoc Cancer Res* **43**, 1081 [abstract].

Wilson, W.R., Li, A.E., Cowan, D.S. and Siim, B.G. (1998). Enhancement of tumor radiation response by the antivascular agent 5,6-dimethylxanthenone-4-acetic acid. *Int J Radiat Oncol Biol Phys* **42**, 905–908.

Yoon, S.S., Eto, H., Lin, C.M., Nakamura, H., Pawlik, T.M., Song, S.U. and Tanabe, K.K. (1999). Mouse endostatin inhibits the formation of lung and liver metastases. *Cancer Res* **59**, 6251–6256.

8

Vasculature-targeting Therapies and Hyperthermia

Michael R. Horsman and **Rumi Murata**

Abstract

A major hindrance to the routine application of hyperthermia in clinical practice is the failure to adequately heat tumours. Since blood flow is probably the most important biological factor controlling the ability to heat a tumour it should be possible to improve tumour heating by targeting the tumour vascular supply. A number of vascular targeting agents (VTAs) are available and many of them have already been combined with hyperthermia in preclinical studies. In this chapter we will review how such VTAs and hyperthermia have been combined and discuss the potential for using such combinations for improving clinical outcome

Keywords

Vascular targeting, Vascular disrupting agents, Hyperthermia, PDT, DMXAA, Combretastatin

8.1   Introduction

Hyperthermia is often considered as an experimental modality with no realistic future in clinical cancer therapy. This is not a valid evaluation. Although hyperthermia *per se* is probably only useful in palliative situations and has no role to play in the curative treatment of human tumors (Overgaard, 1985), there is definitive evidence that when hyperthermia is combined with other therapies, especially radiation, significant improvements in clinical outcome are possible (Horsman and Overgaard, 2002). However, many such clinical studies failed to show any improvement, which probably reflects the fact that current technology cannot deliver adequate power to effectively heat human tumors of all sites

Vascular-targeted Therapies in Oncology   Edited by Dietmar W. Siemann
© 2006 John Wiley & Sons, Ltd.

(Dewhirst *et al.*, 1997). Advances in technology will improve this situation, but an alternative approach that may be easier to exploit is to concentrate on the tumor biology, especially blood flow.

Blood flow is one of the major vehicles by which heat is dissipated from tissues, thus the blood supply of the tumor will have a significant influence on the ability to heat that tumor. The relationship between blood flow and tumor heating has been examined (Jain, Grantham and Gullino, 1979; Patterson and Strang, 1979), and in general the lower the rate of blood flow then the easier it is to heat the tissue. This is illustrated in Figure 8.1, in which a single intra-venous injection of the anti-hypertensive drug hydralazine resulted in a 50 per

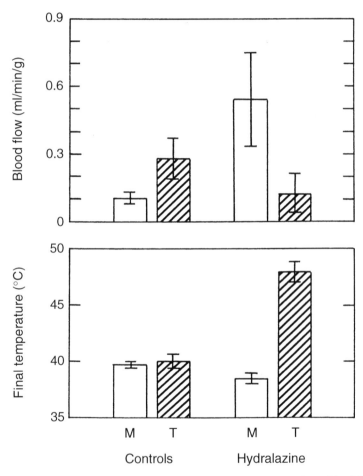

Figure 8.1 The effect of intravenously injecting hydralazine (0.5 mg kg⁻¹) on blood flow and the ability to heat transmissible venereal tumors (T) subcutaneously implanted in the hind limbs of dogs and the underlying normal muscle (M). Blood flow was measured using radioactively labeled microspheres. Heating was achieved by inductive diathermy and tissue temperatures determined using implanted thermistors. Measurements were made in control animals or 15 min after injecting hydralazine. (Redrawn from Voorhees and Babbs, 1982)

cent decrease in tumor blood flow. When tumors were subsequently heated, the tumor temperature in the hydralazine-treated animals was 8°C higher than in those animals receiving heat alone. Blood flow is also important in determining the microenvironmental conditions found within tumors. In general, tumor blood flow is compromised when compared with that of the normal tissue from which it is derived (Peterson, 1979; Reinhold, 1988; Vaupel, Kallinowski and Okunieff, 1989), which results in areas that are nutrient deprived, low in oxygen and highly acidic (Vaupel, Kallinowski and Okunieff, 1989), and several studies have shown that cells incubated in these adverse conditions are more sensitive to hyperthermia (Overgaard and Bichel, 1977; Gerweck, Nygaard and Burlett, 1979; Overgaard and Nielsen, 1980). The importance of the tumor microenvironment influencing the tumor response to heat has also been shown *in vivo*, and is illustrated in Figure 8.2. In this example, local control was measured in tumors made totally hypoxic by clamping for an 80 minute period and heated at 44.8°C for 15 minutes, before, during or after the clamping period. Not only did clamping increase the tumor response to heat, but also the effect on tumor control was greater as the time interval between applying the clamp and subsequent heating was increased.

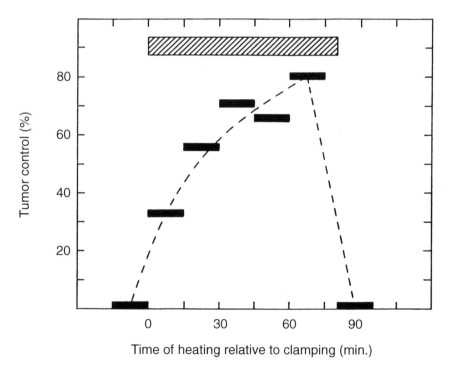

Figure 8.2 Local tumor control in a squamous carcinoma 30 days after treatment. Tumors were heated (44.8°C for 15 min) at various times before, during or after application of a clamp for 80 min. The clamping period is shown by the shaded area and heating by the solid bars. (Redrawn from Hill and Denekamp, 1978)

Numerous other studies have confirmed that decreasing tumor blood flow either by physical clamping (Thrall, Gillette and Dewey, 1975; Dewey, Thrall and Gillette, 1977; Wallen, Colby and Stewart, 1986) or physiological modification using hydralazine (Horsman, Christensen and Overgaard, 1989; Kalmus, Okunieff and Vaupel, 1990; Dewhirst *et al.*, 1990; Honess, Hu and Bleehen, 1991), sodium nitroprusside (Prescott *et al.*, 1992; Krossnes, Mella and Dahl, 1996; Poulson *et al.*, 2004) or glucose (Urano, Montoya and Booth, 1983; Murray, Milas and Meyn, 1984; Osinsky, Bubnovskaja and Gusev, 1989; Hiraoka and Hahn, 1990) is an effective approach for improving tumor response to hyperthermia. However, the clinical applicability of such methods remains questionable. An alternative approach that may be more clinically relevant is the use of agents that specifically target the tumor vasculature: the so-called vascular-targeting agents (VTAs). There are two types of VTA, those that inhibit the angiogenesis process and those that disrupt the already established vasculature, and both these processes are explained more fully elsewhere in this book. The effect that angiogenesis inhibitors (AIs) have on tumor perfusion and the tumor microenvironment is not clear. Recent studies suggest that AIs actually transiently normalize the tumor's vascular network, leading to an improvement in the microenvironmental conditions (Winkler *et al.*, 2004), and as such might not be expected to improve the efficacy of hyperthermia. This is not the case with vascular-disrupting agents (VDAs), in which substantial reductions in tumor blood flow have always been reported (Horsman, Chaplin and Overgaard, 1991; Horsman *et al.*, 1996; Cliffe *et al.*, 1994; Hill, Sampson and Chaplin, 1995; Chaplin *et al.*, 1996; Dark *et al.*, 1997; Lash *et al.*, 1998; Tozer *et al.*, 1999; Murata, Overgaard and Horsman, 2001c) and these agents would clearly be ideal candidates for combining with hyperthermia.

8.2 Enhancing hyperthermia

Despite the fact that one might not expect the combination of AIs and hyperthermia to be beneficial, such a combination has been investigated. TNP-470, the synthetic analogue of fumagillin first isolated from *Aspergillus fumigatus*, is a potent inhibitor of tumor angiogenesis (Ingber *et al.*, 1990). Repeated administration of TNP-470 to mice bearing murine or human tumor xenografts significantly inhibited tumor growth (Yano *et al.*, 1995; Nishimura *et al.*, 1996) and such a schedule given after heating tumors further significantly enhanced the heat response in these same studies. However, this effect was temperature dependent, being observed at 43 and 44°C, but not at 42°C (Yano *et al.*, 1995; Nishimura *et al.*, 1996). This enhancement was attributed to TNP-470 inhibiting angiogenesis that occurred following heat-induced vascular damage, the latter effect being temperature dependent. Similar studies in a BT$_4$An rat glioma model using batimastat, a broad-spectrum inhibitor of metalloproteinases

(Brown, 1993), failed to show any enhancement of heat damage using a temperature of 44°C, which produced substantial vascular damage (Eikesdal, Bjork-haug and Dahl, 2002). This lack of effect could be attributed to the fact that batimastat alone at the dose and schedule used in this study was ineffective at inhibiting growth in this tumor model. Clearly, AIs can be used to improve the heat response of tumors, but do so via mechanisms that do not involve a tumor sensitization to heat resulting from any AI-induced microenvironmental changes. All that is required is that the heat treatment is sufficient to induce vascular damage and that the AIs are effective as angiogenesis inhibitors. There are a large number of AIs currently in clinical testing as potential anti-cancer agents (National Cancer Institute website), and with such substantial interest it is surprising that there are so few studies combining them with hyperthermia.

This is not the situation with VDAs, and many different agents have been combined with hyperthermia, as shown in Table 8.1. The majority of these studies have involved the combination of photodynamic therapy (PDT) and heat. PDT involves the administration of a photosensitizing dye with subsequent activation by visible light (Kessel, 1984; Dougherty, 1987). Tumor cell killing by PDT *in vivo* has been suggested to be the result of both a direct effect on tumor cells (Nelson, Wright and Berns, 1985; Winther, 1989) as well as a result of damage to tumor vasculature (Selman *et al.*, 1984; Star *et al.*, 1986; Horsman and Winther, 1989). When combined with hyperthermia, different schedules have been used, including simultaneous treatments (Orenstein *et al.*, 1999; Kelleher *et al.*, 2003a, 2003b), the PDT given immediately before or after the heat (Waldow and Dougherty, 1984; Henderson *et al.*, 1985; Matsumoto *et al.*, 1989) or with a short 30 minute (Levendag *et al.*, 1988) or longer 4h (Chen *et al.*, 1996) time interval. Of the four studies in which different schedules were compared (Waldow and Dougherty, 1984; Henderson *et al.*, 1985; Matsumoto *et al.*, 1989; Chen *et al.*, 1996), only two found the PDT before heat to be superior (Henderson *et al.*, 1985; Chen *et al.*, 1996). Furthermore, several studies have shown that PDT and heat are an effective combination in vitro, especially when the PDT is administered prior to heating (Christensen, Wahl and Smedshammer, 1984; Mang and Dougherty, 1985). Thus the role of the vascular damaging component of PDT in the sensitization of tumors to heat remains unclear.

Hyperthermia has also been combined with the cytokine tumor necrosis factor (TNF), and various drugs including arsenic trioxide, vinblastine, flavone acetic acid (FAA), 5,6-dimethylxanthenone-4-acetic acid (DMXAA) and combretastatin A-4 disodium phosphate (CA4DP) as listed in Table 8.1. With all these vascular disrupting drugs there was an enhancement of the heat response, and this effect was time and schedule dependent, with the maximum response generally observed if the heating was started 1–6 hours after VDA injection (Horsman, Chaplin and Overgaard, 1991; Horsman *et al.*, 1996; Sakaguchi *et al.*, 1992; Griffin *et al.*, 2000, 2003; Murata, Overgaard and Horsman, 2001a, 2001b; Eikesdal *et al.*, 2000, 2001b), and this clearly corresponded to the time of maximal reduction in

Table 8.1 Preclinical studies combining VDAs and hyperthermia

VDA[1]	Tumor model[2]	Heat treatment[3] (°C)	Reference
PDT	SMT-F mammary carcinoma	40.5–44.5	Waldow and Dougherty, 1984
	RIF-1 fibrosarcoma	44	Henderson et al., 1985
	R-1 rhabdomyosarcoma*	44	Levendag et al., 1988
	Squamous cell carcinoma	43	Matsumoto et al., 1989
	C3H mammary carcinoma	43.5	Chen et al., 1996
	C26 colon carcinoma	39–43	Orenstein et al., 1999
	DS-carcinosarcoma*	43	Kelleher et al., 2003a, 2003b
TNF	DS-carcinosarcoma*	43 + 44	Kallinowski, Moehle and Vaupel, 1989
	SCK mammary carcinoma	42.5	Lin, Park and Song, 1996
ATO	SCK mammary carcinoma	41.5–42.5	Griffin et al., 2000, 2003
	FsaII fibrosarcoma	42.5	Griffin et al., 2000, 2003
VBL	BT$_4$An glioma*	44	Eikesdal, Bjerkvig and Dahl, 2001a
FAA	C3H mammary carcinoma	40.5–42.5	Horsman, Chaplin and Overgaard, 1991; Horsman et al., 1996; Horsman, Murata and Overgaard, 2001
	B16 melanoma	43	Sakaguchi et al., 1992
DMXAA	C3H mammary carcinoma	40.5–42.5	Murata, Overgaard and Horsman, 2001a
CA4DP	BT$_4$An glioma*	44	Eikesdal et al., 2000, 2001b
	C3H mammary carcinoma	40.5–42.5	Murata, Overgaard and Horsman, 2001b

[1] VDAs were photodynamic therapy (PDT), tumor necrosis factor (TNF), arsenic trioxide (ATO), vinblastine (VBL), flavone acetic acid (FAA), 5,6-dimethylxanthenone-4-acetic acid (DMXAA) and combretastatin A-4 disodium phosphate (CA4DP).
[2] Tumor models were either murine or rat*.
[3] Heat treatments indicate the temperatures used in the studies.

tumor blood flow in those studies. For the TNF studies (Kallinowski, Moehle and Vaupel, 1989; Lin, Park and Song, 1996), the heat was only administered 3–4 h after injecting the VDA, but at this time the decrease in tumor blood flow was substantial. With vinblastine the decrease in tumor blood flow took almost 12 hours to reach a nadir, yet the maximal enhancement of heat response occurred much earlier (Eikesdal, Bjerkvig and Dahl, 2001a). Injecting VDAs after heating has been shown to be substantially less effective in enhancing the heat response (Horsman, Chaplin and Overgaard, 1991; Sakaguchi *et al.*, 1992; Murata, Overgaard and Horsman, 2001a, 2001b), and in most cases did not appear to be greater than a simple additive effect of the VDA and heat alone.

Examples of the types of enhancement obtained when the VDAs are administered at the optimal times before heating are shown in Figure 8.3 using DMXAA and CA4DP, two of the leading small-molecule vascular disrupting drugs currently in clinical development. In this C3H mammary carcinoma there was a linear relationship between the tumor growth time and the time of heating at 42.5°C. Injecting either DMXAA or CA4DP had a small effect on tumor growth time, but if tumors were subsequently heated at the time of maximal blood flow reduction by each of these VDAs there was a significant increase in the slope of the heat response curve. The slope values calculated from these curves are shown in Figure 8.4, along with values obtained at other

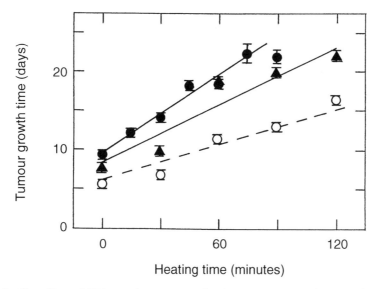

Figure 8.3 The effect of VDAs on the response of a C3H mammary carcinoma to heat. Tumors were locally heated at 42.5°C for the times indicated and the tumor growth time (time taken for tumors to grow from 200 to 1000 mm³) calculated. Mice were given either heat alone (○), or heating started 30 minutes after intraperitoneally injecting CA4DP (▲; 25 mg kg⁻¹) or 6 hours after DMXAA (●; 20 mg kg⁻¹). Results show means (+1 SE) for an average of 12 animals/group. (Modified from Murata, Overgaard and Horsman, 2001a, 2001b)

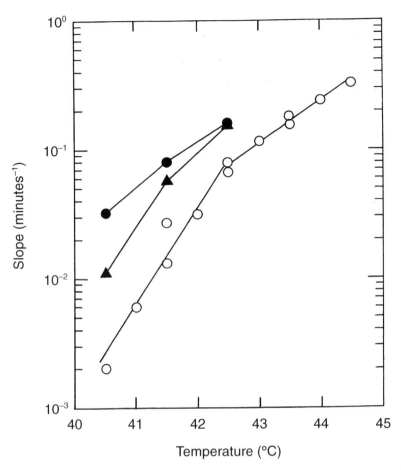

Figure 8.4 Relationship between the temperature at which C3H mammary carcinomas were heated and the slopes of the resulting tumor response curves. The slope values were calculated from data similar to that shown in Figure 8.3. Results are for heat alone ($\bigcirc$), or heating started 30 minutes after intraperitoneally injecting CA4DP ($\blacktriangle$; 25 mg kg^{-1}) or 6 hours after DMXAA ($\bullet$; 20 mg kg^{-1}). (Modified from Horsman, Murata and Overgaard, 2001; Murata, Overgaard and Horsman, 2001a, 2001b)

temperatures. For heat alone there is the typical biphasic response with an inflection point around 42.5°C, which has been suggested to result from thermotolerance developing during heating (Li *et al.*, 1982). With both DMXAA and CA4DP there is a clear enhancement of the heat response at all temperatures. However, while for CA4DP this effect appears to be somewhat independent of temperature, for DMXAA there is a suggestion that this enhancement gets larger as the temperature decreases below the break point of 42.5°C. Identical slope

values to those seen with DMXAA have previously been reported with its analogue FAA (Horsman, Murata and Overgaard, 2001). Why the effects of
DMXAA and FAA are larger than CA4DP at the lower temperatures is not clear,
but may be related to the fact that although the maximal degrees of vascular
shut-down by these drugs are similar in this tumor model the time period for
which this shut-down is maintained is longer for DMXAA and FAA than for
CA4DP (Horsman *et al.*, 1996; Murata, Overgaard and Horsman, 2001c).

The question remains as to the exact mechanism responsible for the enhancement of heat response by these VDAs. The enhanced slope values shown in
Figure 8.4 when using CA4DP are similar to the slope values seen in the same
tumor model when tumors are heated after injecting hydralazine, a transient
physiological modifier of blood flow (Horsman, Christensen and Overgaard,
1989). Additional studies have demonstrated that the hydralazine-induced
reduction in blood flow leads to both a better tumor heating (Horsman, Christensen and Overgaard, 1989; Dewhirst *et al.*, 1990; Honess, Hu and Bleehen,
1991) and an increase in tumor damage (Horsman, Christensen and Overgaard,
1989; Honess, Hu and Bleehen, 1991; Kalmus, Okunieff and Vaupel, 1990),
the latter effect presumably occurring because the reduction in tumor blood flow
results in an increase in tumor hypoxia and associated tumor acidosis, and
several *in vitro* studies have shown that prolonged oxygen deprivation of cells
will increase their sensitivity to heat, an effect that is due to hypoxia-induced
metabolic perturbations (leading to a decrease in pH) rather than hypoxia *per
se* (Overgaard and Bichel, 1977; Gerweck, Nygaard and Burlett, 1979). With
the VDAs there is evidence that similar mechanisms are operating, since studies
with FAA and CA4DP have shown both an improved tumor heating (Sakaguchi
et al., 1992; Eikesdal, Bjerkvig and Dahl, 2001a) and a decrease in tumor pH
(Sakaguchi *et al.*, 1992; Maxwell *et al.*, 1998). However, the studies with
CA4DP and heat (Murata, Overgaard and Horsman, 2001b) revealed that no
enhancement of heat response was observed with a 6 h interval between injecting
a $250\,mg\,kg^{-1}$ dose of CA4DP and the start of heating, despite perfusion still
being decreased by 60 per cent. Furthermore, when a 30 min interval was used
the maximal enhancement of heat damage was independent of drug dose from
25 to $250\,mg\,kg^{-1}$, even though the reduction in tumor perfusion was 20 and
66 per cent at these doses, respectively. This suggests that unlike the situation
with physiological modifiers of tumor blood flow, the enhancement of heat
damage by VDAs involves other factors unrelated to a simple reduction in tumor
blood flow. Whatever the mechanism, the most significant finding in Figure 8.4
is that a heat treatment of around 41.5°C combined with a VDA has an antitumor effect that is equivalent to that seen with a temperature of 42.5–43°C
alone. Clinically, temperatures of around 43°C are generally considered to be
necessary for efficacy, but it is often difficult to achieve this temperature and
less effective mild temperatures of around 41.5°C are often seen (Dewhirst *et
al.*, 1997). The use of VDAs appears to be an effective method for converting
the mild temperatures into a more efficient therapy.

Enhancing tumor response is of no therapeutic benefit if the same effect occurs in normal tissues. Unfortunately, this important aspect has not been investigated to a large degree with respect to the combination of VDAs and hyperthermia. Studies using rats indicated that the uptake of the photosensitizer was greater in a DS-sarcoma than various normal tissues and this would be expected to reduce the effect of PDT in those normal tissues, as well as any enhancement of heat damage (Kelleher *et al.*, 2003a). Indeed, in an additional study in which cortical lesions in rat brains were measured following PDT treatment, absolutely no increase was seen with heat, albeit using a mild temperature of 41°C (Dereski, Madigan and Chopp, 1995). Eikesdal and colleagues reported on the incidence of lethality and the development of edema in heat-treated feet of rats given CA4DP and 44°C heating (Eikesdal *et al.*, 2000, 2001b). Lethality was not influenced by the combination. A moderate increase in edema was seen within 1–2 days after treatment, but this had fully recovered by day 5. Results from additional experiments into the development of skin damage in the normal foot of the mouse are illustrated in Figure 8.5. In these studies, some of the animals were also implanted with a tumor in the opposite untreated foot. This was done because previous studies with FAA had demonstrated that the presence of a tumor could influence the level of normal skin damage induced by heating (Horsman *et al.*, 1996). As shown in Figure 8.5, the response of the skin to local heating in normal mice was significantly increased by either CA4DP or DMXAA, the respective enhancement ratios (ERs; ratio of heating times for heat alone and VDA + heat that produce skin damage in 50 per cent of mice) being 1.3 and 1.5. Having a tumor in the opposite foot did influence this response, but while it gave rise to a more prominent reaction in the CA4DP treated animals (ER = 1.5), with DMXAA the skin reactions were surprisingly reduced (ER = 1.3). Neither DMXAA nor CA4DP caused any significant effect on blood perfusion of skin (Murata, Overgaard and Horsman, 2001c), so this cannot explain the enhancement seen. Previous studies with FAA suggested that the increase in skin damage was the result of an FAA-induced increase in the concentration of TNF-α in the circulation, the elevation of which was much larger in tumor-bearing than non-tumor-bearing mice (Horsman *et al.*, 1996). DMXAA similarly increased TNF-α production, but the TNF-α levels in the DMXAA-treated tumor-bearing mice were significantly higher than in the mice without tumors (Murata, Overgaard and Horsman, 2001a), which is contrary to the skin damage results. Furthermore, studies with CA4DP failed to detect stimulation of TNF-α production (Chaplin, Pettit and Hill, 1999). Thus, the role of TNF-α induction in the enhancement of heat damage by VDAs in normal skin is unclear. Although the reasons for the enhanced response of heat in normal skin remain to be elucidated, the most important finding is that the 1.3–1.5 ERs for skin damage are much lower than the ERs of 1.9 (calculated from the slope values in Figure 8.4) seen with the same CA4DP or DMXAA treatments in the C3H mammary carcinoma grown in the same mouse strain, thus combining VDAs with heat does lead to a therapeutic benefit.

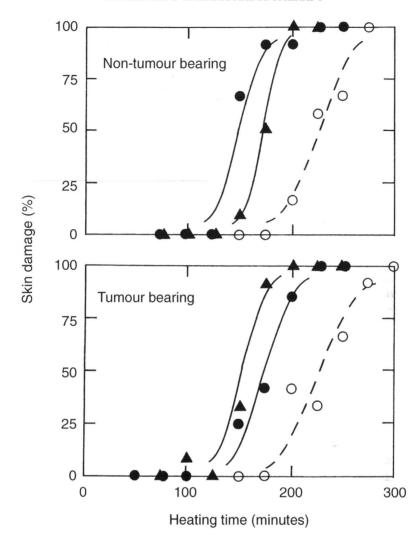

Figure 8.5 The effect of VDAs on the development of normal foot skin damage in CDF1 mice after heating in non-tumor bearing animals or with a 200 mm³ C3H mammary carcinoma in the opposite foot. Results show the percentage of animals in each treatment group showing loss of grasp function and hair in the treated foot, as well as developing redness and edema, plotted against the time of heating at 42.5°C. Mice were given either heat alone (○), or heating started 30 minutes after intraperitoneally injecting CA4DP (▲; 25 mg kg⁻¹) or 6 hours after DMXAA (●; 20 mg kg⁻¹). Each point represents an average of 12 animals/group. (Modified from Murata, Overgaard and Horsman, 2001a, 2001b)

8.3   Enhancing thermoradiotherapy

Hyperthermia on its own has no role to play in the curative treatment of tumors in humans and its clinical potential lies in its use as an adjuvant with other more conventional treatments (Overgaard, 1985). The most widely studied adjuvant use of hyperthermia is with radiation therapy, and numerous studies have demonstrated the ability of heat to enhance the action of radiation in animal tumors (for review see Overgaard, 1978; Field and Bleehen, 1979). Several clinical studies have now also shown the benefit of such a combination (Horsman and Overgaard, 2002). The vascular supply to a tumor is extremely important in the ability of heat to increase the effect of radiation. This is illustrated by the fact that larger tumors show a greater enhancement of radiation damage by heat than do smaller tumors (Overgaard, 1987). Larger tumors are generally less well perfused than smaller tumors and as a result contain a higher proportion of cells that are radiation resistant, yet heat sensitive (Vaupel, Kallinowski and Okunieff, 1989). The increased thermal radiosensitization seen in larger tumors is thus the result of an increase in the cytotoxic action of heat. Indeed, it has been shown that tumor sensitivity to heat alone increases with tumor size (Urano *et al.*, 1980, 1982). This importance of the tumor vasculature for the response to heat and radiation suggests that VDAs could be used to further improve the therapeutic potential.

When combining VDAs with thermoradiotherapy, timing and sequencing of the drug, radiation and heat treatment will be critical to the response obtained. For radiation and heat the greatest anti-tumor effect is obtained when these treatments are given simultaneously, which is primarily because the heat acts as a radiation sensitizer (Horsman and Overgaard, 2002). However, an identical effect is also seen in normal tissues, thus no therapeutic benefit results. When radiation is administered prior to heating in a sequential schedule an enhancement is observed, but since it only results from the heat killing the hypoxic radiation resistant population the overall anti-tumor effect is less than with the simultaneous schedule. The advantage here is that no enhancement of normal tissue damage occurs, thus therapeutically a sequential schedule is superior. A sequential schedule fits very nicely with the application of the VDAs, since one would want to give the VDA prior to heating at a time when vascular shut-down is maximal, but after the radiation treatment to avoid any possible induction of radiation resistant hypoxia. Both DMXAA and CA4DP have been combined with radiation and heat using such a sequential schedule and the results obtained in a C3H mammary carcinoma using the most clinically relevant endpoint of local tumor control are illustrated in Figure 8.6. Although the scheduling was the same with both VDAs, the timing was different, the VDAs being given either 30 or 60 minutes after irradiating for CA4DP and DMXAA respectively, and heating started either 30 minutes after injecting CA4DP or 3 hours after giving DMXAA; these time intervals reflecting the optimal conditions for each VDA. In these studies radiation alone resulted in a TCD50 dose (radiation dose neces-

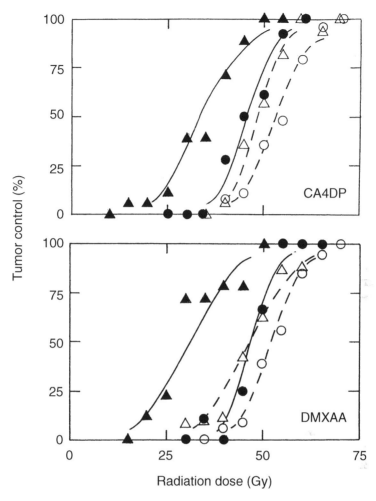

Figure 8.6 The effect of VDAs with or without heating on the radiation response of a C3H mammary carcinoma. Tumors were locally irradiated with graded radiation doses and the percentage of mice in each treatment group showing local tumor control 90 days after treatment was recorded. Mice were given either radiation alone (○), local heating (41.5°C for 60 minutes) started either 1 hour (CA4DP) or 4 hours (DMXAA) after irradiation (●), intraperitoneally injected with CA4DP (25 mg kg^{-1}) or DMXAA (20 mg kg^{-1}) either 30 or 60 minutes after irradiating, respectively (△), or treated with radiation, VDA and heat (▲). Results are from an average of 13 mice/group, with the lines fitted following logit analysis. (Modified from Murata, Overgaard and Horsman, 2001b; Murata and Horsman, 2004)

sary to control 50 per cent of tumors) of 53 Gy. Giving the VDAs or heat alone significantly reduced this TCD50 value to 46–48 Gy. Combining radiation, VDA and heat further significantly reduced the TCD50 values to 30–33 Gy, which is equivalent to ERs of 1.6–1.8 when one compares these TCD50 values with that for radiation alone. The ER obtained with DMXAA at 41.5°C, along with those obtained at a variety of other temperatures, is shown in Figure 8.7. It is clear that for hyperthermia alone one only begins to see any enhancement of radiation response at temperatures above 41.5°C and this effect becomes larger as the temperature increases. With the VDA there is an effect of the drug alone on radiation response, but when combined with heat the radiation response is enhanced at temperatures as low as 40.5°C. In fact, at this temperature the ER is as good as one finds with 43°C alone. An even greater ER was found with the VDA and heat as the temperature increased, and it is interesting to speculate as to what ER could be achieved with temperatures above 41.5°C. Also shown in Figure 8.7 are the ERs obtained with this VDA, heat and radiation combination in normal foot skin. Neither the VDA nor heat alone had any effect on

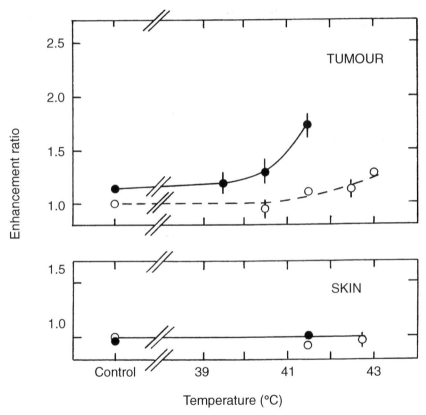

Figure 8.7 The effect of combining radiation, VTAs and hyperthermia on local tumor control in a C3H mammary carcinoma and skin damage in CDF1 mice. Tumors or skin were locally irradiated 4 hours prior to the start of local heating at the indicated temperatures for 60 minutes (○), or mice were intraperitoneally injected with DMXAA (20 mg kg^{-1}) 60 minutes after irradiating and then heated 3 hours later (●). Enhancement ratios (ratios of the response for radiation alone to that for the combined treatments) are taken from the data of Figure 8.6 and from the work of Murata et al. (2001d), Horsman and Murata (2002), and Murata and Horsman (2004), and unpublished observations

radiation response. More importantly, the combination of VDAs with heat also had no influence on radiation response, at least at a temperature of 41.5°C. This means that the enhancement of tumor response at this temperature is a pure therapeutic benefit.

8.4 Conclusions and clinical relevance

VTAs, whether angiogenesis inhibitors or vascular disrupting agents, are not new anti-cancer therapies, but are ones in which there is a renewed interest, especially with the development of less toxic novel agents. However, alone their overall effects on tumor growth are generally considered modest and so for their full potential to be realized they will probably have to be combined with more conventional therapies, in particular radiation or chemotherapy (see other chapters). Hyperthermia is an even older treatment dating back more than 5000 years, and since it not only kills cells directly but also induces vascular damage it is technically a VTA. Like conventional VTAs it also has no future in cancer therapy as a solitary agent. When combined with radiation or chemotherapy significant benefits are often seen. Heat-induced damaged to tumors is also strongly influenced by the extracellular microenvironment, and since this microenvironment is strongly manipulated by VTAs the combination of VTAs and heat is clearly valid.

Numerous preclinical studies have now demonstrated that combining VTAs with heat can be an effective approach for improving tumor response. This effect is clearly dependent on a number of factors including the heat temperature, the VTA dose and the timing and scheduling between the two therapies. For the AIs the best effect is generally seen if the AI follows heat, which could be the result of the AI influencing the repair of cellular damage by heat or preventing angiogenesis occurring after heat-induced vascular damage. Whatever the mechanism, the effect is clearly temperature dependent, only being observed at high temperatures, and appears to require that the dose of AI is sufficient to have anti-tumor activity on its own. With the VDAs, the greatest enhancement is generally seen when the heat is applied at the time of maximal vascular shutdown by the VDA. There is no requirement that the VDA show anti-tumor activity alone and significant enhancements are seen at all hyperthermia temperatures, with the greatest enhancement actually occurring at mild temperatures. Limited normal tissue studies suggest tumor specificity.

Preclinical studies have extensively shown that radiation and hyperthermia are an effective combination. Since VTAs work with either heat or radiation, the combination of all three modalities should be beneficial. No such combinations have been investigated with AIs. A few studies have looked at VDAs with radiation and heat, and substantial improvements in local tumor control reported. This is seen without any influence on normal tissue response, although this is only in early responding skin and clearly needs to be confirmed in more clinically relevant late responding normal tissues. Timing and scheduling are clearly critical issues for the maximal benefit and would certainly need to be considered when clinically relevant fractionated schedules are employed. VDA dose and heating temperature do not appear to be so critical.

Clinical testing of a whole range of different VTAs is ongoing (van Hillegersberg, Kort and Wilson, 1994; National Cancer Institute website; Siemann, Chaplin and Horsman, 2004) and many of these would be suitable candidates for combination with heat and radiation. In fact, several of the VTAs in clinical development are those that have been shown to be the most effective in preclinical studies. Hyperthermia has already undergone extensive clinical evaluation and a number of studies have demonstrated significant improvements in local control and survival when combined with radiation in specific tumor sites (Horsman and Overgaard, 2002). Unfortunately, most studies show little benefit and this is most likely the result of a failure to adequately heat tumors to effective temperatures; while mild hyperthermia temperatures of around 40.5–41.5°C are easier to obtain clinically, such temperatures are not very efficient at enhancing radiation damage and temperatures of around 42.5–43°C are required (Horsman and Overgaard, 2002). However, the preclinical data clearly demonstrates that when VDAs were included in the treatment schedule the tumor response to a temperature of only 40.5°C was as good as that seen with a much higher temperature of 43°C in the absence of any VDA, and a far greater enhancement of radiation damage was seen with the VDAs when the temperature was increased to only 41.5°C. This suggests that if future clinical trials with hyperthermia and radiation were to include a VDA in the treatment regime, we may overcome the problem of ineffective heating of tumors and many more trials should be beneficial.

Acknowledgments

The authors thank the Danish Cancer Society and the Danish Medical Research Council for financial support.

References

Brown, P.D. (1993). Matrix metalloproteinase inhibitors: a new class of anticancer agents. *Curr Opin Invest Drug* **2**, 617–626.

Chaplin, D.J., Pettit, G.R. and Hill, S.A. (1999). Anti-vascular approaches to solid tumor therapy: evaluation of combretastatin A4 phosphate. *Anticancer Res* **19**, 189–196.

Chaplin, D.J., Pettit, G.R., Parkins, C.S. and Hill, S.A. (1996). Antivascular approaches to solid tumor therapy: evaluation of tubulin binding agents. *Br J Cancer* **74** (Suppl. XXVII), S86–S88.

Chen, Q., Chen, H., Shapiro, H. and Hetzel, F. (1996). Sequencing of combined hyperthermia and photodynamic therapy. *Radiat Res* **146**, 293–297.

Christensen, T., Wahl, A. and Smedshammer, L. (1984). Effects of haematoporphyrin derivative and light in combination with hyperthermia on cells in culture. *Br J Cancer* **50**,
85–89.

Cliffe, S., Taylor, M.L., Rutland, M., Baguley, B.C., Hill, R.P. and Wilson WR. (1994).
Combining bioreductive drugs (SR 4233 or SN 23862) with the vasoactive agents flavone
acetic acid or 5,6-dimethylxanthenone acetic acid. *Int J Radiat Oncol Biol Phys* **29**,
373–377.

Dark, G.D., Hill, S.A., Prise, V.E., Tozer, G.M., Pettit, G.R., and Chaplin, D.J. (1997).
Combretastatin A-4, an agent that displays potent and selective toxicity towards tumor
vasculature. *Cancer Res* **57**, 1829–1834.

Dereski, M., Madigan, L. and Chopp, M. (1995). The effect of hypothermia and hyperthermia on photodynamic therapy of normal brain: experimental study. *Neurosurgery* **36**,
141–146.

Dewey, W.C., Thrall, D.E. and Gillette, E.L. (1977). Hyperthermia and radiation – a selective
thermal effect on chronically hypoxic tumor cells in vivo. *Int J Radiat Oncol Biol Phys*
2, 99–103.

Dewhirst, M.W., Prescott, D.M., Clegg, S. *et al.* (1990). The use of hydralazine to manipulate
tumor temperatures during hyperthermia. *Int J Hyperthermia* **6**, 971–983.

Dewhirst, M.W., Prosnitz, L., Thrall, D. *et al.* (1997). Hyperthermic treatment of malignant
diseases: current status and a view toward the future. *Semin Oncol* **24**, 616–625.

Dougherty, T.J. (1987). Photosensitizers: therapy and detection of malignant tumors. *Photochem Photobiol* **45**, 879–889.

Eikesdal, H.P., Bjerkvig, R. and Dahl, O. (2001a). Vinblastine and hyperthermia target the
neovasculature in BT₄AN rat gliomas: therapeutic implications of the vascular phenotype.
Int J Radiat Oncol Biol Phys **51**, 535–544.

Eikesdal, H.P., Bjerkvig, R., Mella, O. and Dahl, O. (2001b). Combretastatin A-4 and
hyperthermia; a patent combination for the treatment of solid tumors. *Radiother Oncol*
60, 147–154.

Eikesdal, H.P., Bjorkhaug, S.T. and Dahl, O. (2002). Hyperthermia exhibits anti-vascular
activity in the BT₄An rat glioma: lack of interaction with the angiogenesis inhibitor
batimastat. *Int J Hyperthermia* **18**, 141–152.

Eikesdal, H.P., Schem, B.C., Mella, O. and Dahl O. (2000). The new tubulin inhibitor combretastatin A-4 enhances thermal damage in the BT₄An rat glioma. *Int J Radiat Oncol
Biol Phys* **46**, 645–652.

Field, S.B. and Bleehen, N.M. (1979). Hyperthermia in the treatment of cancer. *Cancer Treat
Rev* **6**, 63–94.

Gerweck, L.E., Nygaard, T.G. and Burlett, M. (1979). Response of cells to hyperthermia
under acute and chronic hypoxic conditions. *Cancer Res* **39**, 966–972.

Griffin, R.J., Lee, S.H., Rood, K.L. *et al.* (2000). Use of arsenic trioxide as an antivascular
and thermosensitizing agent in solid tumors. *Neoplasia* **2**, 555–560.

Griffin, R.J., Monzen, H., Williams, B.W., Park, H., Lee, S.H. and Song, C.W. (2003). Arsenic
trioxide induces selective tumor vascular damage via oxidative stress and increases thermosensitivity of tumours. *Int J Hyperthermia* **19**, 575–589.

Henderson, B.W., Waldow, S.M., Potter, W.R. and Dougherty, T.J. (1985). Interaction of
photodynamic therapy and hyperthermia: tumor response and cell survival studies after
treatment of mice in vivo. *Cancer Res* **45**, 6071–6077.

Hill, S.A. and Denekamp, J. (1978). The effect of vascular occlusion on the thermal sensitization of a mouse tumor. *Br J Radiol* **51**, 997–1002.

Hill, S.A., Sampson, L.E. and Chaplin, D.J. (1995). Anti-vascular approaches to solid tumor
therapy: evaluation of vinblastine and flavone acetic acid. *Int J Cancer* **63**, 119–123.

Hiraoka, M. and Hahn, G.M. (1990). Changes in pH and blood flow induced by glucose, and their effects on hyperthermia with or without BCNU in RIF-1 tumours. *Int J Hyperthermia* 6, 97–103.

Honess, D.J., Hu, D.E. and Bleehen, N.M. (1991). A study of the mechanism of hydralazine enhancement of thermal damage in the KHT tumour. *Int J Hyperthermia* 7, 667–679.

Horsman, M.R., Chaplin, D.J. and Overgaard, J. (1991). The effect of combining flavone acetic acid and hyperthermia on the growth of a C3H mammary carcinoma. *Int J Radiat Biol* 60, 385–388.

Horsman, M.R., Christensen, K.L. and Overgaard, J. (1989). Hydralazine-induced enhancement of hyperthermic damage in a C3H mammary carcinoma *in vivo*. *Int J Hyperthermia* 5, 123–136.

Horsman, M.R. and Murata, R. (2002). Combination of vascular targeting agents with thermal or radiation therapy. *Int J Radiat Oncol Biol Phys* 54, 1518–1523.

Horsman, M.R., Murata, R. and Overgaard, J. (2001). Improving local tumor control by combining vascular targeting drugs, mild hyperthermia and radiation. *Acta Oncol* 40, 497–503.

Horsman, M.R. and Overgaard, J. (2002). Overcoming tumor radioresistance resulting from hypoxia. In *Basic Clinical Radiobiology for Radiation Oncologists*, 3rd edn, G.G. Steel (ed.). Arnold, London, pp. 169–181.

Horsman, M.R., Sampson, L.E., Chaplin, D.J. and Overgaard, J. (1996). The *in vivo* interaction between flavone acetic acid and hyperthermia. *Int J Hyperthermia* 12, 779–789.

Horsman, M.R. and Winther, J. (1989). Vascular effects of photodynamic therapy in an intraocular retinoblastoma-like tumour. *Acta Oncol* 28, 693–697.

Ingber, D., Fujita, T., Kishimoto, S. *et al.* (1990). Synthetic analogues of fumagillin that inhibit angiogenesis and suppress tumor growth. *Nature* 348, 555–557.

Jain, R.K., Grantham, F.H. and Gullino, P.M. (1979). Blood flow and heat transfer in Walker 256 mammary carcinoma. *J Natl Cancer Inst* 62, 927–933.

Kallinowski, F., Moehle, R. and Vaupel, P. (1989). Substantial enhancement of tumor hyperthermic response by tumor necrosis factor. In *Hyperthermic Oncology*, Vol. 1, T. Sugahara and M. Saito (eds). Taylor and Francis, London, pp. 258–259.

Kalmus, J., Okunieff, P. and Vaupel, P. (1990). Dose-dependent effects of hydralazine on microcirculatory function and hyperthermic response of murine FSaII tumors. *Cancer Res* 50, 15–19.

Kelleher, D.K., Bastian, J., Thews, O. and Vaupel, P. (2003a). Enhanced effects of aminolaevulinic acid-based photodynamic therapy through local hyperthermia in rat tumours. *Br J Cancer* 89, 405–411.

Kelleher, D.K., Thews, O., Scherz, A., Salomon, Y. and Vaupel, P. (2003b). Combined hyperthermia and chlorophyll-based photodynamic therapy: tumor growth and metabolic microenvironment. *Br J Cancer* 89, 2333–2339.

Kessel, D. (1984). Hematoporphyrin and HPD. Photophysics, photo-chemistry and phototherapy. *Photochem Photobiol* 39, 851–859.

Krossnes, B.K., Mella, O. and Dahl, O. (1996). Use of the vasodilator sodium nitroprusside during local hyperthermia: effects on tumor temperature and tumor response in a rat tumor model. *Int J Radiat Oncol Biol Phys* 36, 403–415.

Lash, C.J., Li, A.E., Rutland, M., Baguley, B.C., Zwi, L.J. and Wilson, W.R. (1998). Enhancement of the anti-tumour effects of the antivascular agent 5,6-dimethylxanthenone-4-acetic acid (DMXAA) by the combination with 5-hydroxytryptamine and bioreductive drugs. *Br J Cancer* 78, 439–445.

Levendag, P.C., Marijnissen, H.P.A., de Ru, V.J., Versteeg, J.A.C., van Rhoon, G.C. and Star, W.M. (1988). Interaction of interstitial photodynamic therapy and interstitial hyperthermia in a rat rhabdomyosarcoma – a pilot study. *Int J Radiat Oncol Biol Phys* **14**, 139–145.

Li, G.C., Cameron, R.B., Sapareto, S.A. and Hahn, G.M. (1982). Reinterpretation of Arrhenius analysis of cell activation by heat. *Natl Cancer Inst Mono* **61**, 111–113.

Lin, J.C., Park, H.J. and Song, C.W. (1996). Combined treatment of IL-α and TNF-α potentiates the antitumour effect of hyperthermia. *Int J Hyperthermia* **12**, 335–344.

Mang, T.S. and Dougherty, T.J. (1985). Time and sequence dependent influence of in vitro photodynamic therapy (PDT) survival by hyperthermia. *Photochem Photobiol* **42**, 533–540.

Matsumoto, N., Miyoshi, N., Saito, H. and Fukuda, M. (1989). Combination therapy of microwave hyperthermia and photodynamic therapy on squamous cell carcinoma in vivo. In *Hyperthermic Oncology*, Vol. 1, T. Sugahara and M. Saito M (eds). Taylor and Francis, London, pp. 363–364.

Maxwell, R.J., Nielsen, F.U., Breidahl, T., Stødkilde-Jørgensen, H. and Horsman, M.R. (1998). Effects of combretastatin on murine tumours monitored by ^{31}P MRS, ^{1}H MRS and ^{1}H MRI. *Int J Radiat Oncol Biol Phys* **42**, 891–894.

Murata, R. and Horsman, M.R. (2004). Tumour-specific enhancement of thermoradiotherapy at mild temperatures by the vascular targeting agent 5,6-dimethylxanthenone-4-acetic acid. *Int J Hyperthermia* **20**, 393–404.

Murata, R., Overgaard, J. and Horsman, M.R. (2001a). Potentiation of the anti-tumor effect of hyperthermia by combining with the vascular targeting agent 5,6-dimethylxanthenone-4-acetic acid. *Int J Hyperthermia* **17**, 508–519.

Murata, R., Overgaard, J. and Horsman, M.R. (2001b). Combretastatin A-4 disodium phosphate: a vascular targeting agent that improves the anti-tumor effects of hyperthermia, radiation and mild thermoradiotherapy. *Int J Radiat Oncol Biol Phys* **51**, 1018–1024.

Murata, R., Overgaard, J. and Horsman, M.R. (2001c). Comparative effects of combretastatin A-4 disodium phosphate and 5,6-dimethylxanthenone-4-acetic acid on blood perfusion in a murine tumor and normal tissues. *Int J Radiat Biol* **77**, 195–204.

Murata, R., Siemann, D.W., Overgaard, J. and Horsman, M.R. (2001). Improved tumor response by combining radiation and the vascular-damaging drug 5,6-dimethylxanthenone-4-acetic acid. *Radiat Res* **156**, 503–509.

Murray, D., Milas, L. and Meyn, R.E. (1984). DNA damage produced by combined hyperglycemia and hyperthermia in two mouse fibrosarcoma tumors in vivo. *Int J Radiat Oncol Biol Phys* **10**, 1679–1682.

National Cancer Institute website: www.cancer.gov/clinicaltrials

Nelson, J.S., Wright, W.H. and Berns, M.W. (1985). Histopathological comparison of the effects of hematoporphyrin derivative on two different murine tumors using computer-enhanced digital video fluorescence microscopy. *Cancer Res* **45**, 5781–5786.

Nishimura, Y., Murata, R. and Hiraoka, M. (1996). Combined effects of an angiogenesis inhibitor (TNP-470) and hyperthermia. *Br J Cancer* **73**, 270–274.

Orenstein, A., Kostenich, G., Kopolovic, Y., Babushkina, T. and Malik, Z. (1999). Enhancement of ALA-PDT damage by IR-induced hyperthermia on a colon carcinoma model. *Photochem Photobiol* **69**, 703–707.

Osinsky, S.P., Bubnovskaja, L.N. and Gusev, A.N. (1989). Enhancement of hyperthermic anti-tumor effect by selective alteration of tumor cells environment. In *Hyperthermic Oncology*, Vol. 1, T. Sugahara T and M. Saito (eds). Taylor and Francis, London, pp. 146–147.

Overgaard, J. (1978). The effect of local hyperthermia alone and in combination with radiation on solid tumors. In *Cancer Therapy by Hyperthermia and Radiation*. C. Streffer (ed.). Urban and Schwarzenberg, Baltimore, MD, pp. 49–62.

Overgaard, J. (1985). Rationale and problems in the design of clinical trials. In *Hyperthermic Oncology*, Vol. 2, J. Overgaard (ed.). Taylor and Francis, London, pp. 325–338.

Overgaard, J. (1987). The design of clinical trials in hyperthermia. In *Physics and Technology of Hyperthermia*, S.B. Field and C. Franconi (eds). Martinus Nijhoff, Amsterdam, pp. 598–620.

Overgaard, J. and Bichel, P. (1977). The influence of hypoxia and acidity on the hyperthermic response of malignant cells *in vitro*. *Radiology* **123**, 511–514.

Overgaard, J. and Nielsen, O.S. (1980). The role of tissue environmental factors on the kinetics and morphology of tumor cells exposed to hyperthermia. *Ann NY Acad Sci* **335**, 254–280.

Patterson, J. and Strang, R. (1979). The role of blood flow in hyperthermia. *Int J Radiat Oncol Biol Phys* **5**, 235–241.

Peterson, H.I. (1979). Tumor blood flow compared to normal tissue blood flow. In *Tumor Blood Circulation: Angiogenesis, Vascular Morphology and Blood Flow of Experimental and Human Tumors*. H.I. Peterson (ed.). CRC Press, Boca Raton, FL, pp. 103–114.

Prescott, D.M., Samulski, T.V., Dewhirst, M.W. *et al.* (1992). Use of nitroprusside to increase tissue temperature during local hyperthermia in normal and tumor-bearing dogs. *Int J Radiat Oncol Biol Phys* **23**, 377–385.

Poulson, J.M., Vujaskovic, Z., Gaskin, A.A. *et al.* (2004). Effect of calcitonin gene related peptide vs sodium nitroprusside to increase temperature in spontaneous canine tumours during local hyperthermia. *Int J Hyperthermia* **20**, 477–489.

Reinhold, H.S. (1988). Physiological effects of hyperthermia. In *Recent Results in Cancer Research: Application of Hyperthermia in the Treatment of Cancer*, Vol. 107, R.D. Issels and W. Wilmanns (eds). Springer, Berlin, pp. 32–43.

Sakaguchi, Y., Maehara, Y., Baba, H., Kusumoto, T., Sugimachi, K. and Newman, R.A. (1992). Flavone acetic acid increases the antitumor effect of hyperthermia in mice. *Cancer Res* **52**, 3306–3309.

Selman, S.H, Kreimer-Birnbaum, M., Klaunig, J.E., Goldblatt, P.J., Keck, R.W. and Britton, S.L. (1984). Blood flow in transplantable bladder tumors treated with hematoporphyrin derivative and light. *Cancer Res* **44**, 1924–1927.

Siemann, D.W., Chaplin, D.J. and Horsman, M.R. (2004). Vascular targeting therapies for treatment of malignant disease. *Cancer* **100**, 2491–2499.

Star, W.M., Marijnissen, H.P.A., van den Berg.Blok, A.E., Versteeg, J.A.C., Franken, K.A.P. and Reinhol, H.S. (1986). Destruction of rat mammary tumor and normal tissue microcirculation by hematoporphyrin derivative photoradiation observed in vivo in sandwich observation chambers. *Cancer Res* **46**, 2532–2540.

Thrall, D.E., Gillette, E.L. and Dewey, W.C. (1975). Effect of heat and ionizing radiation on normal and neoplastic tissue of the C3H mouse. *Radiat Res* **63**, 363–377.

Tozer, G.M., Prise, V.E., Wilson, J. *et al.* (1999). Combretastatin A-4 phosphate as a tumor vascular-targeting agent: early effects in tumors and normal tissues. *Cancer Res* **59**, 1626–1634.

Urano, M., Gerweck, L.E., Epstein, R., Cunningham, M. and Suit, H.D. (1980). Response of a spontaneous murine tumor to hyperthermia: factors which modify the thermal response in vivo. *Radiat Res* **83**, 312–322.

Urano, M., Maher, J., Rice, L.C. and Kahn, J. (1982). Response of spontaneous murine tumors to hyperthermia: temperature dependence in two different-sized tumors. *Natl Cancer Inst Monogr* **61**, 299–301.

Urano, M., Montoya, V. and Booth, A. (1983). Effect of hyperglycemia on the thermal response of murine normal and tumor tissue. *Cancer Res* **43**, 453–455.

van Hillegersberg, R., Kort, W.J. and Wilson, J.H. (1994). Current status of photodynamic therapy in oncology. *Drugs* **48**, 510–527.

Vaupel, P., Kallinowski, F. and Okunieff, P. (1989). Blood flow, oxygen and nutrient supply, and metabolic micro-environment of human tumors: a review. *Cancer Res* **49**, 6449–6465.

Voorhees, W.D. and Babbs, C.F. (1982). Hydralazine-enhanced selective heating of transmissible venereal tumor implants in dogs. *Eur J Cancer Clin Oncol* **19**, 1027–1033.

Waldow, S.M. and Dougherty, T.J. (1984). Interaction of hyperthermia and photoradiation therapy. *Radiat Res* **97**, 380–385.

Wallen, C.A., Colby, T.V. and Stewart, J.R. (1986). Cell kill and tumor control after heat treatment with and without vascular occlusion in RIF-1 tumors. *Radiat Res* **106**, 215–223.

Winkler, F., Kozin, S.V., Tong, R.T. *et al.* (2004). Kinetics of vascular normalization by VEGFR2 blockade governs brain tumor response to radiation: role of oxygenation, angiopoietin-1, and matrix metalloproteinases. *Cancer Cell* **6**, 553–563.

Winther, J. (1989). Photodynamic therapy effect in an intraocular retinoblastoma-like tumor assessed by an in vitro colony forming assay. *Br J Cancer* **59**, 869–872.

Yano, T., Tanase, M., Watanabe, A. *et al.* (1995). Enhancement effect of an anti-angiogenic agent, TNP-470, on hyperthermia-induced growth suppression of human esophageal and gastric cancers transplantable to nude mice. *Anticancer Res* **15**, 1355–1358.

9

Flavones and Xanthenones as Vascular-disrupting Agents

Bronwyn G. Siim and Bruce C. Baguley

Abstract

DMXAA (AS1404) is a xanthenone-based vascular disrupting agent developed from FAA via an analogue development programme. DMXAA and FAA produce vascular shutdown selectively in tumours through direct effects on tumour endothelial cells and via induction of cytokines and other bioactive species. The resulting cascade of effects induces prolonged arrest of tumour blood flow, resulting in haemorrhagic necrosis of tumour tissue. DMXAA has antitumour activity as a single agent and marked enhancement of this activity can be obtained by combination with radiation or other cytotoxic agents, especially taxanes. Although DMXAA has a steep dose-response for antivascular and antitumour activity in mice, studies suggest a wider therapeutic index in other species including rats, rabbits, and humans. Clinical trials with DMXAA have shown that it has antivascular activity in human tumours over a wide dose range, and it is currently being evaluated in Phase I/II trials in combination with paclitaxel and carboplatin.

Keywords

DMXAA, AS1404, FAA, vascular, xanthenones, flavones, tumour blood flow

9.1 Development of FAA and DMXAA

LM985, the diethylaminoethyl ester of FAA, was discovered to have high antitumor activity during screening against the murine Colon 38 adenocarcinoma of a series of benzopyran derivatives with anti-inflammatory activity (Atassi *et al.*, 1985; Plowman *et al.*, 1986). LM985 is converted by esterases in the blood to FAA (see structure in Figure 9.1), which was subsequently found to be the active species. Flavonoids, of which FAA is a member, have a large variety of

Vascular-targeted Therapies in Oncology   Edited by Dietmar W. Siemann
© 2006 John Wiley & Sons, Ltd.

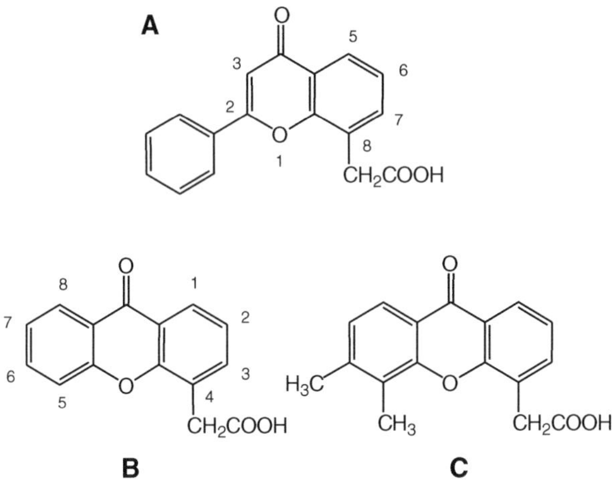

Figure 9.1 Chemical structures of (A) FAA, (B) XAA and (C) DMXAA

biological activities including anti-inflammatory activity (Havsteen, 1983), but FAA differs markedly from most naturally occurring flavonoids by lacking hydroxy functions. Consequently, the investigation of flavonoids with similar antitumor activity to that of FAA has been concerned mainly with analogues with acidic side chains (Aitken *et al.*, 2000; Gobbi *et al.*, 2003; Valenti *et al.*, 2000).

Xanthenone-4-acetic acid (XAA; see the structure in Figure 9.1) was synthesized as a fused ring analogue of FAA and found to have antitumor activity similar to that of FAA (Rewcastle *et al.*, 1989). XAA is a member of the xanthenone series and had previously been synthesized as a potential anti-inflammatory agent (Nakanishi *et al.*, 1975). The antitumor activity of XAA raised the possibility that other polycyclic chromophores attached to acetic acid or other acidic moieties might have activity. This was explored by the synthesis and testing of a number of derivatives containing tricyclic chromophores (Rewcastle *et al.*, 1991c), but almost all were found to be inactive. The rigid structural requirements for activity in the XAA series were borne out by studies on monosubstituted and disubstituted derivatives of XAA, where substitution of even a single methyl or chloro group often led to loss of biological activity. However substitution at the 3-, 5- and 6-positions on the XAA chromophore with methyl groups led to active compounds and DMXAA (Figure 9.1) was developed as the best of the disubstituted derivatives, having substantially increased *in vivo* dose potency as well as greater antitumor activity than FAA or XAA. Derivatives having an ethylene link between the 5- and 6-positions were also highly active (Gobbi *et al.*, 2002). On the other hand, substitution with hydrophilic groups such as hydroxyl or nitro resulted in loss of activity, and replacement of the acidic function of XAA by substituted acetic acid or propionic acid side chains also led to decreased activity (Rewcastle *et al.*, 1991a).

9.2   Antivascular activity of FAA and DMXAA

FAA and DMXAA induce a number of interrelated effects on tumor tissue. It is important to realize that the energy supplies of tumor cells are such that they can withstand deprivation of a blood supply for at least one hour without sustaining a significant decrease in viability (Zwi *et al.*, 1989). Furthermore, the occlusion of vasculature will induce a number of physiological responses, including those caused by hypoxia (Brown, 2002), which will act to restore the blood supply. Effective antivascular treatment may therefore need to incorporate a cascade of effects that induce a prolonged arrest of tumor blood flow (Baguley, 2003). It is therefore not surprising that FAA and DMXAA induce a number of interrelated changes in tumor physiology. The earliest events, occurring within 30 minutes of administration, include a reduction in tumor blood flow (Zwi *et al.*, 1989, 1994), the induction of tumor endothelial cell apoptosis (Ching *et al.*, 2002; Ching, Zwain and Baguley, 2004) and increases in plasma concentrations of serotonin and its metabolite 5-hydroxy-indole acetic acid (5-HIAA) (Baguley, Zhuang and Kestell, 1997; Kestell *et al.*, 2001).

For DMXAA, clear correlations have been demonstrated to link the induction of endothelial cell apoptosis, increased tumor vascular permeability and the induction of 5-HIAA, suggesting a tight mechanistic link (Zhao *et al.*, 2005). DMXAA induces changes to the actin cytoskeleton of tumor endothelial cells but differs from the mitotic poison combretastatin A-4 phosphate in that it does not affect the organization of tubulin in the cytoskeleton (Tozer, Kanthou and Baguley, 2005). DMXAA rapidly induces the expression of von Willebrand factor within tumor blood vessels, which co-localizes with the platelet specific marker CD41 (Siim, unpublished data). This is thought to reflect the recruitment of platelets to tumor endothelium, leading to the release of serotonin and other platelet products important for blood clotting and occlusion of blood vessels. Serotonin itself is an antivascular agent, acting on $5-HT_2$ receptors on vascular endothelial cells to induce stress responses, and may prolong the antivascular effect of DMXAA.

The basis for the selectivity in the targeting of tumor blood vessels by DMXAA is thought to lie in the distinctive features of tumor blood vessels: the capillary network is more permeable and less well organized than that of a normal tissue, and further increase in vascular permeability may cause catastrophic failure (Zhao *et al.*, 2005). Tumor capillaries may also be more immature than those in normal tissues, with many participating in tubulogenesis, a late stage of angiogenesis required in the vascular remodeling of tumors. DMXAA may directly inhibit tubulogenesis, further compromising the permeability of the tumor endothelium. The direct and indirect effects of DMXAA culminate in the breakdown of vascular function and the death of tumor cells through hemorrhagic necrosis.

9.3   Cytokine induction by FAA and DMXAA

A further important property of FAA and DMXAA is an ability to induce the expression of cytokines, particularly of tumor necrosis factor (TNF) (Mace *et al.*, 1990; Philpott, Baguley and Ching, 1995). Cytokine activity increases after a time delay, subsequent to the rapid changes in tumor blood flow, and is therefore not thought to be the initial cause of the antivascular effect (Baguley and Ching, 1997). TNF production is not essential to the activity of DMXAA, since high antitumor activity has been observed in mice lacking the gene either for TNF or the type-1 TNF receptor (Zhao *et al.*, 2002). However, a higher drug dose is required in these TNF$^{-/-}$ or TNFR-1 knockout mice, suggesting that TNF contributes to both the antitumor activity and, at least in mice, the toxicity of DMXAA.

DMXAA induction of cytokines and chemokines such as IP-10 (Cao, Baguley and Ching, 2001) are likely to have significant effects on vascular physiology and might have a major role in extending the duration of the antivascular effects. Initial studies using bioassays for TNF showed large increases in plasma TNF concentrations (Philpott, Baguley and Ching, 1995). However, later studies using ELISA assays showed small increases in TNF in mouse serum but large changes occurring in tumor tissue (Ching *et al.*, 1999). This suggests that tumor-associated cells are the major source of TNF synthesis and that the decrease in tumor blood flow following DMXAA treatment limits release of TNF into the general circulation. Increases in serum TNF have not been observed in clinical trials of DMXAA (Jameson *et al.*, 2000), although TNF synthesis within tumor tissue cannot be excluded.

Tumor tissue is known to contain inflammatory cells and the tumor microenvironment may contribute to the ability of DMXAA to induce TNF. DMXAA requires a second signal such as lipopolysaccharide for efficient TNF induction both in isolated murine splenocytes (Wang *et al.*, 2004) and in isolated human peripheral blood leucocytes (Philpott, Ching and Baguley, 2001), and it is possible that this signal is provided by the tumor microenvironment, contributing to the selectivity of the DMXAA effects.

FAA and DMXAA also induce the synthesis of nitric oxide, perhaps as a consequence of cytokine production (Thomsen *et al.*, 1991; Veszelovsky *et al.*, 1995), and nitric oxide is a further possible contributor to the overall response. A summary of possible pathways is presented in Figure 9.2. The drugs are hypothesized to target both vascular endothelial cells and macrophages in the tumor. The decreased tumor blood flow is thought to arise from drug effects on tumor vascular endothelial cells such as induced apoptosis and changes in

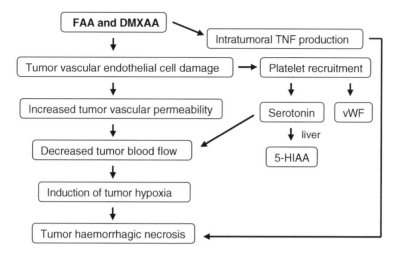

Figure 9.2   A simplified scheme to explain some of the features of FAA and DMXAA

the actin cytoskeleton. Platelets respond to endothelial cell damage by releasing serotonin, which may provide an additional stress response in the tumor. Tumor-associated macrophages or inflammatory/immune cells respond by increased production of cytokines, particularly of TNF, and this can further modify endothelial function and integrity. Nitric oxide may also be induced (not shown) and affect endothelial cell function. Prolonged inhibition of tumor blood flow leads to hemorrhagic necrosis, which may be enhanced by the production of TNF.

9.4   Molecular target

The structure–activity studies on FAA and XAA analogues suggest that their molecular target comprises a lipophilic 'pocket' that will accommodate a tricyclic or phenylbenzopyran structure (Figure 9.1). This pocket probably contains a hydrogen bond donor that interacts with the carbonyl function situated at the 4-position of FAA and the 9-position of DMXAA. It might also contain a region, perhaps a basically charged amino acid, which interacts with the acetic acid group of FAA or DMXAA. The nature of this target, which is presumably a protein, is not yet known.

The induction of natural killer activity in the spleen and the induction of increased TNF concentrations in plasma (Ching and Baguley, 1987; Mace *et al.*, 1990; Philpott, Baguley and Ching, 1995) were two of the earliest features of the action of FAA and DMXAA to be identified, and point to a potential target for these drugs in the regulatory pathways for cytokine induction. *In vitro* studies using murine splenocytes (Wang *et al.*, 2004) and human peripheral leucocytes (Philpott, Ching and Baguley, 2001) suggest that DMXAA acts as a co-inducer rather than an inducer of TNF. In the human system, DMXAA (but not FAA) stimulates TNF production by agents that interact with toll-like receptor-4, or agents that activate the NF-κB transcription factor (Philpott, Ching and Baguley, 2001). NF-κB promoter sites are thought to play an important role in the regulation of cytokine gene expression, but it is also clear that a number of other promoter sites are important in this complex control system to prevent inappropriate activation of cytokine genes. It is of interest that DMXAA itself, like a number of other stress-inducing agents, stimulates the nuclear translocation of NF-κB in a number of cell types (Woon *et al.*, 2002). These results suggest a target in the regulation mechanisms for cytokine synthesis. The ability of DMXAA to co-stimulate TNF production rather than to directly stimulate it suggests that it has a complex role.

Another potential clue to the action of DMXAA is its inhibition of the process of 'vasculogenic mimicry'. When cultured on basement membrane material (Matrigel), some cell lines express a number of genes associated with vascular endothelial cells (Hendrix *et al.*, 2003). Exposure of a human melanoma line, NZM7, to DMXAA at pharmacologically achievable concentrations led to selective inhibition of expression of these genes including ETS1, a transcription factor that is closely involved with activation of genes involved in tubulogenesis (Zhao *et al.*, 2004). These results suggest that DMXAA might modulate the activity of a pathway regulating the expression of ETS1. The relationship between this pathway and the NF-κB pathway is not yet known.

9.5 Preclinical studies: DMXAA as a single agent

DMXAA has shown high activity as a single agent against some tumors, such as the murine Colon 38 tumor (Rewcastle *et al.*, 1991b), although it produces only transient inhibition of tumor growth in others (Siim *et al.*, 2003, 2005). However, the single-agent activity of DMXAA can be improved by multiple dosing. An initial dose of $25\,mg\,kg^{-1}$ i.p. followed 4 and 8 hours later by doses of $5\,mg\,kg^{-1}$ DMXAA resulted in 100 per cent cures of Colon 38 tumors compared with 55 per cent cures for a single $25\,mg\,kg^{-1}$ dose (Zhao *et al.*, 2003). The same study also reported excellent activity against Colon 38 tumors (90 per cent cures) following oral administration of DMXAA ($30\,mg\,kg^{-1}$ followed 4 and 8 hours later by $15\,mg\,kg^{-1}$) (Zhao *et al.*, 2003). A similar administration schedule induced long growth delays and cures of the NZM7 human melanoma line growing as a xenograft in athymic mice (Zhao *et al.*, 2005). Antitumor activity was not a direct function of plasma AUC, but appeared to be dependent on maintaining the plasma drug concentration above a threshold (Zhao *et al.*, 2003).

A weekly schedule where DMXAA ($21\,mg\,kg^{-1}$) was administered on days 0, 7 and 14 resulted in cures of two out of seven WiDr human colon carcinoma

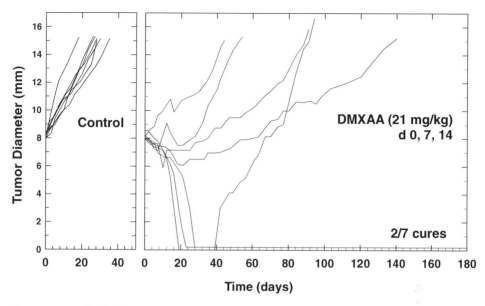

Figure 9.3 Individual growth curves for subcutaneous WiDr human colon carcinoma xenografts, growing in CD-1 nude mice, following treatment with DMXAA (21 mg kg^{-1}) on days 0, 7 and 14

xenografts, with a median tumor growth delay of 65 days (Figure 9.3). Collectively, these studies indicate that DMXAA has significant single-agent activity, and can cure human tumor xenografts when multiple doses are administered.

It should be noted that there are large variations in the response of tumors to single or multiple doses of DMXAA between individual mice (Figure 9.3) (Siim *et al.*, 2003, 2005). Studies with paired tumors growing in contralateral flanks have shown that this variability arises predominantly at the host level rather than the tumor level (Siim *et al.*, 2005). It has been hypothesized that a variable immune response to DMXAA might contribute to these large variations in individual mice, since it has been reported that variations in the inflammatory response of individual patients to cancer may modify the pharmacokinetics, and hence their response to cancer chemotherapy (Slaviero, Clarke and Rivory, 2003).

9.6 Preclinical studies: combination treatments

Histological studies of MDAH-MCa-4 tumors 12 hours after DMXAA treatment have shown that islands of viable tissue survive, particularly in the tumor periphery, with tumors regrowing rapidly from this surviving tissue (Lash *et al.*, 1998). Therefore, in order to obtain the full therapeutic potential of DMXAA, it is necessary to combine it with other therapeutic agents. A number of combinations have been investigated.

Combination with radiation

Baguley and Wilson (2002) proposed that combining DMXAA with agents that preferentially kill well perfused tumor regions should provide therapeutic benefit. This is thought to be the mechanism behind the therapeutic gain obtained from combining DMXAA with radiation (Murata *et al.*, 2001; Wilson *et al.*, 1998): DMXAA kills the poorly perfused tumor regions, while radiation kills the better oxygenated tumor tissue. As expected, the therapeutic gain is lost if DMXAA is administered prior to radiation (Murata *et al.*, 2001; Wilson *et al.*, 1998), presumably through DMXAA-induced hypoxia conferring radioresistance.

Combination with cytotoxic agents

Combination studies with FAA have been limited to studies with mitomycin C (Parkins, Denekamp and Chaplin, 1993) and chlorambucil (Parkins, Chadwick and Chaplin, 1994), where co-administration with FAA produced greater tumor growth delays than either agent alone. The increased antitumor activity for the combinations was attributed, in part, to induced changes in tumor pH.

More extensive studies have been carried out with DMXAA where complementary killing of different tumor regions is thought to account for the excellent antitumor activity obtained from combining DMXAA with conventional chemotherapy agents. Therapeutic gain has been obtained from combining DMXAA with cisplatin or cyclophosphamide against murine KHT tumors or human SKBr3 breast and OW1 ovarian tumor xenografts (Siemann *et al.*, 2002). Enhancement of DMXAA activity against MDAH-MCa-4 murine mammary tumors was observed from combination with several conventional chemotherapy drugs, with the exception of 5-fluorouracil (Siim *et al.*, 2003). The therapeutic gain was most marked for the combination of DMXAA with paclitaxel, for which cures of advanced MDAH-MCa-4 tumors (Siim *et al.*, 2003) and human colon carcinoma WiDr and non-small-cell lung cancer NCI-H460 xenografts (Kelland, 2005; Siim *et al.*, 2005) have been observed. Although there was a broad optimum for the timing of administration for paclitaxel from 4 hours before to 2 hours after DMXAA, antitumor activity was lost if paclitaxel was administered 4 hours after DMXAA, which was attributed to DMXAA-induced vascular shutdown inhibiting delivery of paclitaxel (Siim *et al.*, 2003). Co-administration of DMXAA and paclitaxel, or carboplatin, did not alter the pharmacokinetics of either agent (Siim *et al.*, 2003). However, pharmacokinetic interactions have been observed for some drug combinations with DMXAA.

DMXAA-induced vascular shutdown has been shown to result in entrapment of other therapeutic agents within tumors. This mechanism contributes to the therapeutic interaction between DMXAA and melphalan in KHT tumors (Pruijn *et al.*, 1997), where the maximum potentiation of antitumor activity was achieved when melphalan was administered 2 hours after DMXAA. Induction of tumor acidosis was also thought to contribute to the enhanced antitumor activity obtained from combining DMXAA and melphalan (Pruijn *et al.*, 1997).

Combination with radioimmunotherapy

An entrapment mechanism is also though to contribute to the synergy between DMXAA and antibody-based therapies such as radioimmunotherapy (Pedley *et al.*, 1994, 1996). Again, scheduling of the agents was important, with the greatest antitumor effects obtained when DMXAA was administered 24 or 48 hours after the ^{131}I antiCEA antibody, i.e. at the time of maximum tumor levels of the antibody (Pedley *et al.*, 1994, 1996).

Combination with hypoxia-selective agents

Induction of tumor hypoxia by FAA was inferred from studies with KHT tumors where FAA treatment resulted in loss of radiosensitivity (Edwards, Bremner and Stratford, 1991a). A more direct method, the non-invasive hypoxia marker Prognox (^{99m}Tc-labeled HL-91), was used to demonstrate that DMXAA-induced vascular shutdown results in tumor hypoxia in murine tumors and human tumor xenografts (Siim *et al.*, 2000). FAA has been shown to enhance the antitumor activity of the hypoxia-selective bioreductive drug tirapazamine (Chaplin *et al.*, 1996; Edwards, Bremner and Stratford, 1991b; Sun and Brown, 1989), but not of the bioreductive alkylating agents RSU 1069 or mitomycin C (Edwards, Bremner and Stratford, 1991b). DMXAA enhances the antitumor activity of hypoxia-selective bioreductive drugs including tirapazamine, the dinitrobenzamide mustards SN 23862 and SN 23816 and the 2-nitroimidazole alkylating agent CI-1010 (Cliffe *et al.*, 1994; Lash *et al.*, 1998; Vincent *et al.*, 1997; Wilson and Pruijn, 1995). The antitumor activity of these combinations could be further enhanced by potentiation of the tumor blood flow inhibition using high-dose serotonin, which also has antivascular activity (Lash *et al.*, 1998). DMXAA also strongly enhances the activity of the DNA intercalator/topoisomerase II inhibitor prodrug AQ4N against MDAH-MCa-4 tumors (Wilson *et al.*, 1996).

Combination with anti-inflammatory agents

The tumor vascular injury induced by FAA and DMXAA might be expected to induce an inflammatory response to facilitate the repair of such injury. Anti-inflammatory agents, by inhibiting such a response, could enhance the anti-vascular effects of these drugs. Most studies have involved combination with the agent thalidomide (Ching *et al.*, 1995) but combination with cyclo-oxy-genase inhibitors has also been investigated (Baguley *et al.*, 2004). Both classes of agents augment DMXAA-induced activity against Colon 38 tumors. Co-administration of DMXAA and thalidomide to Colon 38 tumor-bearing mice resulted in a significant increase in AUC values for DMXAA in both plasma and tumor (Kestell *et al.*, 2000). The enhanced antitumor activity of this com-bination (Cao *et al.*, 1999; Ching *et al.*, 1995) presumably results at least partially from this pharmacokinetic interaction, although it is not clear whether this alone leads to the observed increased production of intra-tumoral TNF production (Cao *et al.*, 1999). No pharmacokinetic interaction was observed in rats co-administered DMXAA and thalidomide, indicating that the interac-tion is species dependent (Zhou *et al.*, 2001a). In the case of the cyclo-oxy-genase inhibitor diclofenac in mice, the augmentation of antitumor activity does not appear to be a result of a pharmacokinetic interaction (Baguley *et al.*, 2004).

Combination with hyperthermia

A therapeutic interaction between DMXAA and hyperthermia against C3H mouse mammary tumors results from improved local heat retention (Murata, Overgaard and Horsman, 2001). Although DMXAA also increased heat damage to normal skin, the heat enhancement ratio was greater for tumors (1.9) than for skin (1.3–1.5). Interestingly, potentiation of antitumor activity by DMXAA was greater at the clinically achievable mild hyperthermia temperatures of 40.5 and 41.5 than at 42.5°C (Murata, Overgaard and Horsman, 2001).

Combination with photodynamic therapy

DMXAA has also been shown to enhance the antitumor activity of photo-dynamic therapy against murine RIF-1 tumors, with the maximal effect achieved when DMXAA was administered 1–3 hours before local illumination of the tumors (Bellnier *et al.*, 2003). The rationale for combining DMXAA and pho-todynamic therapy was that TNF had been shown to potentiate the antitumor effects of photodynamic therapy (Bellnier, 1991), and that DMXAA-induced tumor-selective synthesis of TNF would avoid the toxicity associated with sys-temic administration of TNF. However, the contribution of this mechanism is unclear, as photodynamic therapy *decreased* the amount of TNF produced by DMXAA alone in RIF-1 tumors while increasing antitumor activity (Bellnier *et al.*, 2003).

Combination with vasoactive agents

Administration of serotonin to mice with Colon 38 tumors induces hemorrhagic necrosis but little tumor growth delay. However, co-administration of serotonin with a suboptimal dose of DMXAA enhanced tumor necrosis and growth delay in Colon 38 tumors (Baguley et al., 1993). In a further study, co-administration of DMXAA and serotonin substantially increased DMXAA-induced vascular shutdown, tumor necrosis and growth delay in MDAH-MCa-4 tumors, without compromising the maximum tolerated dose of DMXAA (Lash et al., 1998). Unexpectedly, co-administration of cyproheptadine, an antagonist of the 5-HT$_2$ vascular receptor for serotonin, with a sub-optimal dose of DMXAA potentiated its induction of tumor necrosis and tumor growth delay (Zhao et al., 2001). Cyproheptadine alone had no activity and its potentiation of DMXAA activity was shown to result from a pharmacokinetic interaction, increasing both the plasma and tumor half-life of DMXAA (Zhao et al., 2001).

Nitric oxide (NO) is a potent biological messenger and induces a multitude of effects, including vasodilation, inhibition of platelet aggregation and enhanced vascular permeability. The NO donor trinitroglycerine, administered to mice, had no antitumor effect but co-administration enhanced the tumor growth delay induced by DMXAA (Baguley, unpublished data). Both FAA and DMXAA have been shown to induce NO in mice, with maximal concentrations occurring 12 hours after treatment (Thomsen et al., 1991), and DMXAA has been shown to induce NO synthase in mice (Moilanen et al., 1998). Taken together, these results suggest that NO production may contribute to the antitumor activity of DMXAA. On the other hand, the NO-synthase inhibitor, L-nitro-arginine, was found to enhance the antitumor effect of a suboptimal dose of DMXAA in Colon 38 tumor-bearing mice (Baguley, unpublished data). Since toxicity was also increased, it is likely that this is a result of a pharmacokinetic interaction.

9.7 Species differences

An important feature of DMXAA is the difference in dose potency among different species, particularly the 12-fold difference in MTD between mice and rats (Table 9.1). In contrast, the MTD of FAA in rats is comparable to that in mice (O'Dwyer et al., 1987). Nevertheless, FAA has been reported to have antitumor activity in rats (Bowler and Pearson, 1992), and activity of DMXAA against rat tumors has also been observed in this laboratory (M. McKeage, personal communication).

The dose–response curves for both antivascular and antitumor activity of DMXAA in mice are steep and non-linear, with a threshold for activity at about 15 mg kg^{-1} (Lash et al., 1998; Siim et al., 2000). Antitumor activity is observed only at doses close to the maximum tolerated dose, providing a narrow ther-

Table 9.1 Maximum tolerated single doses of DMXAA between species

Species	DMXAA ($mg\,kg^{-1}$)	Reference
Mice	27.5	Zhao *et al.* (2002)
TNF$^{-/-}$ mice	>100	Ching, Zwain and Baguley (2004)
TNFR-1$^{-/-}$ mice	>100	Zhao *et al.* (2002)
Rats	330	Kestell *et al.* (1999)
Rabbits	99	Kestell *et al.* (1999)
Humans	*ca.* 120	Jameson *et al.* (2003)

apeutic window. This is often cited as a major limitation of DMXAA. However, studies with other species suggest that mice might be particularly sensitive to DMXAA.

The steep dose–response curve for DMXAA in mice may be a function of the induction of TNF. Studies with TNF receptor knockout (TNFR-1$^{-/-}$) mice suggest that the toxicity of DMXAA is related to DMXAA-induced production of TNF (Zhao *et al.*, 2002). The maximum tolerated dose of DMXAA in TNFR-1$^{-/-}$ mice (>100 $mg\,kg^{-1}$) was approximately four times higher than in wild-type mice (27.5 $mg\,kg^{-1}$) (Zhao *et al.*, 2002). It was interesting that administration of DMXAA (50 $mg\,kg^{-1}$) to TNFR-1$^{-/-}$ mice produced necrosis and growth delays of Colon 38 tumors equivalent to that produced by a lower dose (25 $mg\,kg^{-1}$) in wild-type mice, suggesting that although TNF contributes, it is not essential for the response of tumors to DMXAA (Zhao *et al.*, 2002).

There are also species differences in the plasma pharmacokinetics of DMXAA. In both rats and mice FAA is metabolized predominantly to the acyl glucuronide derivative (Cummings *et al.*, 1989), while DMXAA is extensively metabolized mainly by glucuronidation of its acetic acid side chain, and 6-methylhydroxylation, to give species that are excreted into bile and urine (Zhou *et al.*, 2002a, 2001c). Plasma pharmacokinetics are non-linear, presumably due to saturation of elimination mechanisms and of plasma protein binding. The effects differ among species, with the highest rate of plasma clearance observed in rabbits, followed by humans, rats and mice (Kestell *et al.*, 1999; Zhou *et al.*, 2002a). Similar differences in rates of DMXAA metabolism were observed *in vitro* using mouse, rat and rabbit microsomes (Zhou *et al.*, 2002c). The interspecies differences in pharmacokinetics of DMXAA could not account for the observed interspecies differences in maximum tolerated dose (Kestell *et al.*, 1999). In addition, gender differences have been reported in rats for plasma pharmacokinetics of DMXAA, with the rate of clearance 1.6 times higher in males than in females (Zhou *et al.*, 2002b), although no such gender differences were observed in mice (Zhou *et al.*, 2001b).

The above studies suggest that some species, particularly mice, might not be good models for the effects of DMXAA, especially in relation to host toxicity.

It is possible that in humans, and perhaps in species other than mice, DMXAA may have a wider therapeutic window. In Phase I clinical trials, DMXAA reduced DCE-MRI parameters related to blood flow over a wide dose range, consistent with a shallow dose–response curve for antivascular activity (Galbraith *et al.*, 2002).

9.8 Clinical studies

The unique preclinical antitumor spectrum of anticancer activity of FAA acid ester (LM985) led to high expectations of clinical activity. However, no responses were found in Phase I trials and reversible hypotension and neurological toxicity were the main side effects. Once FAA had been identified as the active product of hydrolysis of LM985 subsequent trials concentrated on FAA. A number of administration schedules were tested, generally comprising intravenous infusions for different times. Dose-limiting toxicities included hypotension, diarrhea, fatigue and an intense feeling of warmth (Kerr *et al.*, 1987). The maximum tolerated dose was approximately $13 \, \mathrm{g\,m^{-2}}$ when the drug was infused over 12 hours. One patient with renal cell cancer had a partial response of 3 months (Olver *et al.*, 1992) and a response in non-small-cell lung cancer was also reported (Siegenthaler *et al.*, 1992). Combination trials with cytotoxic agents were not reported, but combination trials with recombinant interleukin-2 (IL-2) were conducted. Tumor responses were noted but the response rate was similar to that obtained with IL-2 alone (O'Reilly *et al.*, 1993). FAA was not progressed further in the clinic.

DMXAA was selected for Phase I trial on the basis of its increased dose-potency with respect to FAA, as well as its ability to induce the synthesis of TNF in human cells, unlike FAA (Ching *et al.*, 1994). Two Phase I trials were initiated, where the drug was given by a 20 minute intravenous infusion: one where DMXAA was administered every 3 weeks (Jameson *et al.*, 2003), and one where it was administered weekly (Rustin *et al.*, 2003). At the maximum tolerated dose ($4.9 \, \mathrm{g\,m^{-2}}$), toxicities included confusion, tremor, slurred speech, visual disturbance and anxiety, all of which reversed following completion of the infusion. A partial response, for 24 weeks, was observed in one patient with metastatic cervical carcinoma.

A key feature of the clinical trial of DMXAA was the development of methods for the assessment of antivascular activity. Dynamic contrast-enhanced (DCE) magnetic resonance imaging (MRI) studies were performed in patients treated with DMXAA at doses from 0.5 to $4.9 \, \mathrm{g\,m^{-2}}$ in order to examine changes related to blood flow and permeability in tumor and muscle. Nine of 16 patients had significant reductions in DCE-MRI parameters, implying DMXAA-induced reduction in tumor blood flow (Galbraith *et al.*, 2002). Measurement of changes in plasma concentrations of the serotonin metabolite 5-HIAA, which is correlated with tumor blood flow changes in experimental studies (Ching, Zwain and

Baguley, 2004; Zhao *et al.*, 2005), was used as a second method for assessment of antivascular effects. In both Phase I trials, a dose-dependent increase in 5-HIAA was noted, and the time course of 5-HIAA production generally had a maximum of around 4 hours (Kestell *et al.*, 2001). A further method for assessment of antivascular effects, immunohistological assessment of tumor biopsy samples, was employed in a small number of cases. Induction of tumor endothelial cell apoptosis was observed in one of three patients (Ching *et al.*, 2002) and induction of von Willebrand factor, indicative of platelet activation, was observed in all three patients examined.

Dose-limiting toxicities of DMXAA in Phase I clinical trials appear to be distinct from most other anticancer therapies, providing an argument for combining DMXAA with other therapeutic agents in the clinic. Furthermore, based on excellent preclinical data demonstrating the efficacy of DMXAA in combination with cytotoxic agents (Siim *et al.*, 2003, 2005), DMXAA is being tested in a phase II programme of combination studies. A clinical trial is underway to evaluate DMXAA in combination with paclitaxel and carboplatin for the treatment of non-small-cell lung cancer, and further trials on patients with ovarian (with paclitaxel and carboplatin) and prostate cancer (with docetaxel) are planned.

References

Aitken, R.A., Bibby, M.C., Cooper, P.A., Double, J.A., Laws, A.L., Ritchie, R.B. and Wilson, D.W. (2000). Synthesis and antitumor activity of new derivatives of flavone-8-acetic acid (FAA). Part 4: Variation of the basic structure. *Arch Pharm (Weinheim)* 333 (6), 181–188.

Atassi, G., Briet, P., Berthelon, J.J. and Collonges, F. (1985). Synthesis and antitumor activity of some 8-substituted 4-oxo-4H-1-benzopyrans. *Eur J Medicinal Chem* 5, 393–402.

Baguley, B.C. (2003). Antivascular therapy of cancer: DMXAA. *Lancet Oncol* 4, 141–148.

Baguley, B.C. and Ching, L.M. (1997). Immunomodulatory actions of xanthenone anticancer drugs. *BioDrugs* 8, 119–127.

Baguley, B.C., Cole, G., Thomsen, L.L. and Li, Z. (1993). Serotonin involvement in the antitumor and host effects of flavone-8-acetic acid and 5,6-dimethylxanthenone-4-acetic acid. *Cancer Chemother Pharmacol* 33 (1), 77–81.

Baguley, B.C., Wang, L.C., Ching, L.M., Paxton, J., Ding, Q. and Kestell, P. (2004). Enhancement of the action of the antivascular drug 5,6-dimethylxanthenone-4-acetic acid (DMXAA) by co-administration of non-steroidal anti-inflammatory drugs. *Eur J Cancer, Supplement* 2, 44.

Baguley, B.C. and Wilson, W.R. (2002). Potential of DMXAA combination therapy for solid tumors. *Exp Rev Anticancer Ther* 2 (5), 593–603.

Baguley, B.C., Zhuang, L. and Kestell, P. (1997). Increased plasma serotonin following treatment with flavone-8-acetic acid, 5,6-dimethylxanthenone-4-acetic acid, vinblastine, and colchicine: relation to vascular effects. *Oncol Res* 9 (2), 55–60.

Bellnier, D.A. (1991). Potentiation of photodynamic therapy in mice with recombinant human tumor necrosis factor-alpha. *J Photochem Photobiol B* 8 (2), 203–210.

Bellnier, D.A., Gollnick, S.O., Camacho, S.H., Greco, W.R. and Cheney, R.T. (2003). Treatment with the tumor necrosis factor-alpha-inducing drug 5,6-dimethylxanthenone-4-acetic acid enhances the antitumor activity of the photodynamic therapy of RIF-1 mouse tumors. *Cancer Res* **63** (22), 7584–7590.

Bowler, K. and Pearson, J.A. (1992). Long-term effects of flavone acetic acid on the growth of a rat tumor. *Anticancer Res* **12** (4), 1275–1279.

Brown, J.M. (2002). Tumor microenvironment and the response to anticancer therapy. *Cancer Biol Ther* **1** (5), 453–458.

Cao, Z., Baguley, B.C. and Ching, L.M. (2001). Interferon-inducible protein 10 induction and inhibition of angiogenesis in vivo by the antitumor agent 5,6-dimethylxanthenone-4-acetic acid (DMXAA). *Cancer Res* **61** (4), 1517–1521.

Cao, Z., Joseph, W.R., Browne, W.L., Mountjoy, K.G., Palmer, B.D., Baguley, B.C. and Ching, L.M. (1999). Thalidomide increases both intra-tumoral tumor necrosis factor-alpha production and anti-tumor activity in response to 5,6-dimethylxanthenone-4-acetic acid. *Br J Cancer* **80**, (5/6), 716–723.

Chaplin, D.J., Pettit, G.R., Parkins, C.S. and Hill, S.A. (1996). Antivascular approaches to solid tumor therapy: evaluation of tubulin binding agents. *Br J Cancer* **74** (Suppl. 27), S86–S88.

Ching, L.M. and Baguley, B.C. (1987). Induction of natural killer cell activity by the antitumor compound flavone acetic acid (NSC 347 512). *Eur J Cancer Clin Oncol* **23** (7), 1047–1050.

Ching, L.M., Cao, Z., Kieda, C., Zwain, S., Jameson, M.B. and Baguley, B.C. (2002). Induction of endothelial cell apoptosis by the antivascular agent 5,6-dimethylxanthenone-4-acetic acid. *Br J Cancer* **86** (12), 1937–1942.

Ching, L.M., Goldsmith, D., Joseph, W.R., Korner, H., Sedgwick, J.D. and Baguley, B.C. (1999). Induction of intratumoral tumor necrosis factor (TNF) synthesis and hemorrhagic necrosis by 5,6-dimethylxanthenone-4-acetic acid (DMXAA) in TNF knockout mice. *Cancer Res* **59** (14), 3304–3307.

Ching, L.M., Joseph, W.R., Crosier, K.E. and Baguley, B.C. (1994). Induction of tumor necrosis factor-alpha messenger RNA in human and murine cells by the flavone acetic acid analogue 5,6-dimethylxanthenone- 4-acetic acid (NSC 640488). *Cancer Res* **54** (4), 870–872.

Ching, L.M., Xu, Z.F., Gummer, B.H., Palmer, B.D., Joseph, W.R. and Baguley, B.C. (1995). Effect of thalidomide on tumor necrosis factor production and anti- tumor activity induced by 5,6-dimethylxanthenone-4-acetic acid. *Br J Cancer* **72** (2), 339–343.

Ching, L.M., Zwain, S. and Baguley, B.C. (2004). Relationship between tumor endothelial cell apoptosis and tumor blood flow shutdown following treatment with the antivascular agent DMXAA in mice. *Br J Cancer* **90** (4), 906–910.

Cliffe, S., Taylor, M.L., Rutland, M., Baguley, B.C., Hill, R.P. and Wilson, W.R. (1994). Combining bioreductive drugs (SR 4233 or SN 23862) with the vasoactive agents flavone acetic acid or 5,6-dimethylxanthenone acetic acid. *Int J Radiat Oncol Biol Phys* **29** (2), 373–377.

Cummings, J., Double, J.A., Bibby, M.C., Farmer, P., Evans, S., Kerr, D.J., Kaye, S.B. and Smyth, J.F. (1989). Characterization of the major metabolites of flavone acetic acid and comparison of their disposition in humans and mice. *Cancer Res* **49** (13), 3587–3593.

Edwards, H.S., Bremner, J.C. and Stratford, I.J. (1991a). Induction of hypoxia in the KHT sarcoma by tumor necrosis factor and flavone acetic acid. *Int J Radiat Biol* **59**, 419–32.

Edwards, H.S., Bremner, J.C. and Stratford, I.J. (1991b). Induction of tumor hypoxia by FAA and TNF: interaction with bioreductive drugs. *Int J Radiat Biol* **60**, 373–377.

Galbraith, S.M., Rustin, G.J., Lodge, M.A., Taylor, N.J., Stirling, J.J., Jameson, M., Thompson, P., Hough, D., Gumbrell, L. and Padhani, A.R. (2002). Effects of 5,6-dimethylxanthenone-4-acetic acid on human tumor microcirculation assessed by dynamic contrast-enhanced magnetic resonance imaging. *J Clin Oncol* **20** (18), 3826–3840.

Gobbi, S., Rampa, A., Bisi, A., Belluti, F., Piazzi, L., Valenti, P., Caputo, A., Zampiron, A. and Carrara, M. (2003). Synthesis and biological evaluation of 3-alkoxy analogues of flavone-8-acetic acid. *J Medicinal Chem* **46** (17), 3662–3669.

Gobbi, S., Rampa, A., Bisi, A., Belluti, F., Valenti, P., Caputo, A., Zampiron, A. and Carrara, M. (2002). Synthesis and antitumor activity of new derivatives of xanthen-9-one-4-acetic acid. *J Medicinal Chem* **45** (22), 4931–4939.

Havsteen, B. (1983). Flavonoids, a class of natural products of high pharmacological potency. *Biochem Pharmacol* **32** (7), 1141–1148.

Hendrix, M.J., Seftor, E.A., Hess, A.R. and Seftor, R.E. (2003). Vasculogenic mimicry and tumor-cell plasticity: lessons from melanoma. *Nature Rev Cancer* **3** (6), 411–421.

Jameson, M.B., Thompson, P.I., Baguley, B.C., Evans, B.D., Harvey, V.J., Porter, D.J., McCrystal, M.R. and Kestell, P. (2000). Phase I pharmacokinetic and pharmacodynamic study of 5,6-dimethylxanthenone-4-acetic acid (DMXAA), a novel antivascular agent. *Proc Am Soc Clin Oncol* **19**, 705.

Jameson, M.B., Thompson, P.I., Baguley, B.C., Evans, B.D., Harvey, V.J., Porter, D.J., McCrystal, M.R., Small, M., Bellenger, K., Gumbrell, L., Halbert, G.W. and Kestell, P. (2003). Clinical aspects of a phase I trial of 5,6-dimethylxanthenone-4-acetic acid (DMXAA), a novel antivascular agent. *Br J Cancer* **88** (12), 1844–1850.

Kelland, L.R. (2005). Targeting established tumor vasculature: a novel approach to cancer treatment. *Curr Cancer Ther Rev* **1**, 1–9.

Kerr, D.J., Kaye, S.B., Cassidy, J., Bradley, C., Rankin, E.M., Adams, L., Setanoians, A., Young, T., Forrest, G., Soukop, M. and ••. (1987). Phase I and pharmacokinetic study of flavone acetic acid. *Cancer Res* **47** (24), 6776–6781.

Kestell, P., Paxton, J.W., Rewcastle, G.W., Dunlop, I. and Baguley, B.C. (1999). Plasma disposition, metabolism and excretion of the experimental antitumor agent 5,6-dimethylxanthenone-4-acetic acid in the mouse, rat and rabbit. *Cancer Chemother Pharmacol* **43** (4), 323–330.

Kestell, P., Zhao, L., Baguley, B.C., Palmer, B.D., Muller, G., Paxton, J.W. and Ching, L.M. (2000). Modulation of the pharmacokinetics of the antitumor agent 5,6-dimethylxanthenone-4-acetic acid (DMXAA) in mice by thalidomide. *Cancer Chemother Pharmacol* **46** (2), 135–141.

Kestell, P., Zhao, L., Jameson, M.B., Stratford, M.R., Folkes, L.K. and Baguley, B.C. (2001). Measurement of plasma 5-hydroxyindoleacetic acid as a possible clinical surrogate marker for the action of antivascular agents. *Clinica Chimica Acta* **314** (1/2), 159–166.

Lash, C.J., Li, A.E., Rutland, M., Baguley, B.C., Zwi, L.J. and Wilson, W.R. (1998). Enhancement of the anti-tumor effects of the antivascular agent 5,6-dimethylxanthenone-4-acetic acid (DMXAA) by combination with 5-hydroxytryptamine and bioreductive drugs. *Br J Cancer* **78** (4), 439–445.

Mace, K.F., Hornung, R.L., Wiltrout, R.H. and Young, H.A. (1990). Correlation between in vivo induction of cytokine gene expression by flavone acetic acid and strict dose dependency and therapeutic efficacy against murine renal cancer. *Cancer Res* **50** (6), 1742–1747.

Moilanen, E., Thomsen, L.L., Miles, D.W., Happerfield, D.W., Knowles, R.G. and Moncada, S. (1998). Persistent induction of nitric oxide synthase in tumors from mice treated with the anti-tumor agent 5,6-dimethylxanthenone-4-acetic acid. *Br J Cancer* **77** (3), 426–433.

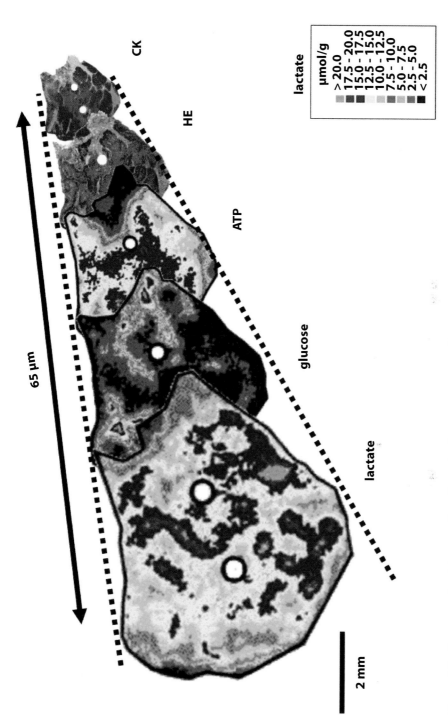

Figure 2.9 Sequence of serial cryosections through a human squamous cell carcinoma of the head and neck (HNSCC) (courtesy of Professor W. Mueller-Klieser and Dr. S. Walenta, Institute of Physiology and Pathophysiology, University of Mainz)

lactate

μmol/g
>20.0
17.5 – 20.0
15.0 – 17.5
12.5 – 15.0
10.0 – 12.5
7.5 – 10.0
5.0 – 7.5
2.5 – 5.0
<2.5

CK

HE

ATP

glucose

lactate

65 μm

2 mm

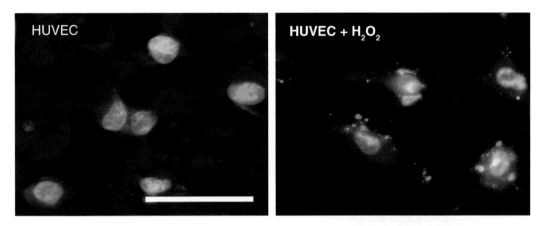

Figure 10.1   Treatment *in vitro* of HUVEC cells leads to exposure of PS on the cell membrane

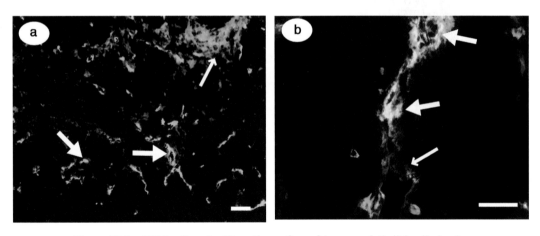

Figure 10.2   3G4 localizes to PS on the surface of tumor endothelial cells *in vivo*

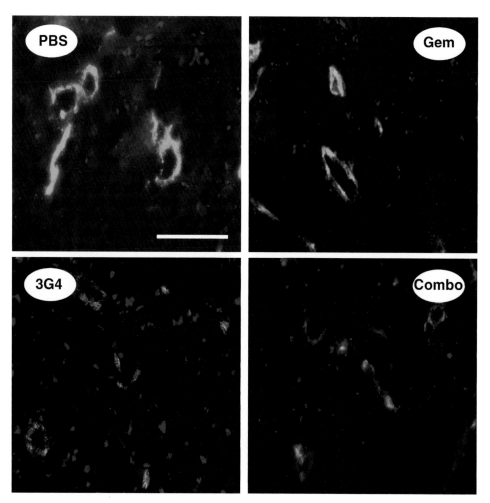

Figure 10.3 Macrophage infiltration is increased in animals treated with both gemcitabine and 3G4

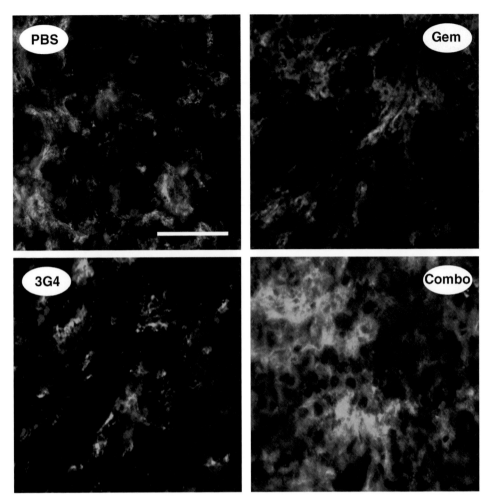

Figure 10.4 Treatment with 3G4 alone decreases microvessel density (MVD) in MiaPaCa-2 pancreatic tumors

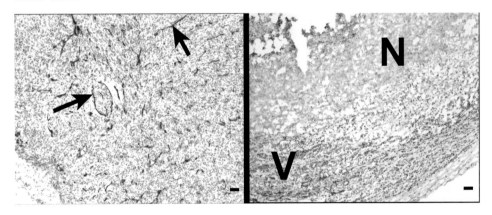

Figure 10.5 Inhibition of tumor vasculature of tumors from 3G4-treated mice

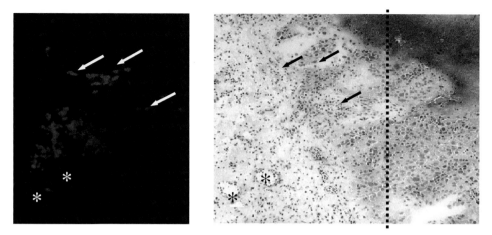

Figure 13.1 Accumulation of tumor imaging agent LipoRed in blood vessels of a patient with bladder cancer. LipoRed is a cationic liposome formulation loaded with the fluorescent dye rhodamine

Normal

Tumor

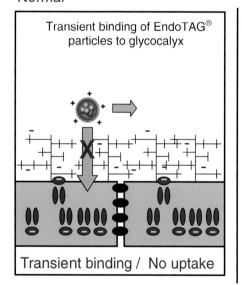

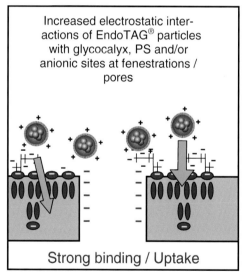

Figure 13.2 Schematic diagram depicting the changes in angiogenic versus quiescent endothelium that are important for understanding the vascular targeting properties of cationic lipid complexes

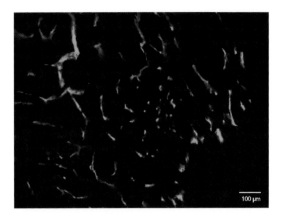

FITC-lectin

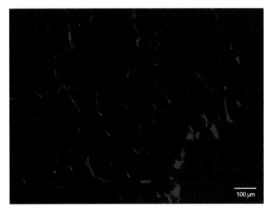

Rh-EndoTAG®-2

Figure 13.3 Vascular localization of rhodamine-labeled EndoTAG-2 in B-16 melanoma (red), 20 min after intravenous administration. Intravenous injected FITC-lectin (green) served as counterstain to label tumor blood vessels

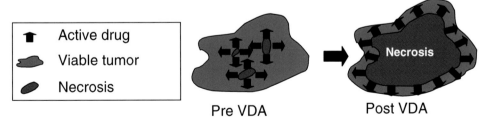

Figure 15.4 Schematic diagram for combination of CDEPT with vascular-disrupting agents (VDAs). Active drug is the anticancer drug generated from its prodrug form by the enzyme expressed in anaerobes

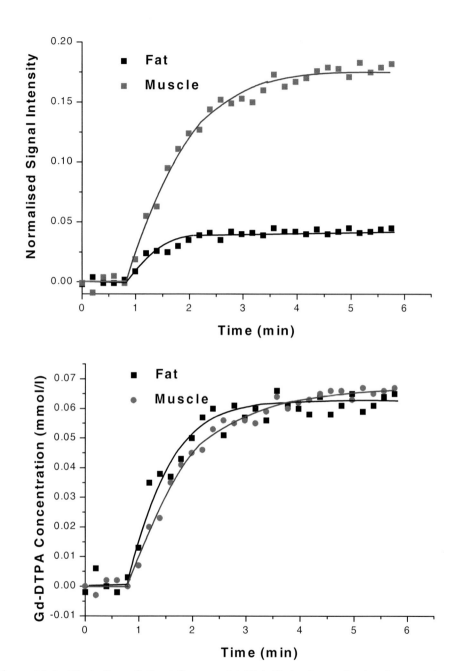

Figure 16.1 Illustration of the influence of initial T1 level on signal enhancement and gradient

Pre treatment 4 hours post 1st dose 24 hours post 1st dose

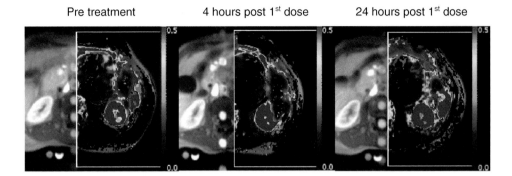

13 days post 3rd dose 13 days post 6th dose

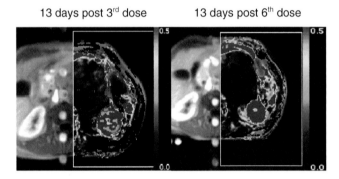

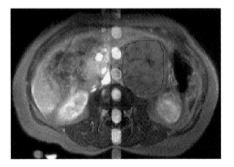

Figure 16.2 Serial K^{trans} parametric maps overlain on transverse T1-weighted images for a patient in the phase I trial of CA4P. Scale = K^{trans} $ml\,ml^{-1}min^{-1}$. Bottom, T2-weighted anatomical image. Note the increase in non-enhancing pixels by the end of treatment

Murata, R., Overgaard, J. and Horsman, M.R. (2001). Potentiation of the anti-tumor effect of hyperthermia by combining with the vascular targeting agent 5,6-dimethylxanthenone-4-acetic acid. *Int J Hyperthermia* **17** (6), 508–519.

Murata, R., Siemann, D.W., Overgaard, J. and Horsman, M.R. (2001). Improved tumor response by combining radiation and the vascular-damaging drug 5,6-dimethylxanthe-none-4-acetic acid. *Radiat Res* **156** (5), 503–509.

Nakanishi, M., Oe, T., Tsuruda, M., Matsuo, H., Sakuragi, S. and Maruyama, Y. (1975). Studies on the synthesis and anti-inflammatory activity of xanthenyl- and benzo-pyranopyridinylacetic acid derivatives. *Studies on Anti-Inflammatory Agents. XXXI.*

O'Dwyer, P.J., Shoemaker, D., Zaharko, D.S., Grieshaber, C., Plowman, J., Corbett, T., Valeriote, F., King, S.A., Cradock, J., Hoth, D.F. and Leyland-Jones, B. (1987). Flavone acetic acid (LM 975, NSC 347512) a novel antitumor agent. *Cancer Chemother Pharma-col* **19**, 6–10.

OReilly, S.M., Rustin, G.J., Farmer, K., Burke, M., Hill, S. and Denekamp, J. (1993). Flavone acetic acid (FAA) with recombinant interleukin-2 (rIL-2) in advanced malignant mela-noma: I. Clinical and vascular studies. *Br J Cancer* **67** (6), 1342–1345.

Olver, I.N., Webster, L.K., Bishop, J.F. and Stokes, K.H. (1992). A phase I and pharmacoki-netic study of 12-h infusion of flavone acetic acid. *Cancer Chemother Pharmacol* **29** (5), 354–360.

Parkins, C.S., Chadwick, J.A. and Chaplin, D.J. (1994). Enhancement of chlorambucil cyto-toxicity by combination with flavone acetic acid in a murine tumor. *Anticancer Res* **14** (4A), 1603–1608.

Parkins, C.S., Denekamp, J. and Chaplin, D.J. (1993). Enhancement of mitomycin-C cyto-toxicity by combination with flavone acetic acid in a murine tumor. *Anticancer Res* **13** (5A), 1437–1442.

Pedley, R.B., Begent, R.H., Boden, J.A., Boxer, G.M., Boden, R. and Keep, P.A. (1994). Enhancement of radioimmunotherapy by drugs modifying tumor blood flow in a colonic xenograft model. *Int J Cancer* **57** (6), 830–835.

Pedley, R.B., Boden, J.A., Boden, R., Boxer, G.M., Flynn, A.A., Keep, P.A. and Begent, R.H. (1996). Ablation of colorectal xenografts with combined radioimmunotherapy and tumor blood flow-modifying agents. *Cancer Res* **56** (14), 3293–3300.

Philpott, M., Baguley, B.C. and Ching, L.M. (1995). Induction of tumor necrosis factor-alpha by single and repeated doses of the antitumor agent 5,6-dimethylxanthenone-4-acetic acid. *Cancer Chemother Pharmacol* **36** (2), 143–148.

Philpott, M., Ching, L. and Baguley, B.C. (2001). The antitumor agent 5,6-dimethylxanthe-none-4-acetic acid acts in vitro on human mononuclear cells as a co-stimulator with other inducers of tumor necrosis factor. *Eur J Cancer* **37** (15), 1930–1937.

Plowman, J., Narayanan, V.L., Dykes, D., Szarvasi, E., Briet, P., Yoder, O.C. and Paull, K. D. (1986). Flavone acetic acid: a novel agent with preclinical antitumor activity against colon adenocarcinoma 38 in mice. *Cancer Treatment Reports* **70** (5), 631–635.

Pruijn, F.B., van Daalen, M., Holford, N.H. and Wilson, W.R. (1997). Mechanisms of enhancement of the antitumor activity of melphalan by the tumor-blood-flow inhibitor 5,6-dimethylxanthenone-4-acetic acid. *Cancer Chemother Pharmacol* **39** (6), 541–546.

Rewcastle, G.W., Atwell, G.J., Baguley, B.C., Boyd, M., Thomsen, L.L., Zhuang, L. and Denny, W.A. (1991a). Potential antitumor agents. 63. Structure–activity relationships for side-chain analogues of the colon 38 active agent 9-oxo-9H-xanthene-4-acetic acid. *J Medicinal Chem* **34** (9), 2864–2870.

Rewcastle, G.W., Atwell, G.J., Baguley, B.C., Calveley, S.B. and Denny, W.A. (1989). Potential antitumor agents. 58. Synthesis and structure–activity relationships of substituted xanthenone-4-acetic acids active against the colon 38 tumor in vivo. *J Medicinal Chem* **32** (4), 793–799.

Rewcastle, G.W., Atwell, G.J., Li, Z.A., Baguley, B.C. and Denny, W.A. (1991b). Potential antitumor agents. 61. Structure–activity relationships for in vivo colon 38 activity among disubstituted 9-oxo-9H-xanthene-4-acetic acids. *J Medicinal Chem* **34** (1), 217–222.

Rewcastle, G.W., Atwell, G.J., Palmer, B.D., Boyd, P.D., Baguley, B.C. and Denny, W.A. (1991c). Potential antitumor agents. 62. Structure–activity relationships for tricyclic compounds related to the colon tumor active drug 9-oxo-9H- xanthene-4-acetic acid. *J Medicinal Chem* **34** (2), 491–496.

Rustin, G.J., Bradley, C., Galbraith, S., Stratford, M., Loadman, P., Waller, S., Bellenger, K., Gumbrell, L., Folkes, L. and Halbert, G. (2003). 5,6-dimethylxanthenone-4-acetic acid (DMXAA), a novel antivascular agent: phase I clinical and pharmacokinetic study. *Br J Cancer* **88** (8), 1160–1167.

Siegenthaler, P., Kaye, S.B., Monfardini, S. and Renard, J. (1992). Phase II trial with flavone acetic acid (NSC.347512, LM975) in patients with non-small cell lung cancer. *Ann Oncol* **3** (2), 169–170.

Siemann, D.W., Mercer, E., Lepler, S. and Rojiani, A.M. (2002). Vascular targeting agents enhance chemotherapeutic agent activities in solid tumor therapy. *Int J Cancer* **99** (1), 1–6.

Siim, B.G., Laux, W.T., Rutland, M.D., Palmer, B.N. and Wilson, W.R. (2000). Scintigraphic imaging of the hypoxia marker (^{99m})technetium-labeled 2,2′-(1,4-diaminobutane)bis(2-methyl-3-butanone) dioxime (^{99m}Tc-labeled HL-91; Prognox): noninvasive detection of tumor response to the antivascular agent 5,6-dimethylxanthenone-4-acetic acid. *Cancer Res* **60** (16), 4582–4588.

Siim, B.G., Lee, A.E., Shalal-Zwain, S., Pruijn, F.B., McKeage, M.J. and Wilson, W.R. (2003). Marked potentiation of the antitumor activity of chemotherapeutic drugs by the anti-vascular agent 5,6-dimethylxanthenone-4-acetic acid (DMXAA). *Cancer Chem Pharmacol* **51** (1), 43–52.

Siim, B.G., Wong, E., Kelland, L. and Wilson, W.R. (2005). Antitumor activity of paclitaxel in combination with the antivascular agent 5,6-dimethylxanthenone-4-acetic acid (DMXAA; AS1404) against murine and human tumor models. submitted.

Slaviero, K.A., Clarke, S.J. and Rivory, L.P. (2003). Inflammatory response: an unrecognised source of variability in the pharmacokinetics and pharmacodynamics of cancer chemo-therapy. *Lancet Oncol* **4** (4), 224–232.

Sun, J.R. and Brown, J.M. (1989). Enhancement of the antitumor effect of flavone acetic acid by the bioreductive cytotoxic drug SR 4233 in a murine carcinoma. *Cancer Res* **49** (20), 5664–5670.

Thomsen, L.L., Ching, L.M., Zhuang, L., Gavin, J.B. and Baguley, B.C. (1991). Tumor-dependent increased plasma nitrate concentrations as an indication of the antitumor effect of flavone-8-acetic acid and analogues in mice. *Cancer Res* **51** (1), 77–81.

Tozer, G.M., Kanthou, C. and Baguley, B.C. (2005). Disrupting tumor blood vessels: com-bretastatins, DMXAA and other low molecular weight drugs. *Nature Rev Cancer* **5**, 423–435.

Valenti, P., Bisi, A., Rampa, A., Belluti, F., Gobbi, S., Zampiron, A. and Carrara, M. (2000). Synthesis and biological activity of some rigid analogues of flavone-8-acetic acid. *Bioorganic Medicinal Chem* **8** (1), 239–246.

Veszelovsky, E., Holford, N.H., Thomsen, L.L., Knowles, R.G. and Baguley, B.C. (1995). Plasma nitrate clearance in mice: modeling of the systemic production of nitrate follow-ing the induction of nitric oxide synthesis. *Cancer Chemother Pharmacol* **36** (2), 155–159.

Vincent, P.W., Roberts, B.J., Elliot, W.L. and Leopold, W.R. (1997). Chemotherapy with DMXAA (5,6-dimethylxanthenone-4-acetic acid) in combination with CI-1010 (1H-imidazole-1-ethanol,alpha-[[(2-bromoethyl)amino]methyl]-2-nitro-,mono hydrobromide (R isomer)) against advanced stage murine colon carcinoma 26. *Oncol Rep* **4**, 143–147.

Wang, L.C., Reddy, C.B., Baguley, B.C., Kestell, P., Sutherland, R. and Ching, L.M. (2004). Induction of tumor necrosis factor and interferon-gamma in cultured murine splenocytes by the antivascular agent DMXAA and its metabolites. *Biochem Pharmacol* **67** (5), 937–945.

Wilson, W.R., Denny, W.A., Pullen, S.M., Thompson, K.M., Li, A.E., Patterson, L.H. and Lee, H.H. (1996). Tertiary amine N-oxides as bioreductive drugs: DACA N-oxide, nitracrine N-oxide and AQ4N. *Br J Cancer Supplement* **27**, S43–S47.

Wilson, W.R., Li, A.E., Cowan, D.S. and Siim, B.G. (1998). Enhancement of tumor radiation response by the antivascular agent 5,6-dimethylxanthenone-4-acetic acid. *Int J Radiat Oncol Biol Phys* **42** (4), 905–908.

Wilson, W.R. and Pruijn, F.B. (1995). Hypoxia–activated prodrugs as antitumor agents: strategies for maximizing tumor cell killing. *Clin Exp Pharmacol Physiol* **22** (11), 881–885.

Woon, S.T., Baguley, B.C., Palmer, B.D., Fraser, J.D. and Ching, L.M. (2002). Uptake of the antivascular agent 5,6-dimethylxanthenone-4-acetic acid (DMXAA) and activation of NF-kappaB in human tumor cell lines. *Oncol Res* **13** (2), 95–101.

Zhao, L., Ching, L.M., Kestell, P. and Baguley, B.C. (2002). The antitumor activity of 5,6-dimethylxanthenone-4-acetic acid (DMXAA) in TNF receptor-1 knockout mice. *Br J Cancer* **87** (4), 465–470.

Zhao, L., Ching, L.M., Kestell, P. and Baguley, B.C. (2003). Improvement of the antitumor activity of intraperitoneally and orally administered 5,6-dimethylxanthenone-4-acetic acid by optimal scheduling. *Clin Cancer Res* **9** (17), 6545–6550.

Zhao, L., Ching, L.M., Kestell, P., Kelland, L.R. and Baguley, B.C. (2005). Mechanisms of tumor vascular shut-down induced by 5,6-dimethylxanthenone-4-acetic acid (DMXAA); increased tumor vascular permeability. *Int J Cancer*, **116**, 322–326.

Zhao, L., Edgar, S., Marshall, E., Kelland, L. and Baguley, B.C. (2004). Inhibition of vasculogenic mimicry in melanoma by the antivascular drug 5,6 dimethylxanthenone-4-acetic acid (DMXAA). *Eur J Cancer Supplement* **2**, 47.

Zhao, L., Kestell, P., Philpott, M., Ching, L.M., Zhuang, L. and Baguley, B.C. (2001). Effects of the serotonin receptor antagonist cyproheptadine on the activity and pharmacokinetics of 5,6-dimethylxanthenone-4-acetic acid (DMXAA). *Cancer Chemother Pharmacol* **47** (6), 491–497.

Zhou, S., Kestell, P., Baguley, B.C. and Paxton, J.W. (2002a). 5,6-dimethylxanthenone-4-acetic acid (DMXAA): a new biological response modifier for cancer therapy. *Invest New Drugs* **20** (3), 281–295.

Zhou, S., Kestell, P., Tingle, M.D., Ching, L.M. and Paxton, J.W. (2001a). A difference between the rat and mouse in the pharmacokinetic interaction of 5,6-dimethylxanthenone-4-acetic acid with thalidomide. *Cancer Chemother Pharmacol* **47** (6), 541–544.

Zhou, S., Kestell, P., Tingle, M.D. and Paxton, J.W. (2002b). Gender differences in the metabolism and pharmacokinetics of the experimental anticancer agent 5,6-dimethylxanthenone-4-acetic acid (DMXAA). *Cancer Chemother Pharmacol* **49** (2), 126–132.

Zhou, S., Paxton, J.W., Kestell, P., Tingle, M.D. and Ching, L.M. (2001b). In vitro and in vivo kinetic interactions of the antitumor agent 5,6-dimethylxanthenone-4-acetic acid with thalidomide and diclofenac. *Cancer Chemother Pharmacol* **47** (4), 319–326.

Zhou, S.F., Paxton, J.W., Tingle, M.D., Kestell, P., Jameson, M.B., Thompson, P.I. and Baguley, B.C. (2001c). Identification and reactivity of the major metabolite (beta-1-

glucuronide) of the anti-tumor agent 5,6-dimethylxanthenone-4-acetic acid (DMXAA) in humans. *Xenobiotica* **31** (5), 277–293.

Zhou, S.F., Tingle, M.D., Kestell, P. and Paxton, J.W. (2002c). Species differences in the metabolism of the antitumor agent 5,6-dimethylxanthenone-4-acetic acid in vitro: implications for prediction of metabolic interactions in vivo. *Xenobiotica* **32** (2), 87–107.

Zwi, L.J., Baguley, B.C., Gavin, J.B. and Wilson, W.R. (1989). Blood flow failure as a major determinant in the antitumor action of flavone acetic acid. *J Nat Cancer Inst* **81** (13), 1005–1013.

Zwi, L.J., Baguley, B.C., Gavin, J.B. and Wilson, W.R. (1994). Correlation between immune and vascular activities of xanthenone acetic acid antitumor agents. *Oncol Res* **6** (2), 79–85.

10

Targeting Inside-Out Phospholipids on Tumor Blood Vessels in Pancreatic Cancer

Adam W. Beck, Rolf A. Brekken and **Philip E. Thorpe**

Abstract

Vascular targeting is currently being explored as a new therapy for pancreatic cancer, and a promising new target is phosphatidylserine (PS). PS is an anionic phospholipid normally located on the inner leaflet of the plasma membrane. Oxidative stress in the microenvironment of tumors causes PS exposure on the surface of endothelial cells. PS-positive endothelial cells are functional and not apoptotic. PS is absent from the endothelium of normal tissues, and is therefore a highly specific marker of tumor vessels.

The antibody 3G4 binds PS and inhibits growth of a variety of tumors in mice. Here we highlight 3G4 as a treatment of pancreatic cancer in a mouse model. Inhibition of primary tumor growth and metastases at all sites was significant with 3G4 alone, and significantly enhanced by combination with gemcitabine. Thus, the combination of PS-targeting and gemcitabine might be an effective new drug combination for treatment of pancreatic cancer.

Keywords

Phosphatidylserine, Pancreatic, Cancer, Vascular, Targeting, Therapy, Oxidative, Antibody, Metastasis, Endothelial

10.1   Vascular targeting

Vascular-targeting agents (VTAs), now called ligand-directed vascular-disrupting agents (VDAs), are designed to damage tumor vasculature and cause a selective shutdown of blood supply to the tumor (Siemann *et al.*, 2005). Unlike

Vascular-targeted Therapies in Oncology   Edited by Dietmar W. Siemann
© 2006 John Wiley & Sons, Ltd.

anti-angiogenic therapies, which are directed at inhibiting the formation of new blood vessels, VDAs are intended to occlude pre-existing tumor blood vessels and cause tumor cell death from decreased delivery of oxygen and nutrients, with subsequent ischemia and hemorrhagic necrosis (Thorpe, 2004). The ideal vascular-targeted therapy should be directed specifically at tumor endothelium, with minimal effect on normal tissue physiology. The pathobiology of tumor endothelium allows for selective targeting of this nature.

Here we examine anionic phospholipids as a potential target for vascular-targeted therapy in pancreatic cancer. The development, progression and spread of pancreatic adenocarcinoma are dependent upon the angiogenic process. In fact, vascularity of pancreatic tumors correlates with metastatic spread of the tumor, while vessel density within pancreatic tumors is an independent predictor of mortality (Karademir *et al.*, 2000). Anionic phospholipids present a unique and novel target for therapy due to their exposure on the outer membrane of vascular endothelium specifically in the tumor microenvironment. *In vivo*, the anionic phospholipids are likely to be complexed with proteins that bind them specifically, including β2-glycoprotein I and prothrombin Factor V, which in turn provide opportunities for tumor vessel targeting.

10.2   Pancreatic cancer: the clinical need

Pancreatic adenocarcinoma is the fourth leading cause of cancer-related death in the United States with the mortality nearly equaling the diagnostic incidence each year. The disease continues to be refractory to all available therapies. Despite multiple experimental manipulations of these therapies, including changes in dose and timing of chemoradiation and performance of extended resections, there has been meager improvement, at best, in the prognosis of the disease. Currently, the overall median survival after diagnosis is 3–5 months; 12 month survival is only 10 per cent and five year survival is about three per cent (Bramhall *et al.*, 1995; Jemal *et al.*, 2002). Chemotherapeutics have provided some improvement in short-term survival of patients with inoperable pancreatic cancer (Palmer *et al.*, 1994; Glimelius 1998), but there has been no improvement in 5 year survival. Additionally, chemotherapy using a newer agent, gemcitabine, a nucleoside analog, has shown some benefit in regards to symptomatology, but has not demonstrated improvement in any objective measures of pancreatic cancer progression, including long-term survival (National Institute for Clinical Excellence, 2004). When technically feasible, surgery remains the primary treatment for the disease and is the only therapy that improves long-term survival. However, only about four per cent of the total population of pancreatic cancer patients is identified as candidates for curative resection. Unfortunately, after potentially curative resection (resection with negative margins), 70–80 per cent of patients will fail therapy due to local recurrence, peritoneal disease or disease in a distant site, especially liver metastases. No therapy is available that decreases the occurrence of metastases or treats them once they are found. Thus, novel therapies are needed to improve survival of this disease.

10.3   Phosphatidylserine

Membrane phospholipids

Anionic phospholipids are generally absent from the outer leaflet of the plasma membrane of resting mammalian cells. Phosphatidylserine (PS) is the most abundant anionic phospholipid and is tightly restricted to the inner leaflet of the plasma membrane in most cell types (Williamson and Schlegel, 1994; Zwaal and Schroit, 1997). Phosphatidylinositol, another major anionic phospholipid, is also located predominantly on the inner plasma membrane (Calderon and DeVries, 1997) along with the minor anionic phospholipids, phosphatidic acid and phosphatidylglycerol (Hinkovska-Galcheva *et al.*, 1989). Neutral phospholipids are also distributed asymmetrically in the plasma membrane with phosphatidylethanolamine (PE) predominantly in the inner leaflet and the choline-containing phospholipids phosphatidylcholine and sphingomyelin mainly in the outer leaflet.

Loss of PS asymmetry

Segregation of PS to the inner leaflet of the plasma membrane is maintained via an ATP-dependent transporter, aminophospholipid translocase (Devaux, 1992). Loss of asymmetry is caused either by inhibition of this translocase (Comfurius *et al.*, 1990) or activation of PS-exporting enzymes such as the ABC-1 floppase and scramblase (Zhou *et al.*, 1997). Loss of PS asymmetry is observed under a number of different pathologic and physiologic conditions, including programed cell death (Bombeli *et al.*, 1997; Blankenberg *et al.*, 1998), cell aging (Herrmann and Devaux, 1990), intercellular fusion of myoblasts (Sessions and Horwitz, 1981) and trophoblasts (Adler *et al.*, 1995), cell migration (Vogt *et al.*, 1996), activation of platelets (Rote *et al.*, 1993) and cell degranulation (Demo *et al.*, 1999). On endothelial cells, PS is externalized in response to calcium fluxes generated by exposure to thrombin (Qu *et al.*, 1996), hyperlipidemia (Lupu *et al.*, 1993), viral infection (van Geelen *et al.*, 1995), non-lytic concentrations of complement proteins C5b-9 (Christiansen *et al.*, 1997), or exposure to the calcium ionophore A23187 and phorbol myristate acetate (PMA) (Julien *et al.*, 1997). Additionally, spontaneous exposure of PS has been noted in malignant cells in the absence of exogenous agents or cellular injury (Utsugi *et al.*, 1991) and has been linked to malignant transformation (Sugimura *et al.*, 1994). A number of consequences result from exposure of PS on the outer surface of the cell. Macrophages recognize, attach and eliminate PS-positive senescent and apoptotic cells (McEvoy *et al.*, 1986; Christiansen *et al.*, 1997) via the PS receptor (PSR) (Fadok *et al.*, 2000). PS is also a mediator in T lymphocyte attachment to thrombin-activated endothelial cells (Qu *et al.*, 1996). The complement cascade is activated by PS and this contributes to the lysis of cells with exposed PS (Test and Mitsuyoshi, 1997). Additionally, PS exposure shifts the normal anti-coagulant nature of vascular endothelial cells to a pro-coagulant nature (Williamson and Schlegel, 1994; Bombeli *et al.*, 1997) by providing a negatively charged surface for coagulation complex assembly and activation (Bevers *et al.*, 1985; Dachary-Prigent *et al.*, 1996).

PS exposure on tumor endothelium

PS exposure is a general feature of tumor vascular endothelium in all tumor models that have been examined. These tumors include human tumors grown subcutaneously (LNCaP prostate, L540 Hodgkin's lymphoma, HT29 colon and NCI-H358 lung), human tumors grown orthotopically (MDA-MB-231 and MDA-MB-435 breast), syngeneic mouse tumors grown subcutaneously (Colo26 colon, 3LL, B16 melanoma, Meth A murine fibrosarcoma) and spontaneous mouse RIP-Tag pancreatic islet cell tumors (Ran *et al.*, 2002, 1998; Ran and Thorpe, 2002). Importantly, PS externalization on vascular endothelium is specific for tumor blood vessels and has not been found on blood vessels in normal tissues regardless of the model used (Ran and Thorpe, 2002). Depending on the tumor type and size, 15–40 per cent of tumor vessels are found to be PS positive (Ran and Thorpe, 2002). The vascular endothelium of PS-positive tumor vessels appears to be viable. The PS-positive endothelial cells lack markers of apoptosis, are morphologically intact, and the vessels are functional at transporting solutes and blood. PS exposure is likely due to stress conditions in the tumor microenvironment including cytokines, leukocytes, metabolites and hypoxia/reoxygenation conditions. These stresses elicit the production of reactive oxygen species, which may oxidize membrane phospholipids and generate calcium fluxes into the cytosol that inhibit aminophospholipid translocase or PS exporters. These conditions can be mimicked in culture by the use of sub-toxic levels of inflammatory cytokines (IL-1, TNF-α, interferon), hypoxia, acidity, thrombin and hydrogen peroxide, which induce PS exposure on endothelial cells without causing apoptosis (Ran and Thorpe, 2002). Taken together, these findings support the pursuit of PS as a target for VDA-based therapy or marker of vasculature in solid tumors. Cells that display PS can be localized *in vivo* with annexin V, a natural ligand for PS and other anionic phospholipids, which has been used to image activated platelets in thrombi, apoptotic cells in actively rejecting cardiac allografts and anti-Fas antibody-treated livers in rodents (Blankenberg *et al.*, 1998). Monoclonal antibodies specific for anionic phospholipids have also been used for localization of PS in animal models. For example,

9D2, a monoclonal antibody targeting anionic phospholipids, specifically localizes to tumor endothelium but not vasculature in normal tissues after intravenous (IV) injection in mice bearing various types of tumor (Ran et al., 2002).

10.4   Proof of concept studies

The '3G4' antibody

3G4, an antibody that binds anionic phospholipids complexed with $\beta2$-glycoprotein 1, is a mouse IgG3 that localizes to tumor vessels as well as individual tumor cells and necrotic regions within solid tumors (Ran et al., 2002; Ran and Thorpe, 2002). 3G4 binds to PS on both endothelial cells and tumor cells in vitro after treatment of the cells with H_2O_2 (Figure 10.1). The morphology of 3G4 binding to intact, non-permeabilized H_2O_2-treated HUVEC was determined by treating adherent cells with H_2O_2, washing the cells and staining them with 3G4 or control mouse IgG_3 followed by FITC-labeled goat anti-mouse IgG antibody (green in figure 10.1). The cytoplasm and nuclei were counterstained with Texas-red labeled phalloidin (red) or DAPI (blue), respectively. 3G4 bound to discrete regions of the plasma membrane, having the appearance of membrane blebs. PS on the surface of the cells using 3G4 (green) before (left) and after (right) treatment with H_2O_2. The scale bar in Figure 10.1 indicates $50\,\mu m$. Although the cells expose PS, they are not apoptotic, and many do not go on to apoptosis after this treatment. A human chimeric version of 3G4 termed Tarvacin^{TM} also binds to and localizes PS-$\beta2$-glycoprotein 1 complexes on tumor endothelial cells in vivo. In previous studies 3G4 has shown significant anti-tumor effects as a stand-alone therapy in multiple xenograft tumor models (Ran et al., 2005). The growth of both small and well established (200–500 mm^3) tumors was inhibited. Specifically, growth of orthotopic human breast tumors (MDA-MB-231 and MDA-MB-435), subcutaneous human prostate cancer (LNCaP) and syngeneic fibrosarcomas (Meth A) were inhibited by 75, 65, 50 and 90 per cent respectively, as compared with control treated animals. Histologic analysis of treated tumors demonstrated localization of 3G4 to tumor endothelium (Figure 10.2), reduced vascularization and disintegration of tumor vessels as well as increased necrosis within the tumors. These findings suggest a direct anti-vascular effect of targeting PS on tumor vascular endothelial cells. Figure 10.2 shows result when SCID mice bearing orthotopic human breast tumors (MDA-MB-435) were injected with $100\,\mu g$ 3G4. Six hours later, the mice were exsanguinated and their tumors removed. Frozen sections were stained with biotinylated goat anti-mouse IgG followed by FITC-streptavidin (green) to detect localized 3G4 and rat anti-mouse CD31 followed by Cy3 goat anti-rat IgG 9 (red) to detect vascular endothelium. A and B demonstrate low and high magnification respectively.

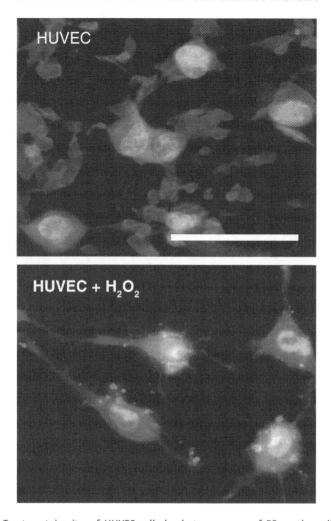

Figure 10.1 Treatment *in vitro* of HUVEC cells leads to exposure of PS on the cell membrane

Yellow staining (bold arrow (a) and (b)) indicates co-localization of PS to endothelial cells. The area with large amounts of FITC staining (thin arrow – A) indicates a necrotic area within the tumor. Areas without colocalized staining on the tumor endothelium (thin arrow – B) demonstrate heterogeneity of PS exposure within tumor endothelium. The scale bar in Figure 10.2 indicates 50 µm.

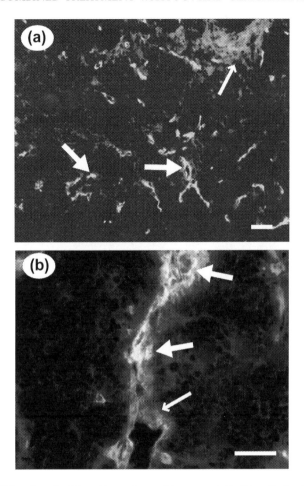

Figure 10.2   3G4 localizes to PS on the surface of tumor endothelial cells *in vivo*

10.5   Combined treatment with 3G4 and gemcitabine in a pancreatic cancer model

Pancreatic cancer modeling in mice

Our studies center around a mouse orthotopic model of pancreatic cancer. Heterotopic flank tumors have been used widely in the study of many cancers in mice, but despite their ease of placement and monitoring, flank tumors do not demonstrate the same growth patterns, angiogenesis, genetic expression or metastasis to distant sites as tumors grown in the pancreas. In our model, pancreatic adenocarcinoma cells stably transfected with enhanced green fluorescent protein (eGFP) are used to form orthotopic pancreatic tumors. Tumors are established in the mouse pancreas by performing a subcapsular injection of tumor cells into the tail of the pancreas at the splenic hilum. Tumors developed with this method reliably metastasize to the same principal sites as do pancreatic tumors in humans, including liver, peritoneum and lymph nodes. Additionally, mice with advanced tumors develop sequelae similar to those of humans, such as biliary obstruction with jaundice, malignant ascites and bowel obstructions from tumor invasion.

Effect of combination treatment on orthotopic pancreatic tumors

MiaPaCa-2 human pancreatic cancer cells expressing eGFP were injected under the capsule of the tail of the pancreas at the splenic hilum in athymic nude mice. Tumors were allowed to grow for 5 days before the onset of therapy. Animals were treated biweekly by intraperitoneal (i.p.) therapy with gemcitabine, 100 μg of 3G4, or a combination of gemcitabine and 3G4.

Final tumor weights were as follows: PBS group, 1440 (+/−165) mg; gemcitabine alone group, 742 (+/−63) mg; 3G4 alone group, 990 (+/−146) mg; combination therapy group 447 (+/−42) mg. The final tumor weights represent a reduced primary tumor growth of 48.4 per cent ($p < 0.001$ versus control) in the gemcitabine group, 31.1 per cent ($p = 0.054$ versus control) in the 3G4 alone group and 69.0 per cent ($p < 0.001$ versus control) in the combination therapy group. Although the 3G4 alone group did not reach statistical significance, the combination of 3G4 with gemcitabine resulted in a reduction of tumor growth that is significantly different from either therapy alone, suggesting that gemcitabine enhances 3G4 function, or *vice versa*.

Effect of combination therapy on metastasis

The most striking finding of this study is that 3G4 significantly reduced metastasis formation. Metastatic burden (liver, lymph node and peritoneal) was evaluated by examination of the abdominal cavity with the naked eye and by using blue light (485 nm) for evaluation of eGFP-expressing tumor cells. Mean visible liver metastases were reduced versus control (PBS group) by 59, 68 and 92 per cent (all $p < 0.001$) by treatment with gemcitabine alone, 3G4 alone or combination therapy, respectively. The incidence of liver metastasis was 4/11 animals in the combination therapy group (36 per cent), and 11/11 in the control group (100 per cent). Mean peritoneal metastatic lesions were reduced versus control by 63 per cent ($p < 0.001$) in the gemcitabine group 56 per cent ($p < 0.001$) in the 3G4 alone group and 83 per cent ($p < 0.001$) in the combination group. The reductions of lymph node metastases versus control were 64 per cent ($p < 0.001$) for the gemcitabine group, 73 per cent ($p < 0.001$) for 3G4 alone and 86 per cent ($p < 0.001$) in the combination therapy group.

Animal health

There were marked differences in the clinical courses of the animals in this study. The control animals had a high incidence of ascites, 9/11 (82 per cent), and generally appeared ill at the end of the experiment. In contrast, the combination therapy group had normal weight gain during the experiment and none of the animals developed ascites. Additionally, the combination therapy animals were well groomed, active and had no signs of distress. Weight gain in the combination therapy animals was normal throughout the duration of the experiment, demonstrating that there was no apparent toxicity to this therapeutic regimen.

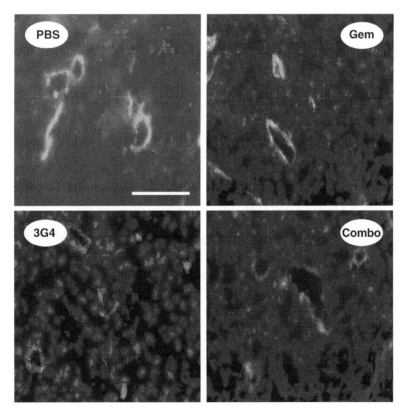

Figure 10.3   Treatment with 3G4 alone decreases microvessel density (MVD) in MiaPaCa-2 pancreatic tumors

10.6 Mechanism of action

Macrophage infiltration of tumors

Prior studies (Ran *et al.*, 2005) have demonstrated increased macrophage infiltration into tumors treated with 3G4, and suggest this as a central portion of the mechanism of action of this therapy. Pancreatic tumors were analyzed for macrophage infiltration by immunohistochemistry using an antibody to a mouse macrophage marker, F4/80. Macrophage infiltration levels were increased over control levels in all groups, with the gemcitabine group having $4.2 \times$ control ($p = 0.06$), 3G4 alone $1.76 \times$ control ($p = 0.22$) and the combination group $14.4 \times$ control levels ($p < 0.01$).

Antivascular effects

The antitumor effects of 3G4 appear to be mediated at least in part by antivascular effects. Treatment with 3G4 decreased the vascular density in the tumors. Microvessel density (MVD) of tumors was evaluated using MECA-32, an antibody to vascular endothelial cells (Figure 10.4). Acetone fixed frozen sections of orthotopic pancreatic tumors harvested from animals treated with PBS (PBS in figure 10.4), gemicitabine (Gem), 3G4 (3G4) or gemcitabine + 3G4 (Combo) were stained with MECA32 (green), an antibody specific for mouse vascular endothelial cells. Tissues were counterstained with the DNA-binding dye Hoechst 33342 (blue). Pixel quantification demonstrated a 63 per cent reduction of MVD over control in the 3G4 group and 64 per cent reduction in the combination group. The scale bar in Figure 10.4 indicates $100 \mu m$. MVD was reduced in all treatment groups, with the 3G4 and combination groups reaching statistical significance. Comparing mean MVD values, 3G4 reduced MVD by 63 per cent ($p < 0.05$) and combination therapy decreased the MVD by 64 per cent ($p < 0.05$) (Figure 10.3). Acetone fixed frozen sections of orthotopic pancreatic tumors harvested from animals treated with PBS (PBS in figure 10.3), gemicitabine (Gem), 3G4 (3G4) or gemcitabine + 3G4 (Combo) were stained with F4/80 (green), an antibody specific for mouse macrophages. Tissues were counterstained with the DNA-binding dye Hoechst 33342 (blue). Pixel quantification demonstrated that tumor macrophage content was 14 times higher in the combination treated animals versus control. The scale bar in Figure 10.3 indicates $100 \mu m$. These results are consistent with findings in previous studies (Ran *et al.*, 2005) showing reduction of vessel density and plasma volume within breast tumors treated with 3G4. In untreated tumors, blood vessel distribution tends to be homogeneous throughout the majority of the tumor. In contrast, tumors treated with 3G4 demonstrate increased necrosis within the central portions of the tumor. Figure 10.5 demonstrates increased necrosis within breast tumors treated with 3G4. SCID mice bearing orthotopic MDA-MB-231 human breast

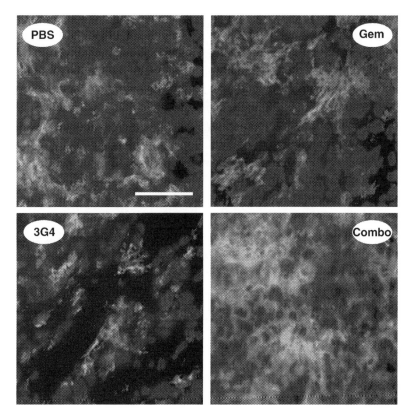

Figure 10.4   Macrophage infiltration is increased in animals treated with both gemcitabine and 3G4

tumors were treated with 3G4 (100 µg per dose) i.p. three times a week for two weeks. Mice were exsanguinated and tumors were removed. Frozen sections were prepared and stained with rat anti-mouse CD31 to detect vascular endothelium. Sections were counterstained with hematoxylin. Left, low magnification view of tumor section from control-treated mouse showing homogeneous distribution of blood vessels (arrows). Right, low magnification view of tumor section from 3G4-treated mouse showing necrotic (**N**) core surrounded by viable (**V**) tumor. The scale bars in Figure 10.5 represent 100 µm.

Role of host leukocytes in vascular damage

In addition to increasing macrophage infiltration into tumors, 3G4 likely enhances macrophage cytotoxicity in tumors through two mechanisms. (1) 3G4 may bind to PS and stimulate binding of macrophages through Fcγ receptors, thereby enhancing antibody-dependent cellular cytotoxicity (ADCC). In support

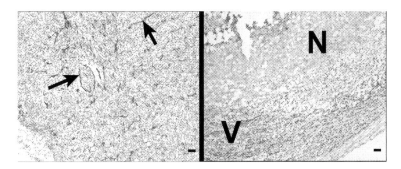

Figure 10.5   Inhibition of tumor vasculature of tumors from 3G4-treated mice

of this, activated macrophages are known to have direct tumoricidal activity, and antiphospholipid antibodies have been shown to facilitate opsonization of PS-expressing cells by macrophages (Manfredi *et al.*, 1998), which leads to induction of TNF-α production. (2) 3G4 may block PS-mediated signals from PS-expressing endothelial cells that would normally lead to a suppression of the inflammatory response. Perhaps binding of 3G4 to tumor endothelial cells causes exposure of the Fc portion of the antibody on the cell surface. This leads to binding of macrophages via an Fc receptor and subsequent pro-inflammatory response, leading to vascular endothelial destruction and ultimately decreased blood flow throughout the tumor. In this regard, 3G4 appears to differ from an agonistic antibody (mAb 217), which identifies PS receptors themselves and supresses inflammatory responses (Fadok *et al.*, 2000). The antitumor action of 3G4 has to be reconciled with the fact that tumor-associated macrophages can induce tumor angiogenesis, which promotes tumor growth. There is probably a balance between the proangiogenic effects of macrophages and their direct cytotoxic effects on tumor vessels and tumor cells that is determined by local conditions (e.g. hypoxia, TGF-β) in the tumor microenvironment. Perhaps 3G4 downregulates TGF-β production by macrophages leading to a downregulation of VEGF production by tumor cells or endothelial cells while simultaneously upregulating the direct cytotoxic activity of macrophages. Simply stated, 3G4 appears to shift the balance of macrophage activity from a pro-angiogenic phenotype to an antitumor inflammatory phenotype.

Enhanced antitumor effects of combination therapy

The effects of combination therapy of 3G4 and gemcitabine appear to be at least additive, if not synergistic, in leading to both decreased primary tumor size and decreased overall metastatic burden (Table 10.1). The mechanism of this improvement over single-drug therapy is potentially mediated by enhanced PS exposure of tumor endothelial cells by gemcitabine. We have found that subtoxic levels of

Table 10.1 3G4 controls the progression and spread of pancreatic cancer in the mouse model

Group	Mean tumor weight (mg)	Mean metastases/mouse			Ascites incidence (%)
		Liver	Peritoneal	LN	
PBS	1440	5.9	10.4	11.8	9/11 (82)
	(+/– 165)	(+/– 0.6)	(+/– 0.9)	(+/– 1.9)	
Gem	740	2.3	3.8	4.2	1/12 (8)
	(+/– 63)	(+/– 0.3)	(+/– 0.5)	(+/– 0.6)	
3G4	990	1.9	4.6	2.8	5/12 (42)
	(+/– 146)	(+/– 0.4)	(+/– 0.6)	(+/– 0.6)	
Combo	447	0.4	1.8	1.7	0/11 (0)
	(+/– 42)	(+/– 0.2)	(+/– 0.6)	(+/– 0.4)	

Animals were inspected at necropsy for final tumor weight, presence of ascites and number of metastatic lesions at the three principal sites of pancreatic cancer metastasis: liver, lymph node and peritoneum. Mean tumor weights and mean number of metastatic lesions in the liver, lymph nodes and peritoneum are shown. The tumor weight data are presented as mean number +/– standard error of the mean. Ascites incidence refers to the number of animals with ascites at necropsy in each group.

gemcitabine induce PS exposure of bovine aortic endothelial cells without inducing apoptosis *in vitro*. It is possible that this happens *in vivo* in tumor endothelial cells, enhancing PS binding and thereby enhancing macrophage infiltration and anti-vascular effects of 3G4. Additionally, treatment with combination therapy decreased metastases at all sites compared to control and single drug therapy. Metastatic dissemination of cancer is a highly selective process, consisting of a series of linked steps in which selected tumor cell(s) detach and are transported within the circulatory system (Fidler and Radinsky, 1990). There are many stresses involved in the steps of metastatic dissemination of tumor cells including shear stress in the vasculature and oxidative stress in the organ of arrest (especially the liver where sinusoidal endothelial cells release reactive oxygen species), as well as internal nitrosative stress in metastasizing cells themselves related to shear stress and 3D growth (Laguinge *et al.*, 2004). We believe that these stresses induce PS exposure on disseminating cells, which is then bound by 3G4 within the vascular system. Gemcitabine may further increase cell stress during metastasis, leading to enhanced PS exposure and binding of 3G4. Bound 3G4 potentiates binding and phagocytosis by macrophages, Kupffer cells and reticuloendothelial cells within the liver and elsewhere.

10.7 Conclusion

In an orthotopic mouse model of pancreatic cancer, combination of gemcitabine with an antibody directed to PS not only decreased primary tumor size, but also metastatic burden. The mechanism of 3G4 is distinct from that of gemcitabine, but appears to be at least additive when the drugs are combined. Currently, surgery provides the only improvement of survival in pancreatic cancer patients. Current available therapies do not improve the ability to resect tumors, and few patients are eligible for surgical resection at presentation due to presence of metastases or local vascular invasion of the primary tumor. In patients with unresectable disease, treatment with the best available therapy, gemcitabine, provides only meager improvements in survival and symptomatology. Translation of therapy consisting of anti-PS antibodies with gemcitabine into the clinical setting may provide improved resectability and potentially decrease the occurrence of or treat metastases.

Additionally, combining these two drugs was well tolerated and without any noticeable ill effects in animals receiving five weeks of twice weekly dosing. Although gemcitabine is a relatively benign drug in the clinical setting, it can cause serious dose-limiting side effects including mucositis and bone marrow suppression. Our results suggest that combination of gemcitabine with 3G4 may lower the required dose of gemcitabine needed to treat tumors. Any improvement in therapy for pancreatic adenocarcinoma patients would be a tremendous advancement in what is currently available for this seemingly impregnable disease.

References

Adler, R.R., Ng, A.K. *et al.* (1995). Monoclonal antiphosphatidylserine antibody inhibits intercellular fusion of the choriocarcinoma line, JAR. *Biol Reprod* **53** (4), 905–910.

Bevers, E.M., Rosing, J. *et al.* (1985). Development of procoagulant binding sites on the platelet surface. *Adv Exp Med Biol* **192**, 359–371.

Blankenberg, F.G., Katsikis, P.D. *et al.* (1998). In vivo detection and imaging of phosphatidylserine expression during programmed cell death. *Proc Natl Acad Sci USA* **95** (11), 6349–6354.

Bombeli, T., Karsan, A. *et al.* (1997). Apoptotic vascular endothelial cells become procoagulant. *Blood* **89** (7), 2429–2442.

Bramhall, S.R., Allum, W.H. *et al.* (1995). Treatment and survival in 13 560 patients with pancreatic cancer, and incidence of the disease, in the West Midlands: an epidemiological study. *Br J Surg* **82** (1), 111–115.

Calderon, R.O. and DeVries, G.H. (1997). Lipid composition and phospholipid asymmetry of membranes from a Schwann cell line. *J Neurosci Res* **49** (3), 372–380.

Christiansen, V.J., Sims, P.J. *et al.* (1997). Complement C5b-9 increases plasminogen binding and activation on human endothelial cells. *Arterioscler Thromb Vasc Biol* **17** (1), 164–171.

Comfurius, P., Senden, J.M. *et al.* (1990). Loss of membrane phospholipid asymmetry in platelets and red cells may be associated with calcium-induced shedding of plasma membrane and inhibition of aminophospholipid translocase. *Biochim Biophys Acta* **1026** (2), 153–160.

Dachary-Prigent, J., Toti, F. *et al.* (1996). Physiopathological significance of catalytic phospholipids in the generation of thrombin. *Semin Thromb Hemost* **22** (2), 157–164.

Demo, S.D., Masuda, E. *et al.* (1999). Quantitative measurement of mast cell degranulation using a novel flow cytometric annexin-V binding assay. *Cytometry* **36** (4), 340–348.

Devaux, P.F. (1992). Protein involvement in transmembrane lipid asymmetry. *Annu Rev Biophys Biomol Struct* **21**, 417–439.

Fadok, V.A., Bratton, D.L. *et al.* (2000). A receptor for phosphatidylserine-specific clearance of apoptotic cells. *Nature* **405** (6782), 85–90.

Fidler, I.J. and Radinsky, R. (1990). Genetic control of cancer metastasis. *J Natl Cancer Inst* **82** (3), 166–168.

Glimelius, B. (1998). Chemotherapy in the treatment of cancer of the pancreas. *J Hepatobiliary Pancreat Surg* **5** (3), 235–241.

Herrmann, A. and Devaux, P.F. (1990). Alteration of the aminophospholipid translocase activity during in vivo and artificial aging of human erythrocytes. *Biochim Biophys Acta* **1027** (1), 41–46.

Hinkovska-Galcheva, V., Petkova, D. *et al.* (1989). Changes in the phospholipid composition and phospholipid asymmetry of ram sperm plasma membranes after cryopreservation. *Cryobiology* **26** (1), 70–75.

Jemal, A., Thomas, A. *et al.* (2002). Cancer statistics, 2002. *CA Cancer J Clin* **52** (1), 23–47.

Julien, M., Millot, C. *et al.* (1997). 12-O-tetradecanoylphorbol-13-acetate inhibits aminophospholipid translocase activity and modifies the lateral motions of fluorescent phospholipid analogs in the plasma membrane of bovine aortic endothelial cells. *Exp Cell Res* **234** (1), 125–131.

Karademir, S., Sokmen, S. *et al.* (2000). Tumor angiogenesis as a prognostic predictor in pancreatic cancer. *J Hepatobiliary Pancreat Surg* **7** (5), 489–495.

Laguinge, L.M., Lin, S. *et al.* (2004). Nitrosative stress in rotated three-dimensional colorectal carcinoma cell cultures induces microtubule depolymerization and apoptosis. *Cancer Res* **64** (8), 2643–2648.

Lupu, F., Moldovan, N. *et al.* (1993). Intrinsic procoagulant surface induced by hypercholesterolaemia on rabbit aortic endothelium. *Blood Coagul Fibrinolysis* **4** (5), 743–752.

Manfredi, A.A., Rovere, P. *et al.* (1998). Apoptotic cell clearance in systemic lupus erythematosus. II. Role of beta2-glycoprotein I. *Arthritis Rheum* **41** (2), 215–223.

McEvoy, L., Williamson, P. *et al.* (1986). Membrane phospholipid asymmetry as a determinant of erythrocyte recognition by macrophages. *Proc Natl Acad Sci USA* **83** (10), 3311–3315.

National Institute for Clinical Excellence. (2004). *Guidance on the Use of Gemcitabine for Pancreatic Cancer.*

Palmer, K.R., Kerr, M. *et al.* (1994). Chemotherapy prolongs survival in inoperable pancreatic carcinoma. *Br J Surg* **81** (6), 882–885.

Qu, J., Conroy, L.A. *et al.* (1996). Phosphatidylserine-mediated adhesion of T-cells to endothelial cells. *Biochem J* **317** (2), 343–346.

Ran, S., Downes, A. *et al.* (2002). Increased exposure of anionic phospholipids on the surface of tumor blood vessels. *Cancer Res* **62** (21), 6132–6140.

Ran, S., Gao, B. *et al.* (1998). Infarction of solid Hodgkins tumors in mice by antibody-directed targeting of tissue factor to tumor vasculature. *Cancer Res* **58** (20), 4646–4653.

Ran, S., He, J., Huang, X., Soares, M., Scothorn, D. and Thorpe, P.E. (2005). Antitumor effects of a monoclonal antibody that binds anionic phospholipids on the surface of tumor blood vessels in mice. *Clin Cancer Res* **11**, 1551–1562.

Ran, S. and Thorpe, P.E. (2002). Phosphatidylserine is a marker of tumor vasculature and a potential target for cancer imaging and therapy. *Int J Radiat Oncol Biol Phys* **54** (5), 1479–1484.

Rote, N.S., Ng, A.K. *et al.* (1993). Immunologic detection of phosphatidylserine externalization during thrombin-induced platelet activation. *Clin Immunol Immunopathol* **66** (3), 193–200.

Sessions, A. and Horwitz, A.F. (1981). Myoblast aminophospholipid asymmetry differs from that of fibroblasts. *FEBS Lett* **134** (1), 75–78.

Siemann, D.W., Bibby, M.C. *et al.* (2005). Differentiation and definition of vascular-targeted therapies. *Clin Cancer Res* **11** (2 Pt 1), 416–420.

Sugimura, M., Donato, R. *et al.* (1994). Annexin V as a probe of the contribution of anionic phospholipids to the procoagulant activity of tumour cell surfaces. *Blood Coagul Fibrinolysis* **5** (3), 365–373.

Test, S.T. and Mitsuyoshi, J. (1997). Activation of the alternative pathway of complement by calcium-loaded erythrocytes resulting from loss of membrane phospholipid asymmetry. *J Lab Clin Med* **130** (2), 169–182.

Thorpe, P.E. (2004). Vascular targeting agents as cancer therapeutics. *Clin Cancer Res* **10** (2), 415–427.

Utsugi, T., Schroit, A.J. *et al.* (1991). Elevated expression of phosphatidylserine in the outer membrane leaflet of human tumor cells and recognition by activated human blood monocytes. *Cancer Res* **51** (11), 3062–3066.

van Geelen, A.G., Slobbe-van Drunen, M.E. *et al.* (1995). Membrane related effects in endothelial cells induced by human cytomegalovirus. *Arch Virol* **140** (9), 1601–1612.

Vogt, E., Ng, A.K. *et al.* (1996). A model for the antiphospholipid antibody syndrome: monoclonal antiphosphatidylserine antibody induces intrauterine growth restriction in mice. *Am J Obstet Gynecol* **174** (2), 700–707.

Williamson, P. and Schlegel, R.A. (1994). Back and forth: the regulation and function of transbilayer phospholipid movement in eukaryotic cells. *Mol Membr Biol* **11** (4), 199–216.

Zhou, Q., Zhao, J. *et al.* (1997). Molecular cloning of human plasma membrane phospholipid scramblase. A protein mediating transbilayer movement of plasma membrane phospholipids. *J Biol Chem* **272** (29), 18 240–18 244.

Zwaal, R.F. and Schroit, A.J. (1997). Pathophysiologic implications of membrane phospholipid asymmetry in blood cells. *Blood* **89** (4), 1121–1132.

11

Cadherin Antagonists as Vasculature-targeting Agents

Orest W. Blaschuk and **Tracey M. Rowlands**

Abstract

Vascular endothelial (VE)- and neural (N)-cadherins play pivotal roles in mediating endothelial cell adhesion, as well as endothelial cell-pericyte adhesion. The function of these two cadherins is compromised in tumor vasculature, thus resulting in defective cell adhesion and unstable blood vessels. This property of the tumor vasculature makes it predisposed to attack by cadherin antagonists. Here we discuss the structures and functions of N- and VE-cadherins, as well as the use of their antagonists to attack the tumor vasculature. The importance of N-cadherin-mediated endothelial cell-pericyte adhesion in the maintenance of stable blood vessels is emphasized.

Keywords

N-cadherin, VE-cadherin, antagonists, endothelial cells, pericytes, tumor vasculature

11.1   Pericytes as regulators of blood vessel stability

Normal, mature microvessels are composed of two cell types: endothelial cells and pericytes (Hirschi and D'Amore, 1996; Gerhardt and Betsholtz, 2003; Betsholtz, Lindblom and Gerhardt, 2005). The endothelial cells line the lumen of the microvessels, whereas the pericytes reside in the stromal compartment and ensheath the endothelial cells. Pericytes are smooth muscle-like cells that are necessary for the formation and maintenance of stable microvessels (Hirschi and D'Amore, 1996; Carmeliet and Jain, 2000; Hellstrom *et al.*, 2001; Gerhardt and Betsholtz, 2003; Hammes *et al.*, 2004; Betsholtz, Lindblom and Gerhardt,

Vascular-targeted Therapies in Oncology   Edited by Dietmar W. Siemann
© 2006 John Wiley & Sons, Ltd.

2005; Jain, 2005). In the absence of pericytes, microvessels are unstable and transendothelial permeability is increased.

Pericytes express platelet-derived growth factor (PDGF)-β receptors and they are recruited to neovessels during angiogenesis (the formation of blood vessels from pre-existing vessels) in response to PDGF-β, which is secreted by the endothelium (Hellstrom *et al.*, 2001; Gerhardt and Betsholtz, 2003; Betsholtz, Lindblom and Gerhardt, 2005). Pericytes are not recruited to microvessels in either PDGF-β null or PDGF-β receptor null mice. These mice die at birth from microvascular hemorrhaging and edema formation, thus emphasizing the importance of pericytes in the maintenance of blood vessel integrity (Hellstrom *et al.*, 2001). In humans, diabetic retinopathy is characterized by a loss of contact between pericytes and endothelial cells, which leads to increased blood vessel permeability and subsequently the formation of microaneurysms (Carmeliet and Jain, 2000; Hammes *et al.*, 2004). These observations provide further support to the contention that pericytes are essential for microvessel stability.

Obviously, cell adhesion is a prerequisite for the formation and maintenance of stable, functional blood vessels. In the absence of proper adhesive contacts between endothelial cells, as well as between endothelial cells and pericytes, blood vessels are unstable, malformed and predisposed to hemorrhage. Two members of the cadherin family of cell adhesion molecules are intimately involved in mediating adhesion between the cells comprising the vasculature. In the subsequent sections, we will discuss the multiple roles of these two cadherins in the formation and preservation of blood vessels.

11.2   Cadherins

Neural (N-) and vascular endothelial (VE-) cadherins are cell adhesion molecules that play essential roles in the formation, stabilization and maintenance of blood vessels (Lampugnani and Dejana, 1997; Dejana, 2004; Paik *et al.*, 2004). Both of these cadherins are calcium-binding, membrane glycoproteins that are indirectly linked to the microfilaments of the cytoskeleton via a supramolecular structure composed of three intracellular proteins: β-catenin, α-catenin and α-actinin (Kemler, 1993; Knudsen *et al.*, 1995; Lampugnani and Dejana, 1997; Rowlands *et al.*, 2000).

N- and VE-cadherins cannot promote the formation of stable cell contacts if they are not linked to the cytoskeleton. Another intracellular protein, p120^{ctn}, binds to the juxtamembrane region of the cytoplasmic tail of N- and VE-cadherin and also influences the strength of cadherin-mediated adhesion (Daniel and Reynolds, 1995; Lampugnani *et al.*, 1997). Furthermore, the strength of N- and VE-cadherin-mediated cell adhesion is regulated by the tyrosine phosphorylation status of these cadherins, as well as β-catenin and p120^{ctn} (Daniel and Reynolds, 1997; Lilien *et al.*, 2002; Dejana, 2004; Xu *et al.*, 2004). In general, increased tyrosine phosphorylation of the cadherin-catenin complex causes decreases in adhesive strength (Daniel and Reynolds, 1997; Lampugnani *et al.*, 1997).

Both N- and VE-cadherin mediate cell adhesion via homophilic interactions, meaning that the two cadherins do not interact with one another (Navarro, Ruco and Dejana, 1998). Although the amino acid sequences of their cytoplasmic domains are similar (thus enabling them both to bind β-catenin), the sequences of their extracellular domains are not well conserved (Tanihara *et al.*, 1994). The structure of N-cadherin is shown in Figure 11.1, N-cadherin is composed of five extracellular domains (EC1-5), a plasmamembrane domain (PM) and two cytoplasmic domains (CP1 and CP2). The first extracellular domain of N-cadherin contains the cell adhesion recognition (CAR) sequence, histidine–alanine–valine (HAV) (Blaschuk, Pouliot and Holland, 1990a; Blaschuk *et al.*, 1990b; Blaschuk and Rowlands, 2002). Linear and cyclic synthetic peptides containing this sequence, as well as antibodies directed against this sequence inhibit N-cadherin-mediated cell adhesion (Blaschuk *et al.*, 1990b; Alexander, Blaschuk and Haselton, 1993; Peluso, Pappalardo and Trolice, 1996; Wilby *et al.*, 1999; Williams *et al.*, 2000; Blaschuk *et al.*, 2003). Monoclonal antibodies directed against the first extracellular domain of VE-cadherin are also capable of blocking cell adhesion (Liao *et al.*, 2000; Corada *et al.*, 2001; Liao *et al.*, 2002; May *et al.*, 2005). Furthermore, electron microscopic studies have demonstrated that the first extracellular domain mediates VE-cadherin homoassociation (Ahrens *et al.*, 2003; Lambert *et al.*, 2005). Collectively, these observations suggest that the first extracellular domain of VE-cadherin contains a CAR sequence.

11.3   Cadherins and the vasculature

In mature microvessels, VE-cadherin is localized to the intercellular junctions (known as adherens junctions) of endothelial cells, whereas N-cadherin is found concentrated in intercellular junctions formed between endothelial cells and pericytes (Figure 11.2(a)) (Gerhardt and Betsholtz, 2003; Paik *et al.*, 2004).

Pericytes of mature microvessels are embedded in the extracellular matrix (ECM) surrounding the endothelium. Pericyte–endothelial cell adhesion is medi-

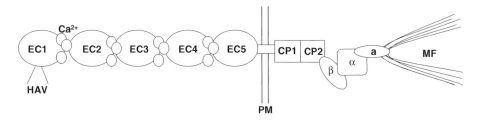

Figure 11.1   Diagram showing the structure of N-cadherin and its association with b-1-catenin (b), arcatenin (a), aractinin (a) and microfilaments of the cytoskeleton (MF)

(a)

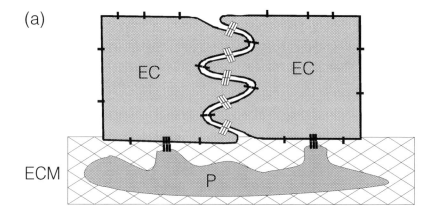

(b)

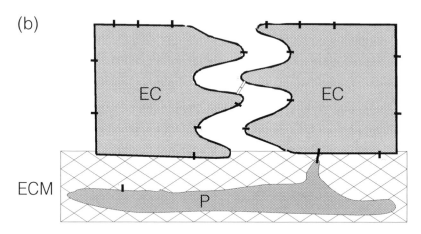

Figure 11.2 Diagram illustrating the relationships between endothelial cells (EC) and pericytes (P) in normal (a) and tumor (b) blood vessels

ated by N-cadherin (black rectangles in Figure 11.2), whereas endothelial cell adhesion is mainly mediated by VE-cadherin (white rectangles). Tumor endothelial cell adhesion, as well as endothelial–pericyte adhesion, is weak in comparison with cell adhesion in normal vasculature (see 11-5) end of paragraph.

N- and VE-cadherin play important roles during vasculogenesis (*de novo* formation of the vasculature) and angiogenesis. Blood vessels do not form in N-cadherin null mice (Radice *et al.*, 1997), whereas the vasculature forms, but is unstable, in VE-cadherin null mice (Carmeliet *et al.*, 1999). These observations suggest that N-cadherin mediates endothelial cell adhesion during the initial stage of vasculogenesis, whereas VE-cadherin is responsible for the establishment of stable intercellular junctions between the endothelial cells at the later stages of vessel maturation. Angiogenesis has also been shown to be dependent on N- and VE-cadherin (Corada *et al.*, 2002; Liao *et al.*, 2002; Paik *et al.*,

2004). Certain monoclonal antibodies directed against VE-cadherin (Liao *et al.*, 2002), cyclic peptides containing the N-cadherin CAR sequence (Blaschuk *et al.*, 2003), and N-cadherin siRNA (Paik *et al.*, 2004) are capable of blocking angiogenesis *in vivo*.

N-cadherin is readily detected by immunohistochemical techniques in normal microvessels, where it is localized to discrete intercellular junctions between endothelial cells and pericytes (Gerhardt and Betsholtz, 2003; Paik *et al.*, 2004). In contrast, only low levels of N-cadherin, diffusely distributed over the endo-thelial cell surface, are present in the pericyte-deficient, unstable microvessels of PDGF-β receptor null mice (Gerhardt and Betsholtz, 2003). Studies utilizing N-cadherin-function-disrupting antibodies have demonstrated the pivotal role of this cell adhesion molecule in mediating the formation and maintenance of stable intercellular junctions between pericytes and endothelial cells (Gerhardt, Wolburg and Redies, 2000). These junctions are disrupted when microvessels are exposed to antibodies directed against N-cadherin. Furthermore, microves-sels treated with these antibodies hemorrhage, thus indicating the necessity of proper N-cadherin function for blood vessel stability. Similarly, a monoclonal antibody directed against VE-cadherin (designated BV13) caused an increase in heart and lung vascular permeability, as well as blood vessel hemorrhage when injected systemically into adult mice (Corada *et al.*, 1999). These observations emphasize the importance of VE-cadherin in the maintenance of blood vessel integrity.

11.4 Tumor vasculature

Tumor and normal, mature blood vessels differ radically from one another (Carmeliet and Jain, 2000; Dvorak, 2003; Lin and Sessa, 2004; Jain, 2005) (Figure 11.2). Studies have shown that tumor blood vessels are deficient in pericytes and, when present, these cells are poorly adherent to the endothelium (Benjamin *et al.*, 1999; Morikawa *et al.*, 2002; Winkler, 2004). The lack of proper pericyte coverage results in tumor blood vessels with an abnormal, poorly formed basement membrane. Endothelial cells of tumor blood vessels are also poorly adherent to one another, often displaying open intercellular junctions (Roberts and Palade, 1997; Carmeliet and Jain, 2000). It is therefore not surprising that tumor blood vessels are hyperpermeable (Dvorak, 2003).

Vascular endothelial growth factor-A (VEGF-A) plays a pivotal role in influ-encing adhesion between endothelial cells, as well as between endothelial cells and pericytes in tumor blood vessels (Dvorak, 2003; Lin and Sessa, 2004; Jain, 2005). This cytokine binds to receptor tyrosine kinases (Dvorak, 2002), thus causing the phosphorylation of tyrosine residues in β-catenin and cadherins, ultimately resulting in unstable cell adhesion (Daniel and Reynolds, 1997; Esser *et al.*, 1998; Lilien *et al.*, 2002; Dejana, 2004; Weis *et al.*, 2004; Xu *et al.*, 2004).

11.5   Manipulation of the tumor vasculature with cadherin antagonists

Many studies have demonstrated that solid tumors require an adequate blood supply for survival and growth (Carmeliet and Jain, 2000; Jain, 2005). Drugs capable of disrupting vasculogenesis and angiogenesis, as well as vascular stability, would therefore be useful tools in the fight against cancer. N- and VE-cadherins expressed by the weakly adherent cells comprising the tumor vasculature represent attractive therapeutic targets. The tumor vasculature appears to be highly susceptible to attack using cadherin antagonists, in comparison to the normal vasculature, which is composed of tightly adherent cells. In view of the observations presented in the preceding sections, it is apparent that N- and VE-cadherin antagonists could conceivably be used to either block the formation (vasculogenesis and angiogenesis), or disrupt the stability (angiolysis) of the tumor vasculature. Furthermore, one cannot exclude the possibility that a cadherin antagonist could simultaneously function as an anti-vasculogenic, anti-angiogenic and angiolytic agent. The action of a cadherin antagonist on the tumor vasculature will likely be affected by many variables, including method of administration, dosing schedule, tumor type, tumor size, tumor vascularity, pericyte coverage, tumor VEGF levels and tumor growth rate. Careful evaluation of the effects of these variables on the ability of cadherin antagonists to act on the tumor vasculature will be needed to maximize the usefulness of these agents in the treatment of cancer.

Studies have shown that certain monoclonal antibodies directed against various extracellular domains of VE-cadherin are capable of blocking angiogenesis and slowing tumor growth in various animal models (Liao *et al.*, 2000; Corada *et al.*, 2002; Liao *et al.*, 2002). In particular, the VE-cadherin function blocking monoclonal antibody designated E4G10 has been shown to have both anti-angiogenic and anti-tumor, but not angiolytic, activities (Liao *et al.*, 2002). This monoclonal antibody recognizes VE-cadherin on the surface of endothelial cells involved in angiogenesis, but not VE-cadherin concentrated in adherens junctions present in mature endothelium. As such, E4G10 does not cause normal blood vessels to hemorrhage, unlike other monoclonal antibodies directed against VE-cadherin (for example, the monoclonal antibody designated BV13) (Corada *et al.*, 1999). It is likely that E4G10 recognizes an epitope that is exposed when VE-cadherin is present on the surface of non-adherent endothelial cells, and that this epitope becomes buried when the cells form adherens junctions (May *et al.*, 2005).

Small cyclic peptides containing the HAV motif have been shown to be capable of acting as N-cadherin antagonists (Williams *et al.*, 2000). The simple cyclic peptide N-Ac-CHAVC-NH$_2$ (also known as ADH-1, or Exherin™) has been shown to disrupt endothelial cell adhesion and cause endothelial cell apoptosis *in vitro* (Erez *et al.*, 2004). This cyclic peptide has also been shown to reduce vascular smooth muscle cell adhesion and cause apoptosis of these cells *in vitro*, thus suggesting that ADH-1 could have similar effects on pericytes

(Koutsouki *et al.*, 2003, 2005). Certain VE-cadherin-function-disrupting mono-clonal antibodies also have similar biological effects on endothelial cells *in vitro* (Carmeliet *et al.*, 1999; Corada *et al.*, 2001). It is therefore not surprising that ADH-1 displays anti-angiogenic properties when tested in various model systems, such as the chick chorioallantoic membrane assay (Blaschuk *et al.*, 2003). More detailed studies on the anti-angiogenic properties of N-cadherin antagonists are clearly warranted.

ADH-1 has also been shown to be capable of acting as an angiolytic agent (Blaschuk *et al.*, 2003; Lepekhin *et al.*, 2003). A single intravenous injection of ADH-1 into tumor-bearing mice has been shown to cause hemorrhage of tumor blood vessels. Importantly, in studies performed thus far, ADH-1 has not been found to affect the vasculature of normal tissues. Like monoclonal antibodies directed against VE-cadherin, ADH-1 has been shown to reduce tumor growth in various animal models. ADH-1 is currently being evaluated in phase IB/II and phase II clinical trials. A phase I safety and pharmacokinetic study found ADH-1 to be well tolerated (Jonker *et al.*, 2004).

11.6   Summary and future directions

The use of cadherin antagonists as vascular targeting agents is in its infancy, although they have shown promise in pre-clinical and clinical studies. These antagonists have been shown to be capable of preferentially targeting the defec-tive, weakly adherent endothelial cells and pericytes of the tumor vasculature. They are also likely to be effective in attacking the abnormal blood vessels that arise in a variety of diseases. Studies are needed in order to better understand the biological activities of such antagonists in various disease states. The realiza-tion that N- and VE-cadherin antagonists can have both anti-angiogenic and angiolytic activities underscores the need to carefully assess the conditions under which they are to be employed. In addition, it may be that N- and VE-cadherin antagonists will need to be used in combination with other drugs to treat cancer. Pre-clinical studies are therefore required to explore these possibilities.

Acknowledgment

The authors express their gratitude to Adherex Technologies Inc. for generous support.

References

Ahrens, T., Lambert, M., Pertz, O., Sasaki, T., Schulthess, T., Mege, R.-M., Timpl, R. and Engel, J. (2003). Homoassociation of VE-cadherin follows a mechanism common to 'classical' cadherins. *J Mol Biol* **325**, 733–742.

Alexander, J.S., Blaschuk, O.W. and Haselton, F.R. (1993). An N-cadherin-like protein contributes to solute barrier maintenance in cultured endothelium. *J Cell Physiol* **156**, 610–618.

Benjamin, L.E., Golijanin, D., Itin, A., Pode, D. and Keshet, E. (1999). Selective ablation of immature blood vessels in established human tumors follows vascular endothelial growth factor withdrawl. *J Clin Invest* **103**, 159–165.

Betsholtz, C., Lindblom, P. and Gerhardt, H. (2005). Role of pericytes in vascular morphogenesis. *EXS* **94**, 115–125.

Blaschuk, O.W., Gour, B.J., Farookhi, R. and Ali, A. (2003). Compounds and methods for modulating endothelial cell adhesion. *U.S. Patent* 6 610 821.

Blaschuk, O.W., Pouliot, Y. and Holland, P.C. (1990a). Identification of a conserved region common to cadherins and influenza strain A hemagglutinins. *J Mol Biol* **211**, 679–682.

Blaschuk, O.W. and Rowlands, T.M. (2002). Plasma membrane components of adherens junctions. *Mol Memb Rev* **19**, 75–80.

Blaschuk, O.W., Sullivan, R., David, S. and Pouliot, Y. (1990b). Identification of a cadherin cell adhesion recognition sequence. *Dev Biol* **139**, 227–229.

Carmeliet, P. and Jain, R. (2000). Angiogenesis in cancer and other diseases. *Nature* **407**, 249–257.

Carmeliet, P., Lampugnani, M.-G., Moons, L., Brevario, F., Compernolle, V., Bono, F., Balconi, G., Spagnuolo, R., Oosthuyse, B., Dewerchin, M., Zanetti, A., Angellilo, A., Mattot, V., Nuyens, D., Lutgens, E., Clotman, F., de Ruiter, M.C., Gittenberger-de Groot, A., Poelmann, R., Lupu, F., Herbert, J.-M., Collen, D. and Dejana, E. (1999). Targeted deficiency or cytosolic truncation of the *VE-cadherin* gene in mice impairs VEGF-mediated endothelial survival and angiogenesis. *Cell* **98**, 147–157.

Corada, M., Liao F., Lindgren, M., Lampugnani, M.G., Brevario, F., Frank, R., Muller, W. A., Hicklin, D.J., Bohlen, P. and Dejana, E. (2001). Monoclonal antibodies directed to different regions of vascular endothelial cadherin extracellular domain affect adhesion and clustering of the protein and modulate endothelial permeability. *Blood* **97**, 1679–1684.

Corada, M., Mariotti, M., Thurston, G., Smith, K., Kunkel, R., Brockhaus, M., Lampugnani, M.G., Martin-Padura, I., Stoppacciaro, A., Ruco, L., McDonald, D.M., Ward, P.A. and Dejana, E. (1999). Vascular endothelial-cadherin is an important determinant of microvascular integrity *in vivo*. *Proc Natl Acad Sci USA* **96**, 9815–9820.

Corada, M., Zanetta, L., Orsenigo, F., Brevario, F., Lampugnani, M.G., Bernasconi, S., Liao, F., Hicklin, D.J., Bohlen, P. and Dejana, E. (2002). A monoclonal antibody to vascular endothelial-cadherin inhibits tumor angiogenesis without side effects on endothelial permeability. *Blood* **100**, 905–911.

Daniel, J.M. and Reynolds, A.B. (1995). The tyrosine kinase substrate p120cas binds directly to E-cadherin but not to the adenomatous polyposis coli protein or α-catenin. *Mol Cell Biol* **15**, 4819–4824.

Daniel, J.M. and Reynolds, A.B. (1997). Tyrosine phosphorylation and cadherin/catenin function. *BioEssays* **19**, 883–891.

Dejana, E. (2004). Endothelial cell–cell junctions: happy together. *Nature Rev Mol Cell Biol* **5**, 261–270.

Dvorak, H.F. (2002). Vascular permeability factor/vascular endothelial growth factor: a critical cytokine in tumor angiogenesis and a potential target for diagnosis and therapy. *J Clin Oncol* **20**, 4368–4380.

Dvorak, H.F. (2003). How tumors make bad blood vessels and stroma. *Am J Pathol* **162**, 1747–1757.

Erez, N., Zamir, E., Gour, B.J., Blaschuk, O.W. and Geiger, B. (2004). Induction of apoptosis in cultured endothelial cells by a cadherin antagonist peptide: involvement of fibroblast growth factor receptor-mediated signaling. *Exp Cell Res* **294**, 366–378.

Esser, S., Lampugnani, M.G., Corada, M., Dejana, E. and Risau, W. (1998). Vascular endothelial growth factor induces VE-cadherin tyrosine phosphorylation in endothelial cells. *J Cell Sci* **111**, 1853–1865.

Gerhardt, H. and Betsholtz, C. (2003). Endothelial–pericyte interactions in angiogenesis. *Cell Tissue Res* **314**, 15–23.

Gerhardt, H., Wolburg, H. and Redies, C. (2000). N-cadherin mediates pericytic–endothelial interaction during brain angiogenesis in the chicken. *Dev Dyn* **218**, 472–479.

Hammes, H.-P., Lin, J., Wagner, P., Feng, Y., vom Hagen, F., Krzizok, T., Renner, O., Breier, G., Brownlee, M. and Deutsch, U. (2004). Angiopoietin-2 causes pericyte dropout in the normal retina. Evidence of involvement in diabetic retinopathy. *Diabetes* **53**, 1104–1110.

Hellstrom, M., Gerhardt, H., Kalen, M., Li, X., Eriksson, U., Wolburg, H. and Betsholtz, C. (2001). Lack of pericytes leads to endothelial hyperplasia and abnormal vascular morphogenesis. *J Cell Biol* **153**, 543–553.

Hirschi, K.K. and D'Amore, P.A. (1996). Pericytes in the microvasculature. *Cardiovasc Res* **32**, 687–698.

Jain, R.K. (2005). Normalization of tumor vasculature: an emerging concept in antiangiogenic therapy. *Science* **307**, 58–62.

Jonker, D.J., Avruch, L., Stewart, D.J., Goel, R., Goss, G., Dent, S., Reaume, M.N., Spencer, T.A. and Peters, W.P. (2004). A phase I safety and PK study of the novel vascular targeting agent (VTA), Exherin, in patients with refractory solid tumors stratified according to N-cadherin expression. *J Clin Oncol* **22** (14S), 3078.

Kemler, R. (1993). From cadherins to catenins: cytoplasmic protein interactions and regulation of cell adhesion. *Trends Genet* **9**, 317–321.

Koutsouki, E., Aguilera-Garcia, G.B., Newby, A.C. and George, S.J. (2003). Cell–cell contact by cadherins provides an essential survival signal to migrating smooth muscle cells. *Eur Heart J* **24**, 1838.

Koutsouki, E., Beeching, C.A., Slater, S.C., Blaschuk, O.W., Sala-Newby, G.B. and George, S.J. (2005). N-cadherin-dependent cell–cell contacts promote human saphenous vein smooth muscle cell survival. *Arterioscler Thromb Vasc Biol* **25**, 982–988.

Knudsen, K.A., Peralta Soler, A., Johnson, K.R. and Wheelock, M.J. (1995). Interaction of α-actinin with the cadherin/catenin cell–cell adhesion complex via α-catenin. *J Cell Biol* **130**, 67–77.

Lambert, O., Taveau, J.-C., Him, J.L.K., Al Kurdi, R., Gulino-Debrac, D. and Brisson, A. (2005). The basic framework of VE-cadherin junctions revealed by cryo-EM. *J Mol Biol* **346**, 1193–1196.

Lampugnani, M.G., Corada, M., Andriopoulou, P., Esser, S., Risau, W. and Dejana, E. (1997). Cell confluence regulates tyrosine phosphorylation of adherens junction components in endothelial cells. *J Cell Sci*, **110**, 2065–2077.

Lampugnani, M.G. and Dejana, E. (1997). Interendothelial junction: structure, signalling and functional roles. *Curr Opin Cell Biol* **9**, 674–682.

Lepekhin, E., Jiang, X., Michaud, S., Tonary, A., Yu, W., Symonds, J.M. and Blaschuk, O. W. (2003). Early and long-term effects of exherin on tumor vasculature. *Proc Am Soc Clin Oncol* **22**, 220.

Liao, F., Doody, J.F., Overhoser, J., Finnerty, B., Bassi, R., Wu, Y., Dejana, E., Kussie, P., Bohlen, P. and Hicklin, D.J. (2002). Selective targeting of angiogenic tumor vasculature by vascular endothelial-cadherin antibody inhibits tumor growth without affecting vascular permeability. *Cancer Res* **62**, 2567–2575.

Liao, F., Li, Y., O'Connor, W., Zanetta, L., Bassi, R., Santiago, A., Overholser, J., Hooper, A., Mignatti, P., Dejana, E., Hicklin, D.J., and Bohlen, P. (2000). Monoclonal antibody to vascular endothelial-cadherin is a potent inhibitor of angiogenesis, tumor growth and metastasis. *Cancer Res* **60**, 6805–6810.

Lilien, J., Balsamo, J., Arregui, C. and Xu, G. (2002). Turn-off, drop-out: functional state switching of cadherins. *Dev Dyn* **224**, 18–29.

Lin, M.I. and Sessa, W.C. (2004). Antiangiogenic therapy: creating a unique 'window' of opportunity. *Cancer Cell* **6**, 529–531.

May, C., Doody, J.F., Abdullah, R., Balderes, P., Xu, X., Chen, C.P., Zhu, Z., Shapiro, L., Kussie, P., Hicklin, D.J., Liao, F. and Bohlen, P. (2005). Identification of a transiently exposed VE-cadherin epitope that allows for specific targeting of an antibody to the tumor neovasculature. *Blood* **105**, 4337–4344.

Morikawa, S., Baluk, P., Kaidoh, T., Haskell, A., Jain, R.K. and McDonald, D.M. (2002). Abnormalities in pericytes on blood vessels and endothelial sprouts in tumors. *Am J Pathol* **160**, 985–1000.

Navarro, P., Ruco, L. and Dejana, E. (1998). Differential localization of VE- and N-cadherins in human endothelial cells: VE-cadherin competes with N-cadherin for junctional localization. *J Cell Biol* **140**, 1475–1484.

Paik, J.-H., Skoura, A., Chae, S.-S., Cowan, A.E., Han, D.K., Proia, R.L. and Hla, T. (2004). Sphingosine 1-phosphate receptor regulation of N-cadherin mediates vascular stabilization. *Genes Dev* **18**, 2392–2403.

Peluso, J.J., Pappalardo, A. and Trolice, M.P. (1996). N-cadherin-mediated cell contact inhibits granulosa cell apoptosis in a progesterone-independent manner. *Endocrinology* **137**, 1196–1203.

Radice, G.L., Rayburn, H., Matsunami, H., Knudsen, K.A., Takeichi, M. and Hynes, R.O. (1997). Developmental defects in mouse embryos lacking N-cadherin. *Dev Biol* **181**, 64–78.

Roberts, W.G. and Palade, G.E. (1997). Increased microvascular permeability and endothelial fenestration induced by vascular endothelial growth factor. *J Cell Sci* **108**, 2369–2379.

Rowlands, T.M., Symonds, J.M., Farookhi, R. and Blaschuk, O.W. (2000). Cadherins: crucial regulators of structure and function in reproductive tissues. *Rev Reprod* **5**, 53–61.

Tanihara, H., Sano, K., Heimark, R.L., St. John, T. and Suzuki, S. (1994). Cloning of five human cadherins clarifies characteristic features of cadherin extracellular domain and provides further evidence for two structurally different types of cadherin. *Cell Adhesion Commun* **2**, 15–26.

Weis, S., Cui, J., Barnes, L. and Cheresh, D. (2004). Endothelial barrier disruption by VEGF-mediated Src activity potentiates tumor cell extravasation and metastasis. *J Cell Biol* **187**, 223–229.

Wilby, M.J., Muir, E.M., Fok-Seang, J., Gour, B.J., Blaschuk, O.W. and Fawcett, J.W. (1999). N-cadherin inhibits Schwann cell migration on astrocytes. *Mol Cell Neurosci* **14**, 66–84.

Williams, E., Williams, G., Gour, B.J., Blaschuk, O.W. and Doherty, P. (2000). A novel family of cyclic peptide antagonists suggests that N-cadherin specificity is determined by amino acids that flank the HAV motif. *J Biol Chem* **275**, 4007–4012.

Winkler, F., Kozin, S., Tong, R.T., Chae, S.-S., Booth, M.F., Garkavtsev, I., Xu, L., Hicklin, D.J., Fukumura, D., di Tomaso, E., Munn, L.L. and Jain, R.K. (2004). Kinetics of vascular normalization by VEGFR2 blockade governs brain tumor response to radiation: role of oxygenation, angiopoietin-1, and matrix metalloproteinases. *Cancer Cell* **6**, 553–563.

Xu, G., Craig, A.W.B., Greer, P., Miller, M., Anastasiadis, P.Z., Lilien, J. and Balsamo, J. (2004). Continuous association of cadherin with β-catenin requires the non-receptor tyrosine-kinase Fer. *J Cell Sci* **117**, 3207–3219.

12

Alphastatin: a Pluripotent Inhibitor of Activated Endothelial Cells

Carolyn A. Staton and Claire E. Lewis

Abstract

As angiogenesis, the development of new blood vessels from the existing vasculature, is crucial for tumour growth, a number of anti-angiogenic agents are currently being tested in anti-cancer clinical trials. Here we detail the discovery of a novel agent, Alphastatin, a 24 amino-acid peptide derived from the amino terminus of the α-chain of human fibrinogen and show that it inhibits both migration and tubule formation of human dermal microvascular endothelial cells in vitro in response to three potent angiogenic factors, bFGF, EGF and VEGF. Moreover, Alphastatin markedly inhibits the growth of tumours *in vivo* by disrupting activated endothelial cells in tumours, leading to formation of intravascular thrombosis and the formation of large areas of tumour necrosis. This was seen to be a selective effect as the vasculature in such healthy tissues as lungs, liver and kidney remained unaffected. We suggest that, as Alphastatin inhibits the actions of multiple growth factors on human endothelial cells and severely disrupts tumour vasculature *in vivo*, it may prove more clinically effective than other agents that inhibit one growth factor alone (e.g. VEGF).

Keywords

anti-angiogenic, haemostasis, angiogenesis, fibrinogen, thrombosis

12.1 Introduction

Angiogenesis is the development of blood vessels from the existing vasculature. During normal physiological processes, such as development of the corpus luteum during ovulation and in wound healing, angiogenesis occurs in a highly regulated manner. Under such circumstances, pro-angiogenic factors stimulate

---

Vascular-targeted Therapies in Oncology Edited by Dietmar W. Siemann
© 2006 John Wiley & Sons, Ltd.

a phase of rapid migration, proliferation and differentiation of endothelial cells and new vessels are formed. Endothelial cells then enter a quiescent phase in the mature vasculature, tightly regulated by the local balance of pro- and anti-angiogenic factors. For tumor growth and metastasis to occur this balance is disturbed in favour of an increase in angiogenic agents.

This role of angiogenesis in tumor growth was first described by Judah Folkman in 1971 (Folkman, 1971). His group showed that tumors implanted into isolated perfused organs failed to develop, whereas those implanted into the ocular chamber within 5 μm of blood vessels became vascularized and grew rapidly (Folkman and Klapsbrun, 1987). These observations led Folkman and co-workers to postulate that solid tumors were dependent on angiogenesis and that anti-angiogenesis might be an effective anti-cancer strategy (Folkman, 1971, 1990).

Anti-angiogenic therapy

The discovery of the importance of angiogenesis to tumor growth and metastasis led directly to the premise that the tumor vasculature could make an ideal and potentially effective target for therapy. Delivery of blood-borne chemotherapeutic agents to tumor cells in solid tumors has proved problematic as abnormalities in tumor blood vessel function, resulting in abnormal blood flow, combined with the lack of lymph drainage, result in high interstitial pressure and poor penetration of externally applied agents (Jain, 1994; Brown and Giaccia, 1998). Tumor cells themselves are a genetically unstable, heterogeneous population, with many quickly becoming resistant to chemotherapy. Indeed, acquired drug resistance has been identified as the major cause of inefficacy of cytotoxic chemotherapies (Gasparini, 1999).

The tumor vasculature is unique, being the only constantly proliferating endothelium within the body of an otherwise healthy adult. Therefore, agents that target this uniquely proliferating vasculature by binding to specific markers can disrupt the tumor vessels, thereby inhibiting blood flow. The added advantage of this mode of therapy is that tumor vascular targeting would also simultaneously affect any disseminated metastases. Given the premise that destruction of the vasculature would lead to the demise of the tumor, by depriving it of oxygen and nutrients essential to its growth, a large number of studies in recent years have focused on developing drugs that target different parts of the angiogenic pathway, followed by testing their safety and efficacy in clinical trials. Of note, the most successful Phase III clinical trial with an angiogenesis inhibitor, to date, has shown that bevacizumab (Avastin, a humanized vascular endothelial growth factor (VEGF) monoclonal antibody), when given in combination with the chemotherapy agents, irinotecan, fluorouracil and leucovorin (IFL), significantly increased survival from 15.6 months in the IFL plus placebo group to 20.3 months in the IFL plus Avastin group (Hurwitz et al., 2004). Avastin was also seen to increase disease free survival from 6.2 months (IFL + placebo) to 10.6 months (IFL + Avastin) and to increase the duration of response to the drugs by 3 months (Hurwitz *et al.*, 2004). However, Avastin is limited in that it targets VEGF alone and many tumors are known to express other pro-angiogenic factors including basic growth factor (bFGF) and epidermal growth factor (EGF) (Suhardja and Hoffman, 2003), which may explain why such tumors escape control after time and disease progresses.

Consequently, work has focused on anti-angiogenic agents that target more than one growth factor as these may have greater therapeutic potential than agents such as Avastin. Interestingly, many endogenous proteins contain cryptic regions, which, when cleaved from the parent molecule, show pro- or anti-angiogenic activity both *in vitro* and *in vivo* not seen in the original protein. Angiostatin, a cleavage product of plasminogen, and endostatin, a cleavage product of collagen type XVIII, have been shown to inhibit endothelial cell migration and tubule formation *in vitro* in response to both bFGF and VEGF, and tumor growth *in vivo* (O'Reilly *et al.*, 1994, 1996, 1997). Despite these encouraging results, and although these agents were well tolerated in clinical trials, there was little evidence of anti-tumor activity in humans (Eder *et al.*, 2002; Twombly, 2002; Beerepoot *et al.*, 2003; Thomas *et al.*, 2003), with, for example, only two out of 25 patients (one with sarcoma, one with, melanoma) demonstrating minor and short-lived anti-tumor activity in response to end-ostatin (Twombly, 2002). This is possibly because anti-angiogenic agents are likely to work better on small tumors that are undergoing active angiogenesis than in large well established tumors. However, invariably only the patients with the latter are available for clinical trials. Also, both agents are large peptides that are unstable in the bloodstream, being easily broken down by enzymes. This compromises their activity over time *in vivo*.

12.2   Discovery of alphastatin

Fibrinogen E-fragment

We have previously demonstrated that when plasmin cleaves the carboxyl termini of the paired α-, β- and γ-chains of human fibrinogen it releases a potent anti-angiogenic factor: the central E-domain (fibrinogen E-fragment, FgnE). Like angiostatin and endostatin, FgnE inhibits the migration and tubule formation of human dermal microvascular endothelial cells in response to VEGF and bFGF *in vitro* (Bootle-Wilbraham *et al.*, 2000). Interestingly, the migration of human dermal microvascular endothelial cells (HuDMEC) was only reduced in the presence of growth factors whereas tubule formation was reduced in both the presence and the absence of these factors. However, within the tubule formation assay on growth factor-reduced Matrigel, endothelial cells are not completely quiescent in the absence of growth factors in the medium, as the matrix itself contains residual levels of growth factors that can stimulate cells. As both bFGF and VEGF have been shown to bind to Fgn (Sahni, Odrljin and Francis, 1998) and the binding sites for these growth factors are not yet known, it remains a possibility that FgnE mediates its effects by binding to growth factors in these assays and preventing them from adhering to the cellular receptors. However, experiments carried out by Sahni and co-workers (Sahni, Sporn and Francis, 1999) have shown that binding of either bFGF or VEGF to Fgn does not prevent growth factors from activating endothelial cells, suggesting that it is unlikely that growth factor binding to FgnE mediates its inhibitory effects. Moreover, it has been shown that exposure of HuDMECs to FgnE for 1 hour prior to addition of the cells to the migration of tubule formation assays *in vitro* (which were then run in the absence of FgnE) was sufficient to significantly inhibit HuDMEC responses in these assays to either bFGF or VEGF (Staton, Brown and Lewis, 2003).

We also examined the effects of FgnE on the formation and function of blood vessels *in vivo* by injecting it daily i.p. into Balb/c mice bearing CT26 tumors (a syngeneic model). FgnE caused widespread damage to blood vessels in tumors, resulting in microvascular thrombosis and occlusion, and causing extensive destruction of tumor cells and retarded growth (Brown *et al.*, 2002). Blood vessels elsewhere within these mice (e.g. liver, lungs and kidneys) were unaffected by these injections of FgnE, indicating that this fragment may target activated endothelium within the growing tumor. Taken together, these findings suggest that FgnE could be used to selectively target tumor blood vessels, causing endothelial cell damage and triggering a hemostatic response that blocks affected blood vessels and leads to inadequate perfusion and widespread tumor death. However, FgnE is a complex protein consisting of six polypeptide chains linked by di-sulfide bridges, which renders it impossible to generate FgnE synthetically for use in the clinic, so our work then focused on identifying the active site of FgnE and synthesizing this as a smaller peptide.

Fibrin E-fragment

Fibrinogen can also be cleaved by thrombin, which removes the amino termini of both the α- and β-chains, termed fibrinopeptide A and B (FpA and FpB) respectively, to yield fibrin monomers (Blomback and Blomback, 1972). These in turn are cleaved by plasmin to produce the fragment closely related to FgnE, namely fibrin E-fragment (FnE) (Lucas *et al.*, 1983). This has been shown to have the opposite effects to FgnE in that it is pro-angiogenic, stimulating proliferation, migration and tubule formation on Matrigel as shown by an increase in tubule number and area (Bootle-Wilbraham *et al.*, 2001). FnE also stimulates vessel formation in the chick chorioallantoic membrane (CAM) assay of angiogenesis (Thompson *et al.*, 1992). As plasmin cleaves the amino terminus of the β-chains between amino acids 42 and 43 in both E-fragments, the only difference between the anti-angiogenic FgnE and pro-angiogenic FnE is that the former contains 16 amino acids at the amino terminus of the α-chains (FpA) (Figure 12.1). These are not present in FnE and this led us to speculate that the anti-angiogenic properties of FgnE may be mediated by FpA. However, a linear form of FpA was found to be inactive *in vitro* in our angiogenesis assays (Bootle-Wilbraham *et al.*, 2001).

The six polypeptide chains of fibrinogen, two α (black in Figure 12.1(a)), two β (dark gray) and two γ (light gray) wrap around each other to form three globular domains, two D and one E. The fibrinopeptides (FpA and FpB) are

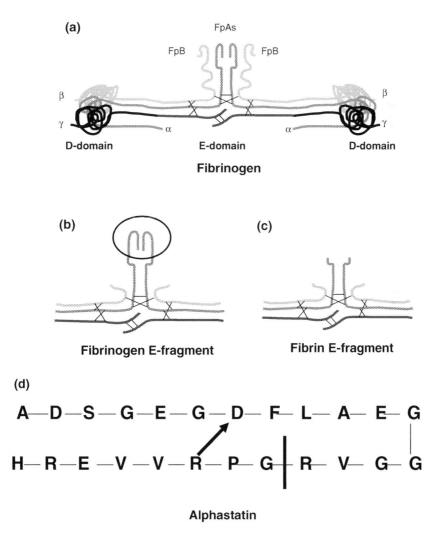

Figure 12.1 Schematic diagrams of (a) fibrinogen; (b) fibrinogen E-fragment (FgnE); (c) fibrin E-fragment (FnE); (d) alphastatin

found at the amino termini of the α- and β-chains within the E-domain. Plasmin cleaves the amino-terminal 42 amino acids of the β-chain and the carboxy-terminus of the α-chain as well as cleaving either side of the central E-domain to release FgnE (Figure 12.1(b)). Initially thrombin cleaves FpA and FpB (shown in the square, Figure 12.1(c)) from the fibrinogen molecule to release a fibrin monomer. Plasmin then cleaves either side of the central E-domain, at position 42 on the β-chain and the carboxy-terminus of the α-chain, to release FnE. Alphastatin (Figure 12.1(d)) is the first 24 amino acids of the α-chain within FgnE (shown in the circle) and consists of a β-bend stabilized by a salt bridge between R19 and D7 (arrow). The thrombin cleavage site is denoted by a vertical line, and the sequence of FpA is from A to R.

Fibrinogen alpha chain structure

The crystal structures of both fibrinogen (Yang *et al.*, 2001) and FgnE (Madrazo *et al.*, 2001) have been described and nuclear magnetic resonance studies by Marsh and co-workers showed that the α-chain amino terminus of fibrinogen contained a β-bend, which was supported by a salt bridge between R19 on the aa17–24 portion of the peptide and residue D7 on the FpA portion of the α-chain (Marsh *et al.*, 1985). We therefore proposed that, when attached to the rest of the FgnE molecule, FpA is held in a β-bend conformation at the end of the α-chains and that this conformation may be essential for the anti-angiogenic activity of FgnE. Therefore, we synthesized the first 24 amino acids of the α-chain of fibrinogen, which includes the D7–R19 salt bridge, for testing *in vitro* and *in vivo*, and called the resultant peptide alphastatin (Staton *et al.*, 2004a).

12.3   Development of alphastatin

Activity of alphastatin *in vitro*

In contrast to FpA, alphastatin exhibited significant anti-angiogenic activity *in vitro* (Staton *et al.*, 2004a), inhibiting bFGF, EGF and VEGF-induced migration of HuDMEC in a dose-dependent manner (Figure 12.2) (Staton *et al.*, 2004b). Migration of HuDMECs treated with alphastatin across a collagen-coated filter in response to medium alone (control) or medium containing $10\,ng\,ml^{-1}$ bFGF, EGF or VEGF is shown in Figure 12.2. Data are shown as mean ± SEM. (*$p <$ 0.03 with respect to relevant 'no alphastatin' group). Tubule formation on GFR-Matrigel was also significantly inhibited in a dose-dependent manner in both the absence and presence of bFGF, EGF and VEGF (Figure 12.3) (Staton *et al.*, 2004b). Tubule formation by HuDMECs in response to alphastatin on GFR-Matrigel in response to medium alone (control) or medium containing $10\,ng\,ml^{-1}$ bFGF, EGF or VEGF measured as area covered by tubules is shown in

Figure 12.3. Data are shown as mean ± SEM. (*$p < 0.04$ with respect to relevant 'no alphastatin' group). Although the reports by Sahni *et al.* (Sahni, Sporn and Francis, 1999; Sahni and Francis, 2000) indicate that Fgn is capable of binding both VEGF and bFGF, it is not known whether this activity is found at the N-terminus of the α-chain. Indeed, it is unlikely that both growth factors will bind to this portion of the protein, as Fgn has the potential to bind both growth factors without apparent steric hindrance, indicating that the growth factor binding sites are found on separate locations on Fgn (Sahni and Francis, 2000). Furthermore, exposure of HuDMECs to alphastatin for 2 hours, prior to the addition of the cells to the GFR-Matrigel assay *in vitro* (which was then run in the absence of

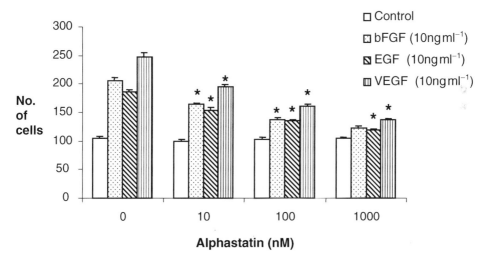

Figure 12.2 *In vitro* effects of alphastatin on HuDMEC migration

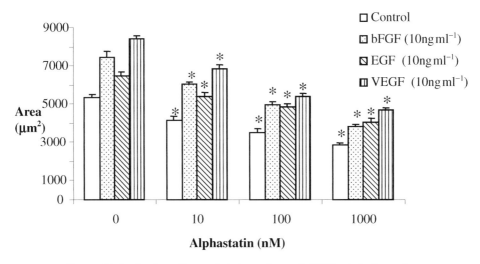

Figure 12.3 *In vitro* effects of alphastatin on HuDMEC tubule formation

Alphastatin), was sufficient to significantly inhibit bFGF and VEGF-induced tubule formation (Staton *et al.*, 2004a). Moreover, alphastatin also inhibits the response of HuDMECs to EGF, a growth factor that does not contain a heparin-binding region necessary for binding to fibrinogen. The fact that alphastatin inhibits the migration and tubule formation of HuDMECs in response to all three growth factors suggests that these effects most likely operate at a post-receptor locus common to the bFGF, VEGF and EGF signalling pathways.

A comparison between the effects mediated by FgnE and alphastatin indicates that FgnE is more effective at inhibiting both migration and tubule formation of endothelial cells than an equivalent dose of alphastatin (Staton *et al.*, 2004a). This may be due to further conformational constraints placed on the amino-terminus of the α-chain when it is bound to the parent FgnE protein (which may not be present in the free peptide). Further electrostatic bonds may be formed between alphastatin and the remainder of the FgnE protein when bound to the parent molecule. An alternative possibility is that within FgnE the amino-termini of the two α-chains are held in close proximity, a property not modelled in the free peptides. 25–30 per cent of α-chains of FgnE are phosphorylated at Ser 3 in the bloodstream, enabling a salt bridge with Arg23 that further stabilizes the β-bend structure (Maurer *et al.*, 1998; Marsh *et al.*, 1985). This configuration is thought to produce a more efficient enzyme–substrate combination, which may lead, in part, to the increased efficacy of FgnE compared with alphastatin, which does not carry this phosphorylation (due to lack of exposure to the relevant enzymes that cause such phosphorylations).

Although anti-angiogenic agents often have a significant effect on endothelial proliferation, alphastatin failed to inhibit HuDMEC proliferation at any of the doses tested (Staton *et al.*, 2004a), whereas FgnE failed to inhibit at the lowest two doses (10 and 100 nM), but at the highest dose tested (1 μM) FgnE showed inhibition of proliferation due, at least in part, to the cytotoxic effect of FgnE at this dose (Bootle-Wilbraham *et al.*, 2000). FgnE was not found to be cytotoxic for other human cell types, including fibroblasts, macrophages and tumor cells, suggesting that this cytotoxicity is a selective effect on endothelial cells. In contrast, alphastatin failed to exhibit a cytotoxic effect on HuDMECs, suggesting that the cytotoxic portion of the protein may be found elsewhere on FgnE and not in the alphastatin region. Therefore, it remains a possibility that FgnE is more efficient in the *in vitro* assay systems at inhibiting endothelial cell function, in part due to its cytotoxic effects.

Activity of alphastatin *in vivo*

Alphastatin, like FgnE, has anti-tumor effects *in vivo* (Staton *et al.*, 2004a, 2004b). In our syngenic CT26/Balb/c tumor model, tumor volumes reached 100–350 mm^3 within 18 days. However, when these tumor-bearing mice were then injected i.p. every day for 12 days with 100 nM alphastatin (0.025 mg kg^{-1}

day^{-1}; $n = 6$) the tumors were significantly smaller than those injected with PBS alone ($n = 8$) by day 12 of injections (Figure 12.4). Colonic adenocarcinoma CT26 cells were implanted on the right flank of Balb/c mice and tumors allowed to reach no more than 350 mm^3 in size (14–18 days). Injections of 0.025 mg kg^{-1} alphastatin in PBS ($n = 5$) or PBS alone (control; $n = 8$) were administered daily i.p. for 12 days. Tumor size was monitored daily using callipers. Tumor volume was significantly ($p < 0.05$) reduced in alphastatin-treated compared with vehicle-treated animals from day 5 of the injection period onwards. When a comparison was carried out between the effects of 100 nM alphastatin (0.025 mg kg^{-1} day^{-1}; $n = 6$) and 100 nM FgnE (0.5 mg kg^{-1} day^{-1}; $n = 7$), the final tumor volumes of the alphastatin- and FgnE-treated tumors were not significantly different by the end of the treatment period (12 days) (Staton, Brown and Lewis, unpublished observations). Although the doses of both alphastatin and FgnE administered were calculated to reach 100 nM in the murine blood-stream (assuming a total blood volume of 2 ml per 20 g mouse), the administration was i.p., so it is possible that the concentration of FgnE or peptide actually reaching the tumor vasculature was lower than this (due to incomplete absorption from the peritoneum and/or enzymatic degradation in the circulation). The pharmacokinetics of the peptide and the fragment are, as yet, undetermined, and it is possible that the final concentrations reaching the tumor site were different. Work is currently underway to establish the pharmacokinetics of both FgnE and alphastatin.

Further work attempting to identify the most efficacious route of administration of alphastatin utilized another syngeneic tumor model, namely 4T1 breast carcinoma cells grown subcutaneously in female Balb/c mice (Stribbling *et al.*, 2004). Again, these tumors were allowed to become established (100–350 mm^3

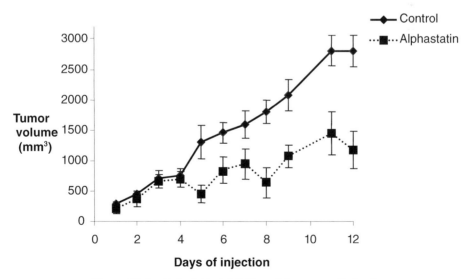

Figure 12.4 Alphastatin inhibition of tumor growth *in vivo*

in volume) before the mice were administered with alphastatin (in PBS) i.p. daily, orally in the drinking water daily (p.o.) or by intravenous injection (i.v.), 3×/ week. Three doses of alphastatin were used, namely 0.0025, 0.025 and 0.25 mg kg^{-1}, and controls received PBS alone. In this tumor model, daily administration of alphastatin i.p. or p.o. had no significant effects on tumor volume over the time course of injections (11 days). However, administration of alphastatin i.v. caused a significant decrease in tumor volume in alphastatin-treated groups compared with controls with the highest dose tested, namely 0.25 mg kg^{-1}, showing a 40 per cent inhibition by day 11 (Stribbling *et al.*, 2004). This suggests that alphastatin behaves slightly differently in different tumor models (i.p. injections significantly inhibited tumor growth in CT26, but not in 4T1 tumors) and that the i.v. route may prove to be the best route for anti-tumor activity in some forms of cancer.

Histological examination of resected control tumors and non-malignant tissues revealed that the endothelial cells formed an intact, continuous, CD31-positive layer lining the blood vessels, indicating that the blood vessels are patent, with no evidence of endothelial disruption (Figure 12.5) (Staton *et al.*, 2004a, 2004b). Figure 12.5(a) shows that alphastatin-treated tumors exhibited increased areas of necrosis (N) and large distended vessels found in areas of viable tumor as well as in areas of necrosis showing a central thrombosis (T) lined with patchy incomplete endothelial cells. By contrast, no effect of alphastatin was evident on the vascular endothelium of (b) lungs, (c) liver and (d)

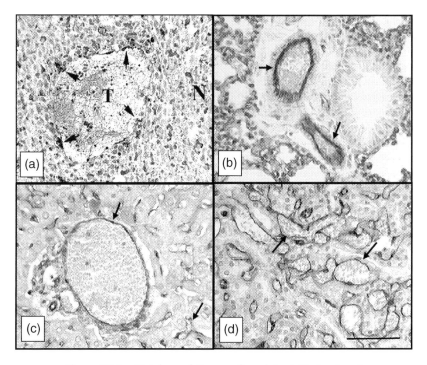

Figure 12.5 Histology of tissues after alphastatin treatment

kidneys, where the CD31$^+$ endothelial cells lining the vessels formed a continuous layer and no thrombosis was evident. Alphastatin treatment resulted in vessel disruption in all but the outermost rim of tumors, characterized by a discontinuous endothelial cell lining with many cells clumped and/or fragmented (Figure 12.5a) (Staton et al., 2004a, 2004b). There was no inflammatory cell accumulation around the disrupted vessels as opposed to unaffected vessels elsewhere in the tumor. In addition, many vessels contained (and were often surrounded by) extensive fibrin deposition, suggesting the formation of extensive thrombosis, and a non-significant increase in tumor thrombosis was seen in alphastatin-treated tumors compared with controls. This resulted in inadequate blood supply to the central areas of the tumor and the formation of large areas of necrosis (Table 12.1). These findings suggest that either Alphastatin is selectively cytotoxic for activated tumor endothelium or that it stimulates the coagulation cascade on endothelial cells directly, leading to formation of thrombosis, which in turn causes the disruption of the endothelial lining. The latter seems the most likely explanation, as there was no evidence in our *in vitro* studies that alphastatin could trigger activated endothelial cells to undergo apoptosis, and morphological analysis of CT26 tumor sections following DAPI (4,6 diamidino-2-phenylindole) staining indicated that apoptosis of endothelial cells had not occurred in treated tumors (Staton et al., 2004a). It therefore appears that alphastatin may up-regulate hemostasis within tumors, thereby blocking the blood vessels, leading to a lack of oxygen and nutrients, which in turn causes necrosis in the centre of the tumors. If the treatment period is extended then a regression in the tumor volumes may be seen as the necrotic regions collapse; however, UK Home Office Regulations do not permit a large tumor burden in mice, so animals in the control groups of our studies had to be killed before this occurred. To allow a direct comparison of tumor histology between treated and control tumors all groups had to be killed on the same day. Studies are currently underway to investigate whether alphastatin mediates its effects via a tumor-specific up-regulation of various hemostatic factors.

Interestingly, alphastatin contains the Gly–Pro–Arg (aa17–19) sequence of the fibrinogen α-chain that is known to bind to CD11c/CD18 on monocytes and neutrophils (Loike et al., 1991). There is some suggestion that CD11c/CD18 may be involved in activation of hemostasis by stimulating tissue factor (TF) expression upon monocyte binding to endothelial cells or smooth muscle cells

Table 12.1 Table showing histological analysis from tumors treated with 100 nM alphastatin. *p < 0.05 with respect to relevant control

Parameter	Control	Alphastatin treated
Tumor volume (mm^3)	2979 ± 264	1174 ± 205*
% necrosis	15.4 ± 3.25	40.6 ± 3.17*
MVD (outer viable rim)	6.23 ± 0.23	6.65 ± 0.42
MVD (inner viable rim)	4.69 ± 0.36	7.25 ± 0.43*

(Marx *et al.*, 1998). It is therefore possible *in vivo* that alphastatin binding to monocytes and neutrophils could cause up-regulation of TF expression, thereby stimulating the thrombosis formation that is seen in the alphastatin-treated tumors. Work is currently underway to investigate this hypothesis.

The blood vessels elsewhere within the mice (e.g. the liver, lungs and kidneys) were not affected by alphastatin treatment (no signs of thrombosis and most vessels were packed with erythrocytes, indicating that the vessels were not occluded), suggesting that alphastatin targets activated endothelium within the tumor rather than quiescent endothelial cells. This confirms that the receptor(s) for alphastatin may be expressed only on activated endothelium within tumor vessels and also supports a possible therapeutic role for alphastatin as an agent to specifically target activated endothelium in areas of angiogenesis, rather than endothelial cells in the quiescent vasculature.

Interestingly, despite the evidence for anti-angiogenic activity of alphastatin *in vitro*, namely inhibition of endothelial cell migration and tubule formation, microvessel density counts on CD31-stained sections of treated and control tumors (Table 12.1) suggest that alphastatin has an anti-vascular rather than anti-angiogenic effect *in vivo*. The vascular counts in the outer rim of the tumors are identical between those treated with alphastatin and control and, although within the inner, less viable rim of tumor cells abutting the areas of necrosis the vascular counts were higher in the alphastatin-treated animals compared with the same region in control tumors, this was not due to an increase in tumor angiogenesis, but a consequence of the dilation of, and thrombosis within, vessels in these tumor areas, causing an increased number of intersections between each vessel and the Chalkley grid. Further work is required to show whether the inhibitory effects of alphastatin on endothelial cells *in vitro* contributes significantly to the anti-vascular effects seen *in vivo*.

As human rather than murine alphastatin was used in our *in vivo* studies, the possibility exists that the effects on the tumor vasculature and growth were due, at least in part, to potential immunogenic effects of human alphastatin in mice. However, this is unlikely because there was no visible microscopic evidence of a peritoneal cellular reaction to alphastatin injections and histologic analysis of lungs, liver and kidneys showed no cellular or structural abnormalities. Moreover, a similar delay in tumor growth and disruption of tumor vessels has been seen in human colon xenografts (HT29; Stribbling, personal communication) and human prostate xenografts (PC3; Fowles, personal communication) grown subcutaneously in immunocompromised (nude) mice, where no such immune response is possible.

Interestingly, within our models of tumor growth, a reduced number of macroscopically visible pulmonary metastases formed by CT26 or 4T1 tumors were observed in immunocompetent (Balb/c) mice treated with alphastatin (Staton and Stribbling, unpublished observations), but these were qualitative observations and further work is continuing to quantify and document any such effect of alphastatin on metastasis.

Alphastatin structure

A number of NMR studies investigating the amino-terminus of the α-chain have suggested/indicated that FpA and the adjoining residues have a defined structure, which is clearly seen when the fibrinogen α-chain is attached to thrombin (Marsh *et al.*, 1985; Ni *et al.*, 1989a, 1989b, 1989c; Malkowski *et al.*, 1997). Interestingly, although in general short linear peptides in solution exist as an ensemble of many conformational states of similar free energy (i.e. they do not adopt a single native, low-energy form), the NMR studies carried out on aa1–23 of the α-chain of fibrinogen (i.e. most of the alphastatin sequence) seem to suggest the presence of secondary structure within this peptide (Ni *et al.*, 1989b). This secondary structure consists of "a single turn of α-helix formed by D7–E11, which is linked via G12 and a type I β-bend, involving residues L9–G12, to an extended chain of residues G13–R16" (Malkowski *et al.*, 1997). This folding produces a compact aliphatic structure with a clustering of hydrophobic side chains of F8, L9 and V15 to form one face (Stubbs *et al.*, 1992). An earlier paper, investigating analogues of FpA binding to thrombin, also provided evidence for a β-bend structure, but suggested that this is found between E11 and G12, and not G12–G13 as previously thought (Nakanishi *et al.*, 1992). Our current work identifying regions of interest in the alphastatin peptide indicates strongly that secondary structure is essential for the activity and that residues from both the FpA and aa17–24 are essential for inhibitory activity (Staton *et al.*, 2004c).

Receptor binding usually involves hydrophobic interactions between the protein and its receptor, often with the receptor containing a hydrophobic pocket into which the hydrophobic portions of the ligand binds. Alphastatin contains a β-turn or loop and hydrophobic residues along one surface of the peptide (Ni *et al.*, 1989b; Stubbs *et al.*, 1992), suggesting that this could be important for receptor binding. Interestingly, bFGF is made up of a series of β-sheets and turns and the receptor binding involves the hydrophobic residues FL on one face of a β-turn in a structure similar to alphastatin (Springer *et al.*, 1994). Similarly, EGF consists of three loops, all of which interact with the EGF receptors via hydrophobic residues (Ogiso *et al.*, 2002). Like bFGF, VEGF consists of β-sheets and turns and the loops are important for the receptor binding (Muller *et al.*, 1997). The region of VEGF responsible for VEGF-R2 binding is not actually a loop of the protein, but does contain hydrophobic residues including phenylalanine, and the VEGF-binding region of VEGF-R2 is a hydrophobic pocket (Muller *et al.*, 1997). As alphastatin inhibits endothelial cell responses to all three growth factors and the structures show some similarity, it is possible that alphastatin could mimic VEGF, EGF and bFGF by binding directly to their receptors. However, our preliminary studies with VEGF and VEGF-R2 show that alphastatin does not affect VEGF binding to its receptor or directly bind the VEGF-R2 (Staton and Lewis, unpublished data), suggesting that alphastatin is more likely to be binding directly to an alternative receptor and inhibiting downstream of the growth factor receptors.

12.4 Conclusions

In conclusion, we have identified a small peptide from the amino-terminus of the α-chain of human fibrinogen – alphastatin. This inhibits both activated endothelial migration and tubule formation *in vitro* and the growth of experimental murine tumors *in vivo*. Moreover, unlike many anti-angiogenics currently in clinical trials (e.g. Avastin), this is a pluripotent inhibitor of activated endothelial cells that inhibits endothelial cell responses to bFGF, VEGF and EGF, and appears to bind directly to endothelial cells. However, the receptor and cellular signalling pathways for alphastatin have yet to be identified. It remains to be seen whether this new anti-angiogenic peptide (or a small-molecule mimetic/smaller/cyclitized peptide derivative) has utility in the treatment of cancer.

References

Beerepoot, L.V., Witteveen, E.O., Groenewegen, G., Fogler, W.E., Sim, B.K., Sidor, C., Zonnenberg, B.A., Schramel, F., Gebbink, M.F. and Voest, E.E. (2003). Recombinant human angiostatin by twice daily subcutaneous injection in advanced cancer: a pharmacokinetic and long-term safety study. *Clin Cancer Res* **9**, 4025–4033.

Blomback, B. and Blomback, M. (1972). The molecular structure of fibrinogen. *Ann NY Acad Sci* **202**, 77–97.

Bootle-Wilbraham, C.A., Tazzyman, S., Marshall, J.M. and Lewis, C.E. (2000). Fibrinogen E-fragment inhibits the migration and tubule formation of human dermal microvascular endothelial cells *in vitro*. *Cancer Res* **60**, 4719–4724.

Bootle-Wilbraham, C.A., Tazzyman, S., Thompson, W.D., Stirk, C.M. and Lewis, C.E. (2001). Fibrin fragment E stimulates the Proliferation, migration and differentiation of human microvascular endothelial cells *in vitro*. *Angiogenesis* **4**, 269–275.

Brown, J.M. and Giaccia, A.J. (1998). The unique physiology of solid tumors: opportunities (and problem) for cancer therapy. *Cancer Res* **58**, 1408–1416.

Brown, N.J., Staton, C.A., Rodgers, G.R., Corke, K.P., Underwood, J.C.E. and Lewis, C.E. (2002). Fibrinogen E fragment selectively disrupts the vasculature and inhibits the growth of tumors in a syngeneic murine model. *Br J Cancer* **86**, 1813–1816.

Eder, J.P., Supko, J.G., Clark, J.W., Puchalski, T.A., Garcia-Carbonero, R., Ryan, D.P., Shulman, L.N., Proper, J., Kirvan, M., Rattner, B., Connors, S., Keogan, M.T., Janicek, M.J., Fogler, W.E., Schnipper, L., Kinchla, N., Sidor, C., Phillips, E., Folkman, J. and Kufe, D.W. (2002). Phase I clinical trial of recombinant human endostatin administered as a short intravenous infusion repeated daily. *J Clin Oncol* **20**, 3772–3784.

Folkman, J. (1971). Tumor angiogenesis: therapeutic implications. *N Engl J Med* **285**, 1182–1186.

Folkman, J. (1990). What is the evidence that tumors are angiogenesis dependent? *J Natl Canc Inst* **82**, 4–6.

Folkman, J. and Klagsbrun, M. (1987). Angiogenic factors. *Science* **235**, 442–447.

Gasparini, G. (1999). The rationale and future potential of angiogenesis inhibition in neoplasia. *Drugs* **58**, 17–38.

Hurwitz, H., Fehrenbacher, L., Novotny, W., Cartwright, T., Hainsworth, J., Heim, W., Berlin, J., Baron, A., Griffing, S., Holmgren, E., Ferrara, N., Fyfe, G., Rogers, B., Ross, R. and Kabbinavar, F. (2004). Bevacizumab plus irinotecan, fluorouracil and leucovorin for metastatic colorectal cancer. *N Engl J Med* **350**, 2335–2342.

Jain, R.K. (1994). Barriers to drug delivery in solid tumors. *Sci Am* **271**, 58–65.

Loike, J.D., Sodeik, B., Cao, L., Leucona, S., Weitz, J.I., Detmers, P.A., Wright, S.D. and Silverstein, S.C. (1991). CD11c/CD18 on neutrophils recognizes a domain at the N-terminus of the A alpha chain of fibrinogen. *Proc Natl Acad Sci USA* **88**, 1044–1048.

Lucas, M.A., Straight, D.L., Fretto, L.J. and McKees, P.A. (1983). The effects of fibrinogen and its cleavage products on the kinetics of plasminogen activation by urokinase and subsequent plasmin activity. *J Biol Chem* **258**, 12171–12217.

Madrazo, J., Brown, J.H., Litvinovich, S., Dominguez, R., Yakovlev, S., Medved, L. and Cohen, C. (2001). Crystal structure of the central region of bovine fibrinogen (E5 fragment) at 1.4 A resolution. *Proc Natl Acad Sci USA* **98**, 11967–11972.

Malkowski, M.G., Martin, P.D., Lord, S.T. and Edwards, B.F. (1997). Crystal structure of fibrinogen-A alpha peptide 1–23 (F8Y) bound to bovine thrombin explains why the mutation of Phe-8 to tyrosine strongly inhibits normal cleavage at Arg-16. *Biochemistry* **326**, 815–822.

Marsh, H.C., Meinwald, Y.C., Lee, S., Martinelli, R.A. and Scheraga, H.A. (1985). Mechanism of action of thrombin on fibrinogen: NMR evidence for a beta-bend at or near fibrinogen A alpha Gly(P5)-Gly(P4). *Biochemistry* **24**, 2806–2812.

Marx, N., Neumann, F-J., Zohlnhofer, D., Dickfeld, T., Fischer, A., Heimerl, S. and Schomig, A. (1998). Enhancement of monocyte procoagulant activity by adhesion on vascular smooth muscle cells and intercellular adhesion molecule-1 transfected Chinese hamster ovary cells. *Circulation* **98**, 906–911.

Maurer, M.C., Peng, J.L., An, S.S., Trosset, J.Y., Henschen-Edman, A. and Scheraga, H.A. (1998). Structural examination of the influence of phosphorylation on the binding of fibrinopeptide A to bovine thrombin. *Biochemistry* **37**, 5888–5902.

Muller, Y.A., Li, B., Christinger, H.W., Wells, J.A., Cunningham, B.C. and deVos, A.M. (1997). Vascular endothelial growth factor: crystal structure and functional mapping of the kinase domain receptor binding site. *Proc Natl Acad Sci USA* **94**, 7192–7197.

Nakanishi, H., Chrusciel, R.A., Shen, R., Bertenshaw, S., Johnson, M.E., Rydel, T.J., Tulinsky, A. and Kahn, M. (1992). Peptide mimetics of the thrombin-bound structure of fibrinopeptide A. *Proc Natl Acad Sci USA* **89**, 1705–1709.

Ni, F., Konishi, Y., Bullock, L.D., Rivetna, M.N. and Scheraga, H.A. (1989a). High resolution NMR studies of fibrinogen like peptides in solution: basis for the bleeding disorder caused by a single mutation of Gly(12) to Val(12) in the Aα chain of human fibrinogen Rouen. *Biochemistry* **28**, 3106–3119.

Ni, F., Konishi, Y., Frazier, R.B. and Scheraga, H.A. (1989b). High resolution NMR studies of fibrinogen like peptides in solution: interaction of thrombin with residues 1–23 of the Aα-chain of human fibrinogen. *Biochemistry* **28**, 3082–3094.

Ni, F., Meinwald, Y.C., Vasquez, M. and Scheraga, H.A. (1989c). High resolution NMR studies of fibrinogen like peptides in solution: structure of a thrombin bound peptide corresponding to residues 7–16 of the Aα chain of human fibrinogen. *Biochemistry* **28**, 3094–3105.

Ogiso, H., Ishitani, R., Nureki, O., Fukai, S., Yamanaka, M., Kim, J.-H., Saito, K., Sakamoto, A., Inoue, M., Shirouzo, M. and Yokoyama, S. (2002). Crystal structure of the complex of human epidermal growth factor and receptor extracellular domains. *Cell* **110**, 775–787.

O'Reilly, M.S., Boehm, T., Shing, Y., Fukai, N., Vasios, G., Lane, W.S., Flynn, E., Birkhead, J.R., Olsen, B.R. and Folkman, J. (1997). Endostatin: an endogenous inhibitor of angiogenesis and tumor growth. *Cell* **88**, 277–285.

O'Reilly, M.S., Holmgren, L., Chen, C. and Folkman, J. (1996). Angiostatin induces and sustains dormancy of human primary tumors in mice. *Nat Med* **2**, 689–692.

O'Reilly, M.S., Holmgren, L., Shing, Y., Chen, C., Rosenthal, R.A., Moses, M., Lane, W.S., Cao, Y., Sage, E.H. and Folkman, J. (1994). Angiostatin: a novel angiogenesis inhibitor that mediates the suppression of metastases by a lewis lung carcinoma. *Cell* **79**, 315–328.

Sahni, A. and Francis, C.W. (2000). Vascular endothelial growth factor binds to fibrinogen and fibrin and stimulates endothelial cell proliferation. *Blood* **96**, 3772–3778.

Sahni, A., Odrljin, T. and Francis, C.W. (1998). Binding of basic fibroblast growth factor to fibrinogen and fibrin. *J Biol Chem* **273**, 7554–7559.

Sahni, A., Sporn, L.A. and Francis, C.W. (1999). Potentiation of endothelial cell proliferation by fibrin(ogen)-bound fibroblast growth factor-2. *J Biol Chem* **274**, 14936–14941.

Springer, B.A., Pantoliano, M.W., Barbera, F.A., Gunyuzlu, P.L., Thompson, L.D., Herblin, W.F., Rosenfeld, S.A. and Book, G.W. (1994). Identification and concerted function of two receptor binding surfaces on basic fibroblast growth factor required for mitogenesis. *J Biol Chem* **269**, 26879–26884.

Staton, C.A., Brown, N.J. and Lewis, C.E. (2003). The role of fibrinogen and related fragments in tumor angiogenesis and metastasis. *Exp Opin Biol Ther* **3**, 1105–1120.

Staton, C.A., Brown, N.J., Rodgers, G., Corke, K.P., Tazzyman, S., Underwood, J.C.E. and Lewis, C.E. (2004a). Alphastatin, a 24-amino acid fragment of fibrinogen, is a potent new inhibitor of activated endothelial cells *in vitro* and *in vivo*. *Blood* **103**, 601–606.

Staton, C.A., Brown, N.J., Rodgers, G., Corke, K.P., Tazzyman, S., Underwood, J.C.E. and Lewis, C.E. (2004b). Alphastatin, a 24-amino acid fragment of fibrinogen is a novel anti-angiogenic and anti-vascular agent. *Microcirculation* **11**, 527–558 (OC9).

Staton, C.A., Garcia-Echeverria, C., Stribbling, S.M., Tazzyman, S., Brown, N.J. and Lewis, C.E. (2004c). Studies on the structure–activity relationship of alphastatin: identification of the minimal essential sequence for anti-angiogenic activity. *Angiogenesis* **7** (Suppl. 1), P12.

Stribbling, S.M., Bury, J.P., Corke, K.P., Lewis, C.E. and Brown, N.J. (2004). The in vivo efficacy of the antiangiogenic peptide alphastatin. *Microcirculation* **11**, 527–558 (P41).

Stubbs, M.T., Oschkinat, H., Mayr, I., Huber, R., Angliker, H., Stone, S.R. and Bode, W. (1992). The interaction of thrombin with fibrinogen. A structural basis for its specificity. *Eur J Biochem* **206**, 187–195.

Suhardja, A. and Hoffman, H. (2003). Role of growth factors and their receptors in proliferation of microvascular endothelial cells. *Microsc Res Tech* **60**, 70–75.

Thomas, J.P., Arzoomanian, R.Z., Alberti, D., Marnocha, R., Lee, F., Friedl, A., Tutsch, K., Dresen, A., Geiger, P., Pluda, J., Fogler, A., Schiller, J.H. and Wilding, C. (2003). Phase I pharmacokinetic and pharmacodynamic study of recombinant human endostatin in patients with advanced solid tumors. *J Clin Oncol* **21**, 223–231.

Thompson, W.D., Smith, E.B., Stirk, C.M., Marshall, F.I., Stout, A.J. and Kocchar, A. (1992). Angiogenic activity of fibrin degradation products is located in fibrin fragment E. *J Pathol* **168**, 47–53.

Twombly, R. (2002). First clinical trials of endostatin yield lukewarm results. *J Natl Cancer Inst* **94**, 1520–1521.

Yang, Z., Kollman, J.M., Pandi, L. and Doolittle, R.F. (2001). Crystal structure of native chicken fibrinogen at 2.7 A resolution. *Biochemistry* **40**, 12515–12523.

13

Cationic Lipid Complexes to Target Tumor Endothelium

Uwe Michaelis and **Michael Teifel**

13.1   Introduction

Vascular disrupting agents (VDAs) for tumor treatment are being developed to attack the pre-existing tumor vasculature. Ultimately this should lead to thrombus formation, blood vessel occlusion and reduction of tumor blood flow. Currently, there are more than a dozen agents under clinical investigation. There are vascular disrupting agents such as the low-molecular-weight cytotoxic drugs that bind and destabilize the tubulin cytoskeleton inside the tumor endothelial cells, thereby inducing rapid changes in endothelial cell shape. Although not directly targeted to the tumor endothelial cells, they are assumed to specifically interact with tumor endothelial tubulin. Others are ligand-directed VDAs, which target specific molecules that are overexpressed on the luminal or abluminal surface of tumor endothelial cells. Among these are highly selective antibodies, peptides or soluble receptors, which are covalently bound to toxins, procoagulant factors or immuno-stimulatory molecules. For an overview on vascular-targeting agents please refer for example to the following recently published reviews: Dass, 2003; Eichhorn, Strieth and Dellian, 2004; Pilat *et al.*, 2004; Siemann, Chaplin and Horsman, 2004; Thorpe, 2004.

Our review focuses on cationic liposomes as a new class of vascular disrupting agents for tumor treatment. We would like to outline recent advances in the understanding of the underlying mode of action for targeting the tumor vasculature. Results from preclinical and early clinical development of cationic liposomes as carriers for cytotoxic drugs will be discussed.

The term 'liposome' is limited to a well defined particle in which a water-filled interior is surrounded by a lipid bilayer. In cases where small-molecular-weight

Vascular-targeted Therapies in Oncology   Edited by Dietmar W. Siemann
© 2006 John Wiley & Sons, Ltd.

compounds are entrapped in the membrane bilayer, thus disturbing the normal regular structure, we prefer to use the more general term 'lipid complex'.

13.2   Tumor vascular targeting by cationic liposomes

Thurston and co-workers were the first to describe that angiogenic blood vessels in tumors preferentially bind and internalize cationic liposomes injected intravenously. They examined binding and uptake of fluorescently labeled cationic liposomes in pancreatic islet cell tumors from RIP-Tag2 transgenic mice (Thurston *et al.*, 1998). This model allows the investigation of cationic liposome targeting at different stages of tumor development in one animal. The angiogenic endothelial cells in the pancreatic islet tumors showed 15–33-fold higher uptake of cationic liposomes than corresponding normal endothelial cells. Anionic, neutral or sterically stabilized neutral liposomes were not bound and internalized. Twenty minutes after injection, electron microscopic studies showed that 85 per cent of the cationic liposomes associated with the tumor vessels were either bound to the luminal surface of the endothelium or taken up by the endothelial cells. Only 15 per cent of the liposomes located at tumor vessels had crossed the endothelium. At this time point, 51 per cent of the liposomes that were found on the luminal endothelial cell surface of tumor vessels were associated with fenestrae, although fenestrae constituted only four per cent of the luminal endothelial cell surface. The authors speculated that the positive charge of the liposomes may be the driving force for binding to the fenestrae, which are assumed to carry a negative charge (Baldwin, Wu and Stein, 1991). Interestingly, accumulation in the tumor blood vessels did not depend on a specific chemical structure of the cationic lipid that was used for the liposome preparation. The commercially available cationic lipids DDAB and DOTAP had similar vascular-targeting effects. Anionic, neutral or sterically stabilized neutral liposomes did not show any uptake by tumor blood vessels, ovaries or other organs 20 minutes after systemic administration. Despite the strong accumulation in tumor vessels cationic liposomes were also taken up by macrophages in the liver and spleen and by endothelial cells in the lung and various other organs.

  The observation that cationic liposomes preferentially target activated tumor endothelium, whereas neutral and anionic liposomes extravasate into the tumor interstitium, was confirmed by several other groups. Campbell and co-workers studied the localization of cationic liposomes by intravital microscopy and biodistribution studies (Campbell *et al.*, 2002). The interstitial localization was low (four per cent of tumor surface area), and was independent of the ratio of cationic lipids used in the formulation. In contrast, the tumor vascular coverage was enhanced compared with the electroneutral liposomes, which served as a control. Liposomes containing 50 mol per cent of cationic lipid associated with 27 per cent of the tumor vascular surface area. In this study, cationic liposomes associated only with approximately four per cent of the vascular surface area in normal tissue. These results were independent of tumor type and its microenvironment (cranial window and dorsal skinfold chamber). Biodistribution studies with ^{111}In-labeled liposomes containing increasing amounts of cationic lipids indicated that the overall uptake in whole-tumor (vascular plus interstitial localization) was not significantly affected by cationic charge. Most probably this is due to the small number of tumor endothelial cells compared to the large tumor cell mass.

The lack of extravasation of cationic liposomes was independently confirmed by several groups in a variety of different tumor models and species. Using high-resolution *in vivo* fluorescence microscopy in an amelanotic hamster melanoma growing in a transparent skinfold chamber preparation, it was shown that localization of fluorescence-labeled cationic liposomes was restricted to intratumoral microvessels. No label could be detected in the tumor extravascular compartment. Endothelial deposition in tumor vessels increased substantially during a continuous 90 min intravenous infusion (Schmitt-Sody et al., 2003). Krasnici and co-workers investigated the time-dependent uptake of cationic liposomes in solid tumors and the interaction of cationic liposomes with angiogenic endothelium in direct comparison with anionic and neutral liposomes (Krasnici et al., 2003). They quantified the distribution of rhodamine-labeled cationic liposomes in histological cryosections of the amelanotic melanoma A-Mel-3 after systemic application. Again, the accumulation of rhodamine fluorescence was highly specific and restricted to tumor blood vessels. The liposomal fluorescence collocalized with the vascular FITC-labeled lectin *lycopersicon esculentum*. Twenty minutes after the end of infusion, there were no signs of extravascular rhodamine fluorescence. Neutral and anionic liposomes extravasated and did not show any significant association with FITC-positive tumor vessels. In contrast to anionic and neutral liposomes, the cationic liposomes were still retained within the tumor vasculature up to six hours after systemic application, but showed a rapid clearance from circulation. The targeting properties were rather independent of the percentage and nature of the colipid in the formulation and mainly determined by the positive charge of the liposomes. Tumor-to-normal tissue fluorescence ratio increased over time in the cationic liposome group. These observations are confirmed by our own studies in animal tumor models, where we consistently observed a collocalization of fluorescence and blood-vessel-wall-specific FITC-lectin staining after intravenous application of fluorescently labeled liposomes.

Neovascular targeting was also demonstrated in biopsies derived from patients from a clinical phase Ib/II tumor imaging trial in bladder cancer. Histological analysis of tumor sections demonstrated that after intravenous infusion of a single low dose of rhodamine-labeled cationic liposomes (0.5 or 2.0 mg total lipid/kg body weight) fluorescence was restricted to capillaries and medium-sized vessels in tumor lesions. Interestingly, stromal capillaries in proximity to tumor area showed the highest fluorescence intensity, indicating an association between binding affinity and neoangiogenesis in the tumor periphery (Knüchel *et al.*, 2003; Figure 13.1). Figure 13.1 shows that uptake of intravenously administered LipoRed is preferentially at the tumor periphery, in regions where many new blood vessels are formed (arrows). Only weak binding is observed in non-tumor blood vessels (stars). Cryosections of the respective area were prepared for histopathology. Left picture: fluorescence microscopy; right picture: bright-field microscopy of the same tissue preparation.

It is worth noting that the targeting of tumor vessels by cationic liposomes does not necessarily mean that the greatest fraction of the administered dose ends up in the tumor. After systemic administration to normal mice, cationic liposomes complexed with DNA or cationic liposomes alone are taken up by endothelial cells, macrophages and intravascular leukocytes (McLean *et al.*, 1997). Furthermore it is known that cationic lipid complexes interact with plasma proteins and surface molecules of circulating blood cells (Nishikawa and Huang, 2001; Eichhorn *et al.*, 2004c; Sakurai *et al.*, 2001a, 2001b). The preferential uptake in tumor vessels compared with that in normal tissue cannot compensate for the high number of weaker-binding regions on quiescent endothelial cells in normal tissue and on circulating blood cells. The vasculature of the tumor occupies only a relatively small area of the total vascular surface in the body. However, systemic administration leads to fast accumulation of two to five per cent of the total administered cationic lipid dose in the intratumoral microvasculature and almost complete coverage of the tumor vessel surface (Campbell *et al.*, 2002; own data, not shown). Therefore cationic liposomes or lipid complexes offer an attractive approach for the physical targeting of highly effective therapeutic drug doses to the angiogenic endothelial cells of solid

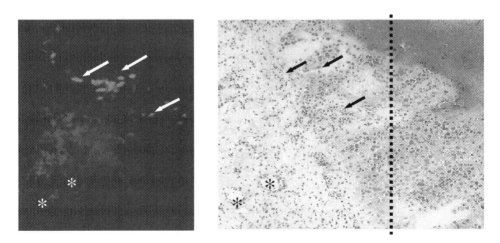

Figure 13.1 Accumulation of tumor imaging agent LipoRed in blood vessels of a patient with bladder cancer. LipoRed is a cationic liposome formulation loaded with the fluorescent dye rhodamine (A color reproduction of this figure can be seen in the color section)

tumors. Finally, this should lead to strong intracellular accumulation of cyto-toxic drugs in the tumor endothelial cells, thereby attacking the tumor at its 'Achilles' heel'. This targeting concept differs fundamentally from conventional therapy with administered free cytotoxic drugs, which are targeting the tumor cells.

13.3 Potential targets for cationic lipid complexes on tumor endothelial cells

It is known that during the process of angiogenesis endothelial cells undergo several dramatic changes affecting endocytotic uptake, receptor expression and the fluidity and charge of the cell surface membrane. In tumors, depending on the tumor type and stage, as many as 1–32 per cent (median value: nine per cent) of the endothelial cells undergo mitosis, whereas endothelial cells from normal tissues hardly divide (0.01–1 per cent; median value: 0.2 per cent) (Denekamp, 1993).

The overall positive charge of the liposomes and lipid complexes is required to enhance the interaction with the tumor endothelium. Therefore, electrostatic interactions between the cationic lipid complexes and the surface of the dividing endothelial cells seem to contribute to the targeting selectivity of cationic liposomes. Nevertheless, the underlying molecular mechanism and structures responsible for enhanced binding and uptake of cationic lipid complexes by tumor endothelial cells are not understood. This raises the question of which characteristic physiological features of endothelial cells lining the blood vessels of tumors or regions of inflammation could potentially attract positively charged particles such as cationic lipid complexes.

Negatively charged cell surface proteoglycans could be an important endothelial cell surface component for the binding and uptake of cationic lipid complexes. Heparan sulfate proteoglycans and dermatan/chondroitin sulfate proteoglycans bind to various components, regulate protein–protein interactions and play a pivotal role in many biological processes including cellular proliferation, differentiation and wound healing (Iozzo and San Antonio, 2001; Trowbridge and Gallo, 2002; Pries, Secomb and Gaehtgens, 2000). Previously it was shown that the expression pattern of proteoglycans can change during angiogenesis. Inflammation-dependent angiogenesis induces the expression of decorin, a chondroitin/dermatan sulfate, in endothelial cells. The exclusive expression of decorin in newly formed blood vessels cells appears to be of direct relevance in angiogenesis (Schönherr et al., 2004). Decorin-positive capillaries are also found in the granulation tissue of healing dermal wounds and capillary neovessels in inflamed temporal artery wall (Nelimarkka et al., 2001). During skin wound healing, the transmembrane heparan sulfate proteoglycans syndecan-1 and syndecan-4 are upregulated. Syndecan-4 is present on endothelial cells and fibroblasts (Echtermeyer et al., 2001), whereas the upregulation of syndecan-1 is restricted to the endothelial cells of the granulation tissue (Gallo *et al.*, 1996).

Immuno-histochemical analysis of human tissue samples has revealed that glypican-1, which is attached to the plasma membrane via a glycosyl phosphoinositol linkage, is dramatically up-regulated in glioma vessel endothelial cells, whereas it is absent in normal brain vessel endothelial cells. In this study, syndecan-1 could not be detected in normal and glioma vessels, whereas low levels of syndecan-4 were seen in both glioma and normal brain vessels. Syndecan-2 was mildly increased in glioma vessel endothelial cells compared with normal brain vessels (Qiao *et al.*, 2003). Enhanced synthesis and deposition of perlecan, an extracellular heparan sulfate proteoglycan, is observed in newly formed blood vessels during tumor development (Iozzo and San Antonio, 2001). There is also experimental evidence that proteoglycans can serve as negatively charged cationic lipid complex receptors *in vivo*. Pretreatment of mice with heparinase I, which cleaves the heparan sulfate proteoglycans, prior to intravenous administration of cationic lipid:DNA complexes, inhibits transfection in several organs (Mounkes *et al.*, 1998). Further evidence that charge interaction between cationic lipid complexes and the proteoglycans plays an important role *in vivo* can be derived from our own studies. Preadministration of polycationic protamin resulted in enhanced accumulation of cationic lipid complexes in the tumor blood vessels, probably by saturation of potential binding sites outside the tumor vasculature (Eichhorn *et al.*, 2004c). The role of specific extracellular negatively charged proteoglycans for enhanced binding and uptake of cationic lipid complexes in newly formed blood vessels needs further examination. Also, it remains to be proven whether the total proteoglycan content is substantially increased at the surface of angiogenic endothelial cells, thereby contributing to an increased exposure of anionic sites.

Recently, other structures were identified that could represent binding sites for the cationic lipid complexes. Anionic phospholipids are known to be largely absent from the surface of resting mammalian cells under normal conditions. It was demonstrated that anionic phospholipids – most likely phosphatidylserine – are exposed on the luminal surface of tumor endothelial cells (Ran, Downes and Thorpe, 2002; Ran and Thorpe, 2002). Up to 40 per cent of the tumor blood vessels were stained positive for anionic phospholipids after systemic administration of Annexin V or a specific antibody directed against anionic phospholipids. The tumor blood vessels appear to be intact and functional. Interestingly, inflammatory cytokines as well as hypoxia/reoxygenation and other stress factors could trigger translocation of negatively charged phospholipids from the inner leaflet to the outer leaflet of the plasma membrane in cultured endothelial cells. None of the blood vessels in other organs examined had detectable anionic phospholipids at the luminal surface of their quiescent endothelium. Most recently, it was shown that the exposure of phosphatidylserine to the luminal plasma membrane was heterogeneous within a single vessel (Ran *et al.*, 2005).

The influence of proteins potentially responsible for enhanced binding and uptake of cationic liposomes needs further investigation. The tumor microenvironment is known to induce distinct protein expression on the endothelial cell surface. Cationic lipid binding proteins at the surface of tumor endothelial cells could be identified by two powerful techniques. For example, by direct proteomic mapping, Schnitzer's group was able to identify tumor-specific endothelial surface proteins that are accessible by the intravenous route (Oh *et al.*, 2004). Also, the *in vivo* phage display screening can identify proteins expressed on the endothelial surface in tumors (see Zurita, Arap and Pasqualini, 2003, for review) or even within focal regions of the microvasculature (Yao *et al.*, 2005).

Augustin and colleagues demonstrated expression of hyperglycosylated and hypersialylated membrane proteins in migrating endothelial cells *in vitro* (Augustin, Kozian and Johnson, 1994). This was probably related to the expression of endosialin, a C-type lectin-like membrane receptor with a core protein that is abundantly sialylated. Several independent investigations have linked the expression of endosialin (tumor endothelial marker 1) to the formation of new vessels in tumors (St Croix *et al.*, 2000; Christian *et al.*, 2001), although the extent of selectivity is controversially discussed (Opavsky *et al.*, 2001). Hyperglycosylation was also found in the corpus luteum *in vivo*, which periodically induces an exceptional rate of angiogenesis (Augustin *et al.*, 1995). Furthermore, TNF-α, which plays an important role in the stimulation of tumor endothelial cells, has been shown to increase negative cell surface charge in cultured human umbilical cord vein endothelial cells (HUVEC) (Kirkpatrick *et al.*, 2003). A schematic diagram depicting the changes in angiogenic versus quiescent endothelium that are important for understanding the vascular-targeting properties of cationic lipid complexes is shown in Figure 13.2. The tight and thick glycocalyx prevents uptake of the transiently bound cationic lipid complexes (left). In the tumor the more negatively charged, less dense glycocalyx and exposure of the negatively charged phosphatidylserine enables strong binding to and uptake into angiogenic endothelial cells (right).

Beside these potential binding molecules at the luminal surface of the endothelial cells, other characteristic features of angiogenic tumor vessels could promote the accumulation of cationic lipid complexes. For example, Campbell *et al.* speculated that the sluggish and irregular tumor blood flow may facilitate charge interaction between cationic liposomes and anionic binding sites on the chaotic tumor vasculature (Campbell *et al.*, 2002).

13.4   Cationic liposomes as drug carriers

Liposomes were first described by Bangham and co-workers (Bangham, Standion and Watkins, 1965). In 1970, Gregoriadis and Ryman described the use of liposomes as a carrier for enzymes or drugs (Gregoriadis and Ryman,

Normal   Tumor

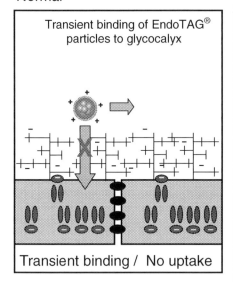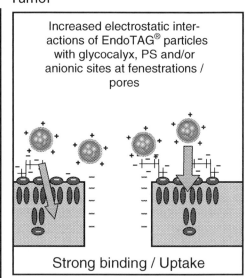

Figure 13.2 Schematic diagram depicting the changes in angiogenic versus quiescent endothelium that are important for understanding the vascular targeting properties of cationic lipid complexes. End TAG® is a registered trademark in Germany (A color reproduction of this figure can be seen in the color section)

1971). The first studies on *in vivo* experiments were subsequently published, describing the fate of liposomally associated proteins after injection into rats (Gregoriadis and Ryman, 1972). Translation of this approach for the delivery of cancer chemotherapy by using liposomes as drug carriers was later discussed by the same group (Gregoriadis *et al.*, 1974).

Gene transfer

In 1987, Felgner and co-workers described the synthesis of the first cationic lipid N-[1-(2,3-dioleyloxy)propyl]-N,N,N-trimethylammonium chloride (DOTMA) for gene transfer to cultured mammalian cells (Felgner *et al.*, 1987). Using cationic liposomes to deliver the polyanionic DNA in form of a lipid: DNA complex was shown to greatly enhance the efficiency of gene transfer to cultured mammalian cells. Since then, a large variety of cationic lipids has been synthesized with the aim of improving the transfection efficiency and reducing the toxicity observed in different types of cell culture (Stamatatos *et al.*, 1988; Behr *et al.*, 1989; Ito *et al.*, 1990; Rose, Buonocore and Whitt, 1991; Gao and Huang, 1991). In parallel, an increasing number of studies has been published describing the use of cationic lipids for gene transfer protocols in animals

(Brigham *et al.*, 1989; Nabel, Plautz and Nabel, 1990; Zhu *et al.*, 1993). In most cases, *in vivo* application of the lipid-complexed nucleic acid was performed by intratumoral administration.

Low transfection efficiencies and observed toxicities were still a major drawback limiting the success of *in vivo* gene transfer using cationic lipids. It was then not until 1993 that Nabel *et al.* undertook the first attempt to use cationic lipids in a clinical setting for the treatment of cancer by means of intratumoral injection or administration via the pulmonary artery (Nabel *et al.*, 1993). In this study, treatment was well tolerated and no signs of toxicity were observed. Subsequently, mechanistic studies were undertaken to evaluate the underlying basis of the observed toxicities. Although mostly published in the context of cationic lipid:DNA complexes, some studies also demonstrated comparable intolerabilities after injection of 'plain' liposomes or such carrying proteins or small-molecular-weight compounds. A detailed summary of these effects will be presented in a subsequent chapter.

The relevance of cationic liposomes in the field of gene therapy as alternatives to viral vectors has been reviewed recently (Smyth-Templeton, 2003; Dass, 2004) and is not the topic of our review.

Chemotherapeutic drugs and proteins

Besides neutral and anionic liposomes, cationic liposomes have been recently used to study their utility as delivery vehicles for several different compounds. Already in the early 1970s, Magee and co-workers described the use of cationic liposomes to enhance the delivery of macromolecules to cultured cells *in vitro* (Magee and Miller, 1972; Magee *et al.*, 1974). In their studies they demonstrated the effective delivery of antibodies or horseradish peroxidase to cultured cells. Further studies have been published concerning the potential to use cationic liposomes as a delivery vehicle for antibiotics to bacteria (Vitas, Diaz and Gamazo, 1997).

Subsequently, several groups evaluated the use of cationic liposomes as delivery vehicles for low-molecular-weight compounds *in vivo*. Arndt *et al.* studied different types of liposome for their utility to encapsulate daunorubicin and to study their antitumor activity (Arndt *et al.*, 1983). Besides neutral and anionic liposomes, they also evaluated liposomes containing less than 10 per cent of stearylamine as a cationic lipid component. The cationic liposomes demonstrated better tolerability, but no improvement in antitumor activity, when compared with the free drug. In a further study, Webb *et al.* used the cationic lipid stearylamine as a colloidal stabilizer in drug-containing liposomes (Webb *et al.*, 1995). It can be assumed that at least some of the beneficial effects originally attributed to the special characteristics of the cationic liposomes can be 'simply' explained by this colloidal stabilization by using small amounts of cationic lipids in the liposomal formulation. In 1997, it was demonstrated for the first time that cationic liposomes are not only able to improve stability or tolerability of a given drug but are also able to yield better efficacy *in vivo* than the non-liposomal drug (Vitas, Diaz and Gamazo, 1997). In their study, encapsulation of gentamicin in cationic liposomes was shown to improve the efficacy against systemic brucellosis. In the following years several studies demonstrated an improvement in therapeutic activity of chemotherapeutic drugs or antibiotics by using cationic liposomal encapsulated drugs (Lee *et al.*, 2002; Sangare *et al.*, 2001; Sengupta *et al.*, 2000, 2001). Sengupta and co-workers clearly demonstrated that the cationic lipid-complexed topoisomerase II inhibitor etoposide had much stronger antitumor efficacy than the corresponding free drug. However, none of these studies described the use of cationic liposomes for delivery of compounds to endothelial cells, nor have they shown the affinity of cationic liposomes for angiogenic endothelial cells. This concept was first published by McDonald and co-workers, who described that angiogenic endothelial cells avidly accumulate cationic liposomes (Thurston *et al.*, 1998).

13.5 Side-effects of intravenously administered cationic lipid complexes

Although considered as relatively safe delivery vehicles, the *in vivo* application of cationic liposomes or cationic lipid:DNA complexes is often associated with side-effects. In fact, numerous reports describe their application as being associated with moderate to severe toxicity (Yew *et al.*, 1999; Tousignant *et al.*, 2000; Audouy *et al.*, 2002; Hirko, Tang and Hughes, 2003; Simberg *et al.*, 2004; Zhang, Liu and Huang, 2005). Besides the activation of the complement system, interaction of cationic liposomes or cationic lipid:DNA complexes with blood components namely serum proteins and blood cells are further possible causes of intolerabilities observed after intravenous administration (Senior, Trimble and Maskiewicz, 1991; Sakurai *et al.*, 2001a, 2001b). Most prominent among the published side-effects is the development of typical symptoms of lung emboli, ranging from temporal difficulties of breathing to shocklike symptoms. Sakurai *et al.* provide evidence that after systemic intravenous application cationic lipid: DNA complexes become transiently bound to normal blood vessels such as lung capillaries (Sakurai *et al.*, 2001a, 2001b).

In general, toxicity associated with cationic lipids is discussed highly controversially within the scientific community. For an understanding of the reported adverse events, it is of critical importance to take the different physicochemical characteristics of the individual formulations (e.g. size, charge/zetapotential, fluidity, lipid composition) and the differences in the experimental conditions into account. Obviously, the route of application, e.g. intravascular versus intratumoral, but also intravenous versus intraarterial, may induce totally different side-effects. Furthermore, variables such as dose and speed of application are factors that strongly influence tolerability.

Some reported reactions are not specifically associated with positively charged lipids or liposomes, but are at least in part related to the colloidal nature of the particles. In fact, comparing the reported findings for intravenously administered neutral liposomal formulations such as Doxil®, Ambisome® or liposomal hemoglobin with those of cationic liposomal formulations or lipid:DNA complexes, it is obvious that these formulations exhibit some overlap in the toxicity profile. Some of the observed intolerabilities may be subsumed under the generic term 'infusion reactions'. Among these, for the approved drugs Ambisome® and Doxil®, are symptoms such as dyspnea, hypertension, hypotension, shocklike symptoms, low body temperature and back pain (Szebeni et al., 2000, 2002).

Already in 1979, a first report described the potential of liposomes to trigger an induction of human complement (Cunningham et al., 1979), which is thought to play a major role in the genesis of various toxic reactions. Subsequently, further studies have been published describing the activation of the complement system by different liposomal formulations, including neutral, anionic and cationic liposomes and also lipid:DNA complexes, in more detail (Mold and Gewurz, 1980; Tsujimoto, Inoue and Nojima, 1981; Chonn, Cullis and Devine, 1991; Plank et al., 1996). Very detailed mechanistic studies on the biochemical processes underlying the toxicities observed after intravenous administration of several liposomal and micellar formulations have been published by Szebeni and co-workers (Szebeni et al., 1994; Szebini, Muggia and Awing, 1998; Szebini et al., 1999, 2000; Szebini, 2001; Szebini, et al., 2002; Szebini, 2004). The activation of the complement system via the alternative pathway has been clearly demonstrated after intravenous administration of neutral liposomes with or without encapsulated hemoglobin in rats (Szebeni et al., 1994). Very comparable effects have subsequently been demonstrated for the Cremophor EL®-containing micellar formulation of Taxol® (Szebeni, Muggia and Awing, 1998) and for the PEGylated liposomal Doxorubicin formulation Doxil® (Szebeni et al., 2002). The effects observed in animal models as well as in patients were at least in part comparable and consisted of a rise in pulmonary arterial pressure (PAP), decline in cardiac output, potential increase in heart rate and pulmonary and systemic vascular resistance (PVR, SVR). In very detailed mechanistic studies in pigs, these side-effects could be attributed to an up to 100-fold rise in plasma thromboxane B2 (Szebeni et al., 1999) and to an induction of complement factors such as C3a, C5a and liposome-complexing antibodies (Szebeni et al., 2000). As the infusion reaction to liposomes arises without prior sensitization (i.e. also at first application), and usually symptoms lessen or disappear after later treatments or upon interruption of the injection, the term 'pseudoallergy' was coined by the authors. To combine his findings with those reported by others, Szebeni also introduced the term 'complement-activation-related pseudoallergy' (CARPA; Szebeni, 2001). However, the extent and severity of these toxicities were strongly dependent on lipid composition, liposome charge and size, the total lipid dose administered and the speed of administration (Szebeni et al., 2000). The strongest side-effects were observed after intravenous bolus injection of high doses

of large multilamellar (1–4 μm in diameter) anionic liposomes with a high cholesterol content. Slow infusions of small unilamellar liposomes (~200 nm in
diameter) with reduced cholesterol content were found to be safe.

The strong dependence of side-effects on the specific nature of cationic lipid
complexes has been confirmed by our own studies. During the development of
EndoTAG®-1,* a cationic liposomal formulation of paclitaxel as a vascular-
disrupting agent for treatment of solid tumors, we have therefore systematically
optimized the lipid composition (including the ratio between cationic and helper
lipid), the size and the overall charge of the cationic lipid complex. Over 100
different formulations were screened in numerous animal models. In these
studies, it also appeared to be of great importance to manufacture well defined
lipid complexes in terms of, e.g., mean diameter, size distribution (polydispersity
index), charge, drug content and lamellarity. We subsequently investigated the
toxicity of EndoTAG®-1 in acute intravenous and subchronic toxicity studies in
mice, rats and beagles. Here, we also experienced that fast intravenous bolus
injection of EndoTAG®-1 can induce shocklike symptoms. However, by reducing the injection speed the tolerability dramatically improved to virtual absence
of side-effects. In summary, EndoTAG®-1 was well tolerated over a wide dose
range.

13.6   Preclinical data

In this section, key preclinical results with EndoTAG-1 and EndoTAG-2 will be
presented.

EndoTAG®-1 and EndoTAG®-2 are cationic lipid formulations of the antimitotic drug paclitaxel and the topoisomerase I inhibitor camptothecin, respectively. Both formulations are designed to carry chemotherapeutic drugs to the
tumor endothelium and thus act as a vascular-disrupting agent able to destroy
existing tumor blood vessels. The overall cationic charge of the liposomal formulation serves as a 'stabilizer' for the colloidal formulation, avoiding aggregation of the liposomes *in vitro*, and most importantly is responsible for targeting
the drug-containing cationic liposomal formulations to the tumor endothelium.
The background for this cationic-charge-mediated vascular targeting has already
been discussed in Section 13.3.

The effective binding to and the absence of leakage through the tumor vasculature was demonstrated using rhodamine-labeled EndoTAG®-2 in the B-16
melanoma model in mice (Brill *et al.*, 2004). FITC-labeled lectin *Lycopersicon
esculentum* was used to label tumor blood vessels (Figure 13.3, upper figure).
Colocalization of rhodamine-labeled EndoTAG®-2 with the tumor blood vessels
and absence of extravasation was demonstrated in the rhodamine fluorescence
mode (Figure 13.3, lower figure). Once bound to the tumor endothelial cell

*EndoTAG-1 and EndoTAG-2 are the new names for MBT-0206 and MBT-0312.

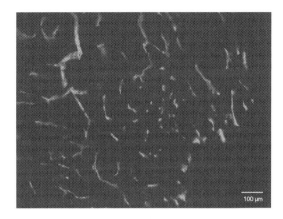

FITC-lectin

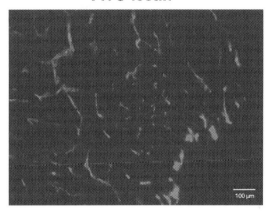

Rh-EndoTAG®-2

Figure 13.3 Vascular localization of rhodamine-labeled EndoTAG®-2 in B-16 melanoma (red), 20 min after intravenous administration. Intravenous injected FITC-lectin (green) served as counterstain to label tumor blood vessels (A color reproduction of this figure can be seen in the color section)

surface, the drug-carrying cationic liposomes are thought to be taken up by an endocytotic process. Thurston *et al.* have used gold-labeled cationic liposomes to study the process of uptake by angiogenic tumor endothelial cells in the RIP-Tag2 model (Thurston *et al.*, 1998). Only 20 min after intravenous application, the gold-labeled cationic liposomes were shown to be taken up into endothelial cells by endocytotic processes.

Subsequently, it was demonstrated that EndoTAG®-1, the cationic liposomal formulation containing paclitaxel, exhibited a drastically different activity profile as compared with the non-liposomal formulation of paclitaxel Taxol® (Kunstfeld *et al.*, 2003). The cationic liposomal paclitaxel formulation showed strongly enhanced anti-tumor activity as compared with Taxol. Furthermore, it was demonstrated that, in contrast to Taxol, EndoTAG®-1 strongly reduced the mitotic rate of tumor endothelial cells, providing another line of evidence for an uptake of intact drug-loaded cationic liposomes into angiogenic tumor endothelial cells. In addition, histochemical analysis using antibodies against von Willebrand factor (vWF) confirmed these observations by demonstrating a reduction in the vessel density after treatment with EndoTAG®-1. Another important finding was that in contrast to Taxol®, EndoTAG®-1 blocked tumor invasion. In the EndoTAG®-1 treatment group, there was a sharp demarcated tumor border, a clear evidence for effective inhibition of tumor invasion. In contrast, in the Taxol® group very aggressive infiltration of the healthy tissue was detected.

Further experimental data supporting this finding was published recently by Dellian and co-workers. Using the syngeneic melanoma A-Mel-3 growing in a skinfold chamber preparation on the back of Syrian golden hamsters, the authors demonstrated that EndoTAG®-1 treatment affected several micro-circulatory parameters (Strieth et al., 2004). In contrast to the Taxol®-, empty-liposome- or vehicle-treated group, EndoTAG®-1 treatment resulted in reduction of the functional vessel density and in impairment of vessel maturation as exemplified by constant vessel diameter and blood flow. In a very recent study, MRI measurements in a solid hamster melanoma model revealed a reduced tumor blood volume and a decreased clearance of the MRI contrast agent from tumors, indicating enhanced leakage of the contrast agent out of the damaged vessels. Further histological studies revealed that treatment with EndoTAG®-1 was able to disrupt tumor blood vessels, leading to a leakage of red blood cells (RBCs), which may lead to thrombotic occlusion of tumor blood vessels, as shown by preliminary results (Eichhorn et al., 2004a, 2004b). Evidence for vessel damage was also presented by Kunstfeld et al. in histological sections. They observed an additional perivascular accumulation of fluorescently labeled liposomes in mice that had previously received treatment with paclitaxel-loaded cationic lipid complexes designed to disrupt the tumor vasculature (Kunstfeld et al., 2003).

These anti-vascular effects in the tumor are thought to represent the basis for pronounced impairment of tumor growth, which was demonstrated by us and several collaborators in various Taxol®-sensitive but most importantly also in Taxol®-resistant tumor models in mice and rats. Strong anti-tumor activity has been demonstrated at different treatment schedules and doses in mouse renal carcinoma (RenCa), mouse B-16 melanoma, human melanoma A-375, mouse Lewis lung carcinoma (LLC), human pancreatic carcinoma (L3.6pl) and others. In the rat glioblastoma 101-8, increased survival rates were observed after monotherapy with EndoTAG®-1. For example, efficacy superior to that of empty liposomes or the free drug Taxol® has been shown in the A-375 melanoma model (Figure 13.4). Male NMRI nude mice ($n = 8$ per group) with A-375 subcutaneous melanoma were treated by six i.v. injections over 2 weeks starting on day 14 after tumor inoculation. The animals received either five

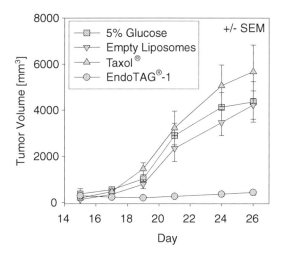

Figure 13.4   Efficacy of EndoTAG®-1 in A-375 melanoma model in NMRI nude mice

per cent glucose, empty liposomes, 12.5 mg lipid-complexed paclitaxel (EndoTAG®-1)/kg b.w. or 12.5 mg paclitaxel (Taxol®)/kg b.w., respectively. Data shown in Figure 13.4 are the mean tumor volumes +/− SEM. In another melanoma model, the A-Mel-3 in Syrian Golden hamsters, Schmitt-Sody *et al.* demonstrated superior inhibition of tumor growth by EndoTAG®-1 treatment (Schmitt-Sody *et al.*, 2003). Furthermore, they observed a delayed onset of metastasis, an effect that was subsequently confirmed in a study by Bruns and co-workers in a strongly metastatic orthotopic human pancreatic cancer model in nude mice (Papyan *et al.*, 2004). Both monotherapy with EndoTAG®-1 and combination therapy with the standard chemotherapeutic drug gemcitabine, in addition to a strong anti-tumor activity, led to a total suppression of the development of liver metastasis. Also, combination therapy of EndoTAG®-1 with cisplatin showed at least additive activity (data not shown), indicating the attractiveness of combining vascular-disrupting approaches with conventional chemotherapy directed against the tumor itself.

In the Taxol®-resistant B-16 melanoma model in C57/BL6 mice, anti-tumor activity was evaluated in comparison to empty liposomes, Taxol® (several doses) and a combination treatment of empty liposomes and Taxol® to demonstrate that the anti-tumor activity of EndoTAG®-1 is mediated by the intact cationic liposomal formulation of paclitaxel targeted to the tumor endothelium. As shown in Figure 13.5, treatment with EndoTAG®-1 was superior to all control groups, providing further evidence of the vascular-disrupting properties of EndoTAG®-1. Treatment starts on day 10; paclitaxel dose 5 mg paclitaxel/kg b.w. (low-dose Taxol and EndoTAG-1), 20 mg paclitaxel/kg b.w. (high-dose Taxol); schedule, days 10, 12 and 14 for all groups except high-dose Taxol (days

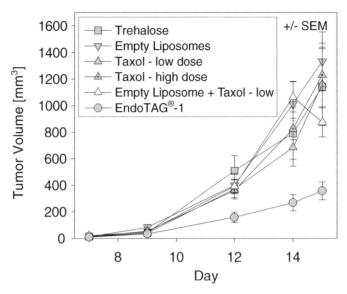

Figure 13.5   Anti-tumor efficacy of EndoTAG®-1 against B-16 melanoma ($n = 8$–10)

10 and 14). Data shown in Figure 13.5 are the mean tumor volumes +/– SEM. In line with these findings, Groner and co-workers published a study where they used the camptothecin-containing cationic liposomal formulation EndoTAG®-2 for the treatment of renal carcinoma (RenCa) and B-16 melanoma in syngeneic mice (Brill *et al.*, 2004). In this study, in contrast to the free drug sodium-camptothecin, EndoTAG®-2 showed strong anti-tumor activity (Figure 13.6). Female C57/BL6 mice ($n = 10$ per group) with subcutaneous B-16 melanoma were treated by six i.v. injections over 2 weeks on a Mon, Wed, Fri schedule. Treatment was initiated at day 7 after tumor cell injection. The animals received 10 per cent trehalose, 2.0 mg/kg b.w. CPT or 2.0 mg/kg b.w. lipid-complexed CPT (EndoTAG®-2), respectively. Data shown in Figure 13.6 are the mean tumor volumes + SEM.

In parallel, the authors evaluated the anti-vascular effects of a single treatment in a very elegant experiment using several immuno-histochemical and ELISA-based methods. For immuno-histochemistry, DAPI was used to label cell nuclei, endothelial-specific antibody CD31 to label endothelial cells and finally the TUNEL stain to detect cells undergoing apoptosis. Using these markers, the authors were able to demonstrate the induction of tumor endothelial cell apoptosis upon treatment with EndoTAG®-2 as early as 8 hours after a single treatment (Figure 13.7). Quantification of the number of tumor endothelial cells undergoing apoptosis revealed that in contrast to free sodium-camptothecin, a single treatment with EndoTAG®-2 induced apoptosis in as much as ~13 per cent of the tumor endothelial cells 8 hours after treatment.

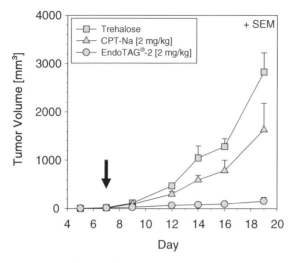

Figure 13.6 Anti-tumor efficacy of EndoTAG®-2 against B-16 melanoma ($n = 8$–10)

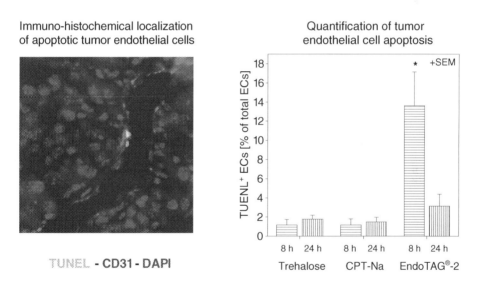

Figure 13.7 Strong and fast induction of tumor endothelial cell apoptosis in B16 melanoma after a single treatment with 10 per cent trehalose, 2.0 mg/kg b.w. CPT or 2.0 mg/kg b.w. lipid-complexed CPT (EndoTAG®-2), respectively. Data shown are mean values + SEM. *$p < 0.05$ versus controls

In parallel, serum levels of soluble E-Selectin (sE-Sel) were measured as a potential surrogate marker for the anti-vascular effects of EndoTAG®-2 treatment. Also, 8 hours after EndoTAG®-2 treatment, the time-point of maximal tumor endothelial cell apoptosis, a strong increase in the serum levels of soluble

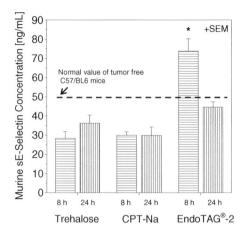

Figure 13.8 Increase of soluble E-Selectin levels in serum of B-16-melanoma-bearing mice after a single treatment with 10 per cent trehalose, 2.0 mg/kg b.w. CPT or 2.0 mg/kg b.w. lipid-complexed CPT (EndoTAG®-2), respectively. Data shown are mean values + SEM. *$p < 0.05$ versus controls

E-Selectin (sE-Sel) was demonstrated (Figure 13.8). This finding supports the further evaluation of soluble E-Selectin as a candidate for a surrogate marker of anti-vascular-targeted treatment regimes.

In summary, vascular-targeted chemotherapeutic drugs on the basis of the EndoTAG® platform showed strong anti-tumor activity in a large variety of tumor models at doses where the free drugs were ineffective. EndoTAG®-1 demonstrated activity in Taxol®-sensitive and most importantly also in Taxol®-resistant tumor models. These observations provide strong evidence that cationic lipid complexes are directing encapsulated drugs against the tumor vasculature. Mechanistic studies confirmed the anti-vascular effects as the underlying mode of action for cationic-lipid-based therapy.

13.7   Clinical data

The toxicity and accumulation of fluorescent cationic lipid complexes (LipoRed) in human tumor microvasculature was investigated in phase I clinical studies on bladder cancer and head and neck squamous cell carcinoma. These studies with LipoRed validated the concept of selectively targeting tumor endothelium with cationic lipid complexes in humans, as shown by histological examination of biopsies (Knüchel *et al.*, 2003, Section 13.2, Figure 13.1). Labeling of tumor blood vessels with intravenously administered LipoRed demonstrated that the targeting effect on tumor blood vessel endothelial cells is consistent in rodents and humans. It is interesting to note that in these diagnostic clinical trials the uptake of the diagnostic label was not strictly limited to the solid tumor area. It also occurred in angiogenic blood vessels in tissue adjacent to the tumor.

Subsequently, EndoTAG®-1, a cationic lipid formulation of paclitaxel, was evaluated in a broad phase I clinical program in several indications including breast, colorectal, prostate and gastro-intestinal cancer. Between June 2002 and July 2003 in total 118 patients with advanced, metastatic cancer were enrolled. The primary goal of these studies was to determine the safety and tolerability of EndoTAG®-1 infusion and to investigate the pharmacokinetics. Varying dosing regimes were investigated, ranging from 2.6 to 63 mg lipid-complexed paclitaxel m^{-2} per single dose. The overall response rate in these patients with advanced, metastatic cancer was 8–14 per cent, which is in the typical range for phase I trials (i.e. 10.6 per cent) according to Horstmann *et al.* (2005). Importantly, long-term treatment seemed to improve the thera-peutic response and there were no signs of resistance or accumulation of tox-icities. It is important to mention that patients in the highest-dose group received up to 48 mg total lipid per kg body weight in a single dose. There were no drug-related deaths and only a low number of serious adverse events, indicative of low organ and bone marrow toxicity. Infusion reactions appeared frequently but were manageable and generally mild. Overall, EndoTAG®-1 appears to be a safe drug and is a promising candidate for further clinical testing.

A large phase II trial for EndoTAG®-1 in combination with gemcitabine in patients with advanced or metastatic adenocarcinoma of the pancreas is cur-rently under preparation.

13.8 Conclusion

Cationic-liposome-based-vascular-targeting agents attack the dividing tumor endothelial cell – a novel cellular target. This is in contrast to other vascular-targeting or anti-angiogenic approaches (e.g. anti-VEGF antibodies or VEGF-receptor antagonists), which interfere with specific molecular targets. This mode of action theoretically offers several advantages. It is not restricted to a certain tumor entity, as the vasculature of all solid tumors investigated so far seems to have a high affinity for the positively charged liposomes. This new mode of action is independent from the redundant molecular angiogenic pathways. Therefore, all tumors and tumor stages, irrespective of the angiogenic factor they depend on, are potential targets for treatment with cationic lipid complexed drugs. Further, cationic liposomes offer an attractive therapeutic concept for the treatment of tumors that have developed resistance against chemotherapeutic drugs.

Acknowledgments

The authors would like to thank Dr. Ulrich Delvos for critically reading the manuscript and for his comments and Christina Padanyi for her help in preparing this manuscript.

References

Arndt, D., Fichtner, I., Reszka, R. and Elbe, B. (1983). Preparation, properties and therapeutic effect of Daunorubicin-containing liposomes. *Pharmazie* **38** (5), 331–335.

Audouy, S.A., de Leij, L.F., Hoekstra, D. and Molema, G. (2002). *In vivo* characteristics of cationic liposomes as delivery vectors for gene therapy. *Pharm Res* **19** (11), 1599–1605.

Augustin, H.G., Braun, K., Telemenakis, I., Modlich, U. and Kuhn, W. (1995). Ovarian angiogenesis. Phenotypic characterization of endothelial cells in a physiological model of blood vessel growth and regression. *Am J Pathol* **147** (2), 339–351.

Augustin, H.G., Kozian, D.H. and Johnson, R.C. (1994). Differentiation of endothelial cells: analysis of the constitutive and activated endothelial cell phenotypes. *Bioessays* **16** (12), 901–906.

Baldwin, A.L., Wu, N.Z. and Stein, D.L. (1991). Endothelial surface charge of intestinal mucosal capillaries and its modulation by dextran. *Microvasc Res* **42** (2), 160–178.

Bangham, A.D., Standish, M.M. and Watkins, J.C. (1965). Diffusion of univalent ions across the lamellae of swollen phospholipids. *J Mol Biol* **13** (1), 238–252.

Behr, J.P., Demeneix, B., Loeffler, J.P. and Perez-Mutul, J. (1989). Efficient gene transfer into mammalian primary endocrine cells with lipopolyamine-coated DNA. *Proc Natl Acad Sci USA* **86** (18), 6982–6986.

Brigham, K.L., Meyrick, B., Christman, B., Magnuson, M., King, G. and Berry, L.C. Jr. (1989). *In vivo* transfection of murine lungs with a functioning prokaryotic gene using a liposome vehicle. *Am J Med Sci* **298** (4), 278–281.

Brill, B., Werner, A., Brunner, C., Michaelis, U., Teifel, M. and Groner, B. (2004). Neovascular targeting by EndoTAG-2 (MBT-0312) inhibits growth of subcutaneous mouse tumors. *Angiogenesis* **7** (1), 29.

Campbell, R.B., Fukumura, D., Brown, E.B., Mazzola, L.M., Izumi, Y., Jain, R.K., Torchilin, V.P. and Munn, L.L. (2002). Cationic charge determines the distribution of liposomes between the vascular and extravascular compartments of tumors. *Cancer Res* **62** (23), 6831–6836.

Chonn, A., Cullis, P.R. and Devine, D.V. (1991). The role of surface charge in the activation of the classical and alternative pathways of complement by liposomes. *J Immunol* **146** (12), 4234–4241.

Christian, S., Ahorn, H., Novatchkova, M., Garin-Chesa, P., Park, J.E., Weber, G., Eisenhaber, F., Rettig, W.J. and Lenter, M.C. (2001). Molecular cloning and characterization of EndoGlyx-1, an EMILIN-like multisubunit glycoprotein of vascular endothelium. *J Biol Chem* **276** (51), 48 588–48 595.

Cunningham, C.M., Kingzette, M., Richards, R.L., Alving, C.R., Lint, T.F. and Gewurz, H. (1979). Activation of human complement by liposomes: a model for membrane activation of the alternative pathway. *J Immunol* **122** (4), 1237–1242.

Dass, C.R. (2003). Improving anti-angiogenic therapy via selective delivery of cationic liposomes to tumour vasculature. *Int J Pharm* **267** (1/2), 1–12.

Dass, C.R. (2004). Lipoplex-mediated delivery of nucleic acids: factors affecting *in vivo* transfection. *J Mol Med* **82** (9), 579–591.

Denekamp, J. (1993). Review article: angiogenesis, neovascular proliferation and vascular pathophysiology as targets for cancer therapy. *Br J Radiol* **66** (783), 181–196.

Echtermeyer, F., Streit, M., Wilcox-Adelman, S., Saoncella, S., Denhez, F., Detmar, M. and Goetinck, P. (2001). Delayed wound repair and impaired angiogenesis in mice lacking syndecan-4. *J Clin Invest* **107** (2), R9–R14.

Eichhorn, M.E., Becker, S., Strieth, S., Werner, A., Sauer, B., Ruhstorfer, H., Michaelis, U., Griebel, J., Brix, G., Jauch, K.W. and Dellian, M. Dynamic magnet resonance tomography for monitoring the efficacy of an anti-vascular tumor therapy by paclitaxel encapsulating cationic lipid complexes (MBT-0206). *Proc AACR* **45**, March 2004a, Abstract 1310.

Eichhorn, M.E., Becker, S., Strieth, S., Werner, A., Sauer, B., Ruhstorfer, H., Michaelis, U., Griebel, J., Brix, G., Jauch, K.W. and Dellian, M. (2004b). Dynamic magnetic resonance tomography for monitoring the efficacy of an anti-vascular tumor therapy by paclitaxel encapsulating cationic lipid complexes. *Angiogenesis* **7** (1), 18.

Eichhorn, M.E., Strieth, S. and Dellian, M. (2004). Anti-vascular tumor therapy: recent advances, pitfalls and clinical perspectives. *Drug Resist Updat* **7** (2), 125–138.

Eichhorn, M.E., Strieth, S., Krasnici, S., Sauer, B., Teifel, M., Michaelis, U., Naujoks, K. and Dellian, M. (2004c). Protamine enhances uptake of cationic liposomes in angiogenic microvessels. *Angiogenesis* **7** (2), 133–141.

Felgner, P.L., Gadek, T.R., Holm, M., Roman, R., Chan, H.W., Wenz, M., Northrop, J.P., Ringold, G.M. and Danielsen, M. (1987). Lipofection: a highly efficient, lipid-mediated DNA-transfection procedure. *Proc Natl Acad Sci USA* **84** (21), 7413–7417.

Gallo, R., Kim, C., Kokenyesi, R., Adzick, N.S. and Bernfield, M. (1996). Syndecans-1 and -4 are induced during wound repair of neonatal but not fetal skin. *J Invest Dermatol* **107** (5), 676–683.

Gao, X. and Huang, L. (1991). A novel cationic liposome reagent for efficient transfection of mammalian cells. *Biochem Biophys Res Commun* **179** (1), 280–285.

Gregoriadis, G. and Ryman, B.E. (1971). Liposomes as carriers of enzymes or drugs: a new approach to the treatment of storage diseases. *Biochem J* **124** (5), 58P.

Gregoriadis, G. and Ryman, B.E. (1972). Fate of protein-containing liposomes injected into rats. An approach to the treatment of storage diseases. *Eur J Biochem* **24** (3), 485–491.

Gregoriadis, G., Wills, E.J., Swain, C.P. and Tavill, A.S. (1974). Drug-carrier potential of liposomes in cancer chemotherapy. *Lancet* **1** (7870), 1313–1316.

Hirko, A., Tang, F. and Hughes, J.A. (2003). Cationic lipid vectors for plasmid DNA delivery. *Curr Med Chem* **10** (14), 1185–1193.

Horstmann, E., McCabe, M.S., Grochow, L., Yamamoto, S., Rubinstein, L., Budd, T., Shoemaker, D., Emanuel, E.J. and Grady, C. (2005). Risks and benefits of phase 1 oncology trials, 1991 through 2002. *N Engl J Med* **352** (9), 895–904.

Iozzo, R.V. and San Antonio, J.D. (2001). Heparan sulfate proteoglycans: heavy hitters in the angiogenesis arena. *J Clin Invest* **108** (3), 349–355.

Ito, A., Miyazoe, R., Mitoma, J., Akao, T., Osaki, T. and Kunitake, T. (1990). Synthetic cationic amphiphiles for liposome-mediated DNA transfection. *Biochem Int* **22** (2), 235–241.

Kirkpatrick, A.P., Kaiser, T.A., Shepherd, R.D. and Rinker, K.D. (2003). Biochemical mediated glycocalyx modulation in human umbilical vein endothelial cells (HUVEC). *Summer Bioengineering Conference*.

Knüchel, R., Bartelheim, K., Reich, O., Oberneder, R., Stepp, H., Michaelis, U., Naujoks, K. and Sauer, B. (2003). Cationic liposomes for tumor imaging: first clinical results. *Proc Am Assoc Cancer Res* (2nd edn), **44**, 5397.

Krasnici, S., Werner, A., Eichhorn, M.E., Schmitt-Sody, M., Pahernik, S.A., Sauer, B., Schulze, B., Teifel, M., Michaelis, U., Naujoks, K. and Dellian, M. (2003). Effect of the surface charge of liposomes on their uptake by angiogenic tumor vessels. *Int J Cancer* **105** (4), 561–567.

Kunstfeld, R., Wickenhauser, G., Michaelis, U., Teifel, M., Umek, W., Naujoks, K., Wolff, K. and Petzelbauer, P. (2003). Paclitaxel encapsulated in cationic liposomes diminishes tumor angiogenesis and melanoma growth in a 'humanized' SCID mouse model. *J Invest Dermatol* **120** (3), 476–482.

Lee, C.M., Tanaka, T., Murai, T., Kondo, M., Kimura, J., Su, W., Kitagawa, T., Ito, T., Matsuda, H. and Miyasaka, M. (2002). Novel chondroitin sulfate-binding cationic liposomes loaded with cisplatin efficiently suppress the local growth and liver metastasis of tumor cells *in vivo*. *Cancer Res* **62** (15), 4282–4288.

Magee, W.E., Goff, C.W., Schoknecht, J., Smith, M.D. and Cherian, K. (1974). The interaction of cationic liposomes containing entrapped horseradish peroxidase with cells in culture. *J Cell Biol* **63** (2 Pt 1), 492–504.

Magee, W.E. and Miller, O.V. (1972). Liposomes containing antiviral antibody can protect cells from virus infection. *Nature* **235** (5337), 339–341.

McLean, J.W., Fox, E.A., Baluk, P., Bolton, P.B., Haskell, A., Pearlman, R., Thurston, G., Umemoto, E.Y. and McDonald, D.M. (1997). Organ-specific endothelial cell uptake of cationic liposome-DNA complexes in mice. *Am J Physiol* **273** (1 Pt 2), H387–H404.

Mold, C. and Gewurz, H. (1980). Activation of human complement by liposomes: serum factor requirement for alternative pathway activation. *J Immunol* **125** (2), 696–700.

Mounkes, L.C., Zhong, W., Cipres-Palacin, G., Heath, T.D. and Debs, R.J. (1998). Proteoglycans mediate cationic liposome–DNA complex-based gene delivery *in vitro* and *in vivo*. *J Biol Chem* **273** (40), 26 164–26 170.

Nabel, E.G., Plautz, G. and Nabel, G.J. (1990). Site-specific gene expression *in vivo* by direct gene transfer into the arterial wall. *Science* **249** (4974), 1285–1288.

Nabel, G.J., Nabel, E.G., Yang, Z.Y., Fox, B.A., Plautz, G.E., Gao, X., Huang, L., Shu, S., Gordon, D. and Chang, A.E. (1993). Direct gene transfer with DNA–liposome complexes in melanoma: expression, biologic activity, and lack of toxicity in humans. *Proc Natl Acad Sci USA* **90** (23), 11 307–11 311.

Nelimarkka, L., Salminen, H., Kuopio, T., Nikkari, S., Ekfors, T., Laine, J., Pelliniemi, L. and Jarvelainen, H. (2001). Decorin is produced by capillary endothelial cells in inflammation-associated angiogenesis. *Am J Pathol* **158** (2), 345–353.

Nishikawa, M. and Huang, L. (2001). Nonviral vectors in the new millennium: delivery barriers in gene transfer. *Hum Gene Ther* **12** (8), 861–870.

Oh, P., Li, Y., Yu, J., Durr, E., Krasinska, K.M., Carver, L.A., Testa, J.E. and Schnitzer, J.E. (2004). Subtractive proteomic mapping of the endothelial surface in lung and solid tumours for tissue-specific therapy. *Nature* **429** (6992), 629–635.

Opavsky, R., Haviernik, P., Jurkovicova, D., Garin, M.T., Copeland, N.G., Gilbert, D.J., Jenkins, N.A., Bies, J., Garfield, S., Pastorekova, S., Oue, A. and Wolff, L. (2001). Molecular characterization of the mouse Tem1/endosialin gene regulated by cell density *in vitro* and expressed in normal tissues *in vivo*. *J Biol Chem* **276** (42), 38 795–38 807.

Papyan, A., Werner, A., Ischenko, I., Teifel, M., Michaelis, U., Jauch, K.W. and Bruns, C.J. (2004). Combination of standard chemotherapy with MBT-0206 enhances the anti-tumor efficacy in a highly metastatic human pancreatic cancer mouse model. *Angiogenesis* **7** (1), 22.

Pilat, M.J., McCormick, J. and LoRusso, P.M. (2004). Vascular targeting agents. *Curr Oncol Rep* **6** (2), 103–110.

Plank, C., Mechtler, K., Szoka, F.C. Jr. and Wagner, E. (1996). Activation of the complement system by synthetic DNA complexes: a potential barrier for intravenous gene delivery. *Hum Gene Ther* **7** (12), 1437–1446.

Pries, A.R., Secomb, T.W. and Gaehtgens, P. (2000). The endothelial surface layer. *Pflugers Arch* **440**, 653–666.

Qiao, D., Meyer, K., Mundhenke, C., Drew, S.A. and Friedl, A. (2003). Heparan sulfate proteoglycans as regulators of fibroblast growth factor-2 signaling in brain endothelial cells. Specific role for glypican-1 in glioma angiogenesis. *J Biol Chem* **278** (18), 16 045–16 053.

Ran, S., Downes, A. and Thorpe, P.E. (2002). Increased exposure of anionic phospholipids on the surface of tumor blood vessels. *Cancer Res* **62**, 6132–6140.

Ran, S., He, J., Huang, X., Soares, M., Scothorn, D. and Thorpe, P.E. (2005). Antitumor effects of a monoclonal antibody that binds anionic phospholipids on the surface of tumor blood vessels in mice. *Clin Cancer Res* **11** (4), 1551–1562.

Ran, S. and Thorpe, P.E. (2002). Phosphatidylserine is a marker for tumor vasculature and a potential target for cancer imaging and therapy. *Int J Radiat Oncol Biol Phys* **54** (5), 1479–1484.

Rose, J.K., Buonocore, L. and Whitt, M.A. (1991). A new cationic liposome reagent mediating nearly quantitative transfection of animal cells. *Biotechniques* **10** (4), 520–525.

Sakurai, F., Nishioka, T., Saito, H., Baba, T., Okuda, A., Matsumoto, O., Taga, T., Yamashita, F., Takakura, Y. and Hashida, M. (2001a). Interaction between DNA-cationic liposome complexes and erythrocytes is an important factor in systemic gene transfer via the intravenous route in mice: the role of the neutral helper lipid. *Gene Ther* **8**, 677–686.

Sakurai, F., Nishioka, T., Yamashita, F., Takakura, Y. and Hashida, M. (2001b). Effects of erythrocytes and serum proteins on lung accumulation of lipoplexes containing cholesterol or DOPE as a helper lipid in the single-pass rat lung perfusion system. *Eur J Pharm Biopharm* **52**, 165–172.

Sangare, L., Morisset, R., Gaboury, L. and Ravaoarinoro, M. (2001). Effects of cationic liposome-encapsulated doxycycline on experimental *Chlamydia trachomatis* genital infection in mice. *J Antimicrob Chemother* **47** (3), 323–331.

Schmitt-Sody, M., Strieth, S., Krasnici, S., Sauer, B., Schulze, B., Teifel, M., Michaelis, U., Naujoks, K. and Dellian, M. (2003). Neovascular targeting therapy: paclitaxel encapsulated in cationic liposomes improves antitumoral efficacy. *Clin Cancer Res* **9** (6), 2335–2341.

Schönherr, E., Sunderkotter, C., Schaefer, L., Thanos, S., Grassel, S., Oldberg, A., Iozzo, R. V., Young, M.F. and Kresse, H.(2004). Decorin deficiency leads to impaired angiogenesis in injured mouse cornea. *J Vasc Res* **41** (6), 499–508.

Sengupta, S., Tyagi, P., Chandra, S., Kochupillai, V. and Gupta, S.K. (2001). Encapsulation in cationic liposomes enhances antitumour efficacy and reduces the toxicity of etoposide, a topo-isomerase II inhibitor. *Pharmacology* **62** (3), 163–171.

Sengupta, S., Tyagi, P., Velpandian, T., Gupta, Y.K. and Gupta, S.K. (2000). Etoposide encapsulated in positively charged liposomes: pharmacokinetic studies in mice and formulation stability studies. *Pharmacol Res* **42** (5), 459–464.

Senior, J.H., Trimble, K.R. and Maskiewicz, R. (1991). Interaction of positively-charged liposomes with blood: implications for their application *in vivo*. *Biochim Biophys Acta* **1070** (1), 173–179.

Siemann, D.W., Chaplin, D.J. and Horsman, M.R. (2004). Vascular-targeting therapies for treatment of malignant disease. *Cancer* **100** (12), 2491–2499.

Simberg, D., Weisman, S., Talmon, Y. and Barenholz, Y. (2004). DOTAP (and other cationic lipids): chemistry, biophysics, and transfection. *Crit Rev Ther Drug Carrier Syst* **21** (4), 257–317.

Smyth-Templeton, N. (2003). Cationic liposomes as *in vivo* delivery vehicles. *Curr Med Chem* **10** (14), 1279–1287.

St Croix, B., Rago, C., Velculescu, V., Traverso, G., Romans, K.E., Montgomery, E., Lal, A., Riggins, G.J., Lengauer, C., Vogelstein, B. and Kinzler, K.W. (2000). Genes expressed in human tumor endothelium. *Science* **289** (5482), 1197–1202.

Stamatatos, L., Leventis, R., Zuckermann, M.J. and Silvius, J.R. (1988). Interactions of cationic lipid vesicles with negatively charged phospholipid vesicles and biological membranes. *Biochemistry* **27** (11), 3917–3925.

Strieth, S., Eichhorn, M.E., Sauer, B., Schulze, B., Teifel, M., Michaelis, U. and Dellian, M. (2004). Neovascular targeting chemotherapy: encapsulation of paclitaxel in cationic liposomes impairs functional tumor microvasculature. *Int J Cancer* **110** (1), 117–124.

Szebeni, J. (2001). Complement activation-related pseudoallergy caused by liposomes, micellar carriers of intravenous drugs, and radiocontrast agents. *Crit Rev Ther Drug Carrier Syst* **18** (6), 567–606.

Szebeni, J. (2004). Hypersensitivity reactions to radiocontrast media: the role of complement activation. *Curr Allergy Asthma Rep* **4** (1), 25–30.

Szebeni, J., Baranyi, L., Savay, S., Bodo, M., Morse, D.S., Basta, M., Stahl, G.L., Bunger, R. and Alving, C.R. (2000). Liposome-induced pulmonary hypertension: properties and mechanism of a complement-mediated pseudoallergic reaction. *Am J Physiol Heart Circ Physiol* **279** (3), H1319–1328.

Szebeni, J., Baranyi, L., Savay, S., Milosevits, J., Bunger, R., Laverman, P., Metselaar, J.M., Storm, G., Chanan-Khan, A., Liebes, L., Muggia, F.M., Cohen, R., Barenholz, Y. and Alving, C.R. (2002). Role of complement activation in hypersensitivity reactions to doxil and hynic PEG liposomes: experimental and clinical studies. *J Liposome Res* **12** (1/2), 165–172.

Szebeni, J., Fontana, J.L., Wassef, N.M., Mongan, P.D., Morse, D.S., Dobbins, D.E., Stahl, G.L., Bunger, R. and Alving, C.R. (1999). Hemodynamic changes induced by liposomes and liposome-encapsulated hemoglobin in pigs: a model for pseudoallergic cardiopulmonary reactions to liposomes. Role of complement and inhibition by soluble CR1 and anti-C5a antibody. *Circulation* **99** (17), 2302–2309.

Szebeni, J., Muggia, F.M. and Alving, C.R. (1998). Complement activation by Cremophor EL as a possible contributor to hypersensitivity to paclitaxel: an *in vitro* study. *J Natl Cancer Inst* **90** (4), 300–306.

Szebeni, J., Wassef, N.M., Spielberg, H., Rudolph, A.S. and Alving, C.R. (1994). Complement activation in rats by liposomes and liposome-encapsulated hemoglobin: evidence for anti-lipid antibodies and alternative pathway activation. *Biochem Biophys Res Commun* **205** (1), 255–263.

Thorpe, P.E. (2004). Vascular targeting agents as cancer therapeutics. *Clin Cancer Res* **10** (2), 415–427.

Thurston, G., McLean, J.W., Rizen, M., Baluk, P., Haskell, A., Murphy, T.J., Hanahan, D. and McDonald, D.M. (1998). Cationic liposomes target angiogenic endothelial cells in tumors and chronic inflammation in mice. *J Clin Invest* **101** (7), 1401–1413.

Tousignant, J.D., Gates, A.L., Ingram, L.A., Johnson, C.L., Nietupski, J.B., Cheng, S.H., Eastman, S.J. and Scheule, R.K. (2000). Comprehensive analysis of the acute toxicities induced by systemic administration of cationic lipid: plasmid DNA complexes in mice. *Hum Gene Ther* **11** (18), 2493–2513.

Trowbridge, J.M. and Gallo, R.L. (2002). Dermatan sulfate: new functions from an old glycosaminoglycan. *Glycobiology* **12** (9), 117R–125R.

Tsujimoto, M., Inoue, K. and Nojima, S. (1981). Reactivity of human C-reactive protein with positively charged liposomes. *J Biochem (Tokyo)* **90** (5), 1507–1514.

Vitas, A.I., Diaz, R. and Gamazo, C. (1997). Protective effect of liposomal gentamicin against systemic acute murine brucellosis. *Chemotherapy* **43** (3), 204–210.

Webb, M.S., Wheeler, J.J., Bally, M.B. and Mayer, L.D. (1995). The cationic lipid stearylamine reduces the permeability of the cationic drugs verapamil and prochlorperazine to lipid bilayers: implications for drug delivery. *Biochim Biophys Acta* **1238** (2), 147–155.

Yao, V.J., Ozawa, M.G., Trepel, M., Arap, W., McDonald, D.M. and Pasqualini, R. (2005). Targeting pancreatic islets with phage display assisted by laser pressure catapult microdissection. *Am J Pathol* **166** (2), 625–636.

Yew, N.S., Wang, K.X., Przybylska, M., Bagley, R.G., Stedman, M., Marshall, J., Scheule, R.K. and Cheng, S.H. (1999). Contribution of plasmid DNA to inflammation in the lung after administration of cationic lipid: pDNA complexes. *Hum Gene Ther* **10** (2), 223–234.

Zhang, J.S., Liu, F. and Huang, L. (2005). Implications of pharmacokinetic behavior of lipoplex for its inflammatory toxicity. *Adv Drug Deliv Rev* **57** (5), 689–698.

Zhu, N., Liggitt, D., Liu, Y. and Debs, R. (1993). Systemic gene expression after intravenous DNA delivery into adult mice. *Science* **261** (5118), 209–211.

Zurita, A.J., Arap, W. and Pasqualini, R. (2003). Mapping tumor vascular diversity by screening phage display libraries. *J Control Release* **91** (1/2), 183–186.

14

Development of Vasculature-targeted Cancer Gene Therapy

Graeme J. Dougherty, Peter D. Davis and
Shona T. Dougherty

Abstract

Vascular-targeted gene therapy, although less well developed than equivalent small molecule-based approaches, shows great promise as a modality in the treatment of cancer. There is no shortage of genes that are potentially capable of inducing vessel occlusion if expressed at a high enough level within the tumor vasculature. Importantly, a number of strategies have been developed through which such genes can be selectively targeted to and/or expressed within tumor-associated endothelial cells. While absolute specificity for tumor sites may be difficult to achieve using any single mechanism, there is increasing optimism that vectors incorporating multiple independent control elements will ultimately prove a safe and effective means of inducing tumor-restricted vascular occlusion. Initial pre-clinical studies have been encouraging and there is an expectation that as further insights are gained into the molecular and biochemical nature of the changes induced in endothelial cells as a result of exposure to the unique tumor microenvironment, additional improvements will be made with respect to the tissue specificity of vascular-targeted gene therapy.

Keywords

gene therapy, vascular targeting, transductional targeting, transcriptional targeting, functional targeting

14.1 Introduction

As with the small-molecule- and antibody-based approaches described elsewhere in this volume, the primary objective of vascular-targeted cancer gene therapy

Vascular-targeted Therapies in Oncology Edited by Dietmar W. Siemann
© 2006 John Wiley & Sons, Ltd.

is to interrupt the delivery of oxygen and/or nutrients to a tumor site for a period of time long enough to induce a necrotic response of sufficient magnitude to impact on the course of disease when used either alone or in combination with other modalities. The power of gene therapy, and the reason the approach remains so attractive in the face of the substantial developmental and regulatory obstacles that need to be overcome to produce a viable cancer treatment, lies in the specificity for tumor sites that can potentially be achieved through the use of molecular approaches. Thus, by employing rational vector design it should ultimately be possible to specifically target the delivery and/or expression of therapeutic genes to the vascular cells of tumors, thereby minimizing the damage inflicted on various normal tissues. The benefits gained with respect to both efficacy and toxicity would more than justify the effort involved.

14.2   Advantages of tumor vasculature as a target in cancer gene therapy

While most current cancer gene therapy approaches target the malignant cell population, there are practical advantages in directing therapy to vascular endothelial cells instead. Thus, the major limitation of most tumor-cell-directed strategies relates to the generally poor levels of gene transduction that are normally achieved upon direct intratumoural or locoregional injection. Systemically administered vectors are even less efficient, reflecting in part the impact of poor and/or intermittent blood flow and high interstitial pressure on the entry of vectors into solid tumors as well as their subsequent diffusion through the tumor mass (Jain, 1990; Bilbao et al., 2000). In contrast to the situation with tumors, the direct contact that exists between endothelial cells and the blood stream obviously serves to facilitate transduction with intravenously administered vectors. More importantly, perhaps, it can be argued that the transduction efficiencies that need to be achieved in relation to endothelial cell targeting in order to produce therapeutic benefit may be far less than those required for equivalent tumor-cell-directed approaches since even modest damage to vasculature may translate to substantial tumor cell death if gene expression results in the cessation of blood flow and a subsequent inhibition in the delivery of oxygen and/or nutrients to the tumor site. Of more practical note, while it is appreciated that the particular microenvironment that exists within solid tumors may induce unique phenotypic characteristics that could prove useful in the development of targeting strategies, the continued survival and growth of essentially all solid tumors depends upon the presence of a vascular supply. Thus, any vascular-targeted approach is likely to prove applicable and effective in the treatment of a broad spectrum of tumors, irrespective of histological type or tissue location. Furthermore, in contrast to tumor cells, which are often genetically unstable and highly adaptive, endothelial cells are both non-transformed and diploid, suggesting that resistance to therapy is less likely to develop, at least in the short term. Optimistically, when taken together, these arguments suggest that rather than having to tailor therapy to address the characteristics of a particular tumor one may require only a limited number of vascular-targeting vectors in order to meet most needs.

14.3 Genes of value in vascular-targeted cancer gene therapy

The range of genes of potential value in vascular-targeted cancer gene therapy is large. Among the most obvious are those that simply kill endothelial cells if expressed at a high enough level. Examples include the bacterial toxins *Pseudomonas* exotoxin A and diphtheria toxin, both of which posses potent ADP ribosyltransferase activity and inhibit protein synthesis by attacking elongation factor 2. Genes that play a role in the regulation of cell survival and apoptosis as well as those that sensitize cells to the cytotoxic effects of chemotherapeutic agents or ionizing radiation or that activate prodrugs are also attractive. The temporal and spatial control offered by radiotherapy suggests that its use in combination with gene therapy may prove especially powerful in the context of vascular targeting. Genes that regulate complement activation or the coagulation cascade also have potential if their effects can be localized to the tumor microenvironment. Finally, although little studied to date, given the success of small-molecule vascular-disrupting agents such as combretastatin A4 and ZD6126 that target tubulin, there is obvious merit in exploring the therapeutic potential of genes involved in the regulation of endothelial cell shape and adhesion to the basement membrane. As emphasized above, it is important to keep in mind when considering which gene might ultimately prove most effective that, unlike many other cancer gene therapy approaches, it may be possible to achieve a dramatic anti-tumor effect even if a gene is expressed only transiently in a subset of endothelial cells in a tumor-associated vessel.

14.4 Targeting gene therapy to tumor vasculature

It is over ten years since the delivery of genes to vascular endothelial cells *in vivo* was first demonstrated (Nabel, Plautz and Nabel, 1991). In these and other early studies, targeting to vasculature was achieved through the use of vessel dwell procedures, catheterization, direct injection or *ex vivo* transduction of veins prior to re-engraftment. Although local delivery to tumor vasculature may be feasible in some rare circumstances, it is generally envisaged that vascular-targeted cancer gene therapy will be administered systemically. Indeed, as emphasized above, this is perceived as an important advantage of the approach. However, since intravenously administered vectors will rapidly distribute throughout the body, it is essential that efforts be made to restrict the delivery, expression and/or function of therapeutic genes to the desired target site if normal tissue toxicity is to be avoided. Generally speaking, the approaches that have been employed in an effort to achieve this goal fall into four main categories: transductional targeting, functional targeting, transcriptional targeting and post-transcriptional targeting.

Transductional targeting

The term 'transductional targeting' describes the use of vectors that are designed to deliver a DNA construct specifically to a desired cell type and not other cells that they may come into contact with. We, and others, have recently reviewed this approach in detail with respect to vasculature targeting, and it will be covered here only briefly (Dougherty, Davis and Dougherty, 2004; Baker et al., 2005).

Although the situation may well change in the future as new technologies are developed, to date viruses have proven the most efficient and robust vehicles for in vivo gene delivery. While endothelial cells are transduced in the course of infection with a surprisingly large number of pathogenic viruses, including Ebola, CMV, Hepatitis C, HIV, HTLV-1 and certain arboviruses, specificity for the vasculature is at best relative and may only occur at certain defined stages in the disease process. In any event, many other cell types are also infected in the course of disease progression, preventing the use of unmodified viruses in vascular-targeted cancer gene therapy applications. Recently, it has been suggested that PVC-211, a murine leukemia virus (MuLV) that induces a neuro-pathogenic condition in neonatal (but not adult) mice and rats, exhibits tropism for capillary endothelial cells (CEC) in the brain and certain other organs including kidney, liver and heart (Masuda et al., 1996, 1997; Jinno-Oue, Oue and Ruscetti, 2001). Interestingly, the relationship between age and susceptibility to viral transduction was lost in vitro, suggesting that PVC-211 might provide insights into endothelial cell tropism that may prove useful in the further development of vascular-targeted vectors (Masuda et al., 1997; Jinno-Oue, Oue and Ruscetti, 2001).

The viral vectors generally employed in cancer and other gene therapy applications are based upon retroviruses, adenoviruses or adeno-associated viruses. While interest in replication competent viruses is increasing, in most cases key genes involved in viral replication are deleted, producing vectors that are not further propagated after initial target cell infection. Importantly, the counter-receptors recognized by these various viruses are widely distributed, and as a result they exhibit little in the way of cellular targeting specificity. Indeed, although both retroviruses and adenoviruses are capable of infecting endothelial cells, serotype-2-based adeno-associated viruses (AAV-2) are relatively poor in this regard. Thus, when blood vessels are perfused with an AAV-2 vector, gene expression is seen in the surrounding smooth muscle cells but not the endothelial cells that line the vessel (Richter *et al.*, 2000). Recent studies suggest that this finding can be attributed to both sequestration of virus by extracellular matrix components associated with endothelial cells and by rapid and efficient degradation via a proteasome-dependent mechanism of any viral particles that are taken up (Nicklin *et al.*, 2001a; Pajusola *et al.*, 2002). Although other AAV serotypes appear to show an enhanced ability to transduce certain tissues, including the liver (Gao *et al.*, 2002; Sarkar *et al.*, 2004) and heart (Gregorevic *et al.*, 2004) none of those tested to date are efficient at infecting endothelial cells.

In any event, the broad distribution of the viral counter receptors suggests that in order to achieve vascular-endothelial-cell-specific gene delivery it will be necessary to both abrogate the binding of vectors to their natural ligands, then redirect them to alternative surface structures differentially expressed on endothelial cells. Of course, these alternative ligands are required to possess the unique and often ill defined characteristics necessary to function as receptors for the corresponding virus. Moreover, the changes that one introduces in order to inactivate binding to the natural ligand must not interfere with the subsequent steps involved in virus uptake, transport and gene expression. At least in the case of adenoviruses, what has proven particularly encouraging is that a remarkably large number of surface proteins appear capable of substituting for the natural coxsackie and adenovirus receptor protein (CAR) in studies employing various bispecific crosslinkers. Even more surprising is the finding that in cells that lack both CAR and the integrins (principally $\alpha v\beta 3$ and $\alpha v\beta 5$) that contribute to subsequent viral uptake via recognition of an Arg–Gly–Asp/RGD motif in the viral penton base protein (Wickham *et al.*, 1993; Greber *et al.*, 1993; Wang *et al.*, 1998; Bergelson, 1999) infection can, in at least some circumstances, be facilitated through binding to a single cell surface protein (Wickham *et al.*, 1997).

While these studies provide evidence that the cellular tropism of viral vectors can be altered, successful vascular targeting depends upon the presence on tumor-associated endothelial cells of differentially expressed surface structures that can function as ligands for appropriately engineered viruses. Fortunately, however, there are good grounds to be optimistic that such molecules will be found. There are, for example, obvious structural and functional differences between normal vasculature and the vasculature of tumors that might confidently be expected to reflect phenotypic heterogeneity (Denekamp, 1990). Thus, while the endothelial cells that line normal vessels are essentially quiescent, dividing only once every 1000 or so days, a significant proportion of the equivalent cells present in tumor-associated vessels proliferate rapidly, dividing every 1–2 days (Denekamp, 1993). Thus cell surface proteins upregulated in response to stimulation with various pro-angiogenic cytokines such as vascular endothelial growth factor (VEGF) or fibroblast growth factor (FGF) are obvious candidates for targeting with tropism-modified viral vectors. cDNA array analysis has identified a number of such molecules including the receptor tyrosine kinases

Tie-1 and Tie-2 (angiopoietin-1 receptor), neural (N-) cadherin and vascular endothelial (VE-) cadherin, follistatin and the αv, α5, β1 and β5 integrin sub-units (Zhang et al., 1999; Kozian and Augustin, 1995; Prols, Loser and Marx, 1998). Monoclonal antibody (mAb) staining studies have confirmed that at least some of these molecules are indeed differentially expressed at sites of active angiogenesis (Zhang et al., 1999; Fabbri et al., 1996; Enenstein and Kramer, 1994). Moreover, confirming an important role in the angiogenic process, antag-onists of αvβ1, α1β1 and α2β2 have been shown to inhibit VEGF-induced new vessel formation in various model systems (Brooks et al., 1994, 1995; Senger et al., 1997).

Although practical considerations have tended to focus interest on proteins induced in response to proliferative signals, a number of molecules upregulated at later stages in the angiogenic process have also been identified and may also prove useful in the future development of targetable viral vectors. Notable examples include osteopontin and a molecule designated PC4, both of which are significantly upregulated as endothelial cells differentiate and organize into tubelike structures in vitro (Prols, Loser and Marx, 1998).

It is essential to keep in mind when considering targeting such molecules that angiogenesis is involved in a broad range of normal physiological processes, including, most notably, the menstrual cycle and wound repair, and that it also occurs in association with various pathologic conditions including coronary vascular disease, primary pulmonary hypertension, Kawasaki disease and peripheral vascular disease. Thus targeting tumor vasculature based solely on proliferative status will result in specificity that is relative rather than absolute. Structures induced on proliferating endothelial cells do however have the impor-tant advantage of being common to many different malignancies. Thus, while the unique microenvironment generated within a solid tumor may also modulate the phenotype of the endothelial cells associated with the mass, the particular spectrum of changes induced will probably vary from tumor to tumor, reflecting differences in cytokine milieu etc. Targeting such molecules may be less desirable as it requires therapy to be individualized in response to prior analysis of biopsied tumor tissue.

While antibodies and other bispecific crosslinkers might facilitate the targeting of engineered viral vectors to determinants differentially expressed on tumor endothelial cells in vitro, their use in vivo is fraught with potential problems. A far better approach would be to directly incorporate targeting moieties into the vector itself. Of course, as indicated above, this has to be achieved without compromising either the structural integrity of the virus or the function of other viral proteins, both of which could have a negative impact on titer.

In the case of adenoviral vectors a simple pseudotyping approach in which the fiber protein from one serotype is replaced with that derived from another that possess a preferred cellular tropism has proven effective. It is the knob portion of the fiber coat protein that mediates initial attachment of virus to cellular counter-receptors. Thus replacement of the Ad5 fiber protein, which recognizes and binds to CAR, with the fiber protein from the subgroup B virus Ad16, which utilizes CD46 as a receptor, produces a psuedotyped virus that exhibits an enhanced ability to transduce CD46-positive vascular cells both *in vitro* and in venous explants (Gaggar, Shayakhmetov and Lieber, 2003).

Although encouraging, the usefulness of pseudotyping is obviously limited by the narrow range of receptors that are recognized by naturally occurring viral strains. An alternative experimental approach with far greater potential is to engineer defined peptide sequences directly into the Ad5 fiber protein (Krasnykh *et al.*, 1998). Peptide sequences with the necessary specificity can be rapidly identified using phage display techniques without any prior knowledge of the distribution of the molecules with which they interact. Cloning such peptides into the H1 loop of the fiber protein is relatively straightforward, and in vectors where both the CAR-binding function of the fiber protein and the interaction of the penton base protein with heparin are compromised, specificity for the cognate receptor defined by the peptide ligand can be achieved. A recent example illustrating the power of this approach in a vascular setting can be seen in a study from Nicklin *et al.* (2004), in which 12-mer peptides with binding specificity for endothelial cells identified by screening a phage display library *in vitro*, dramatically enhanced the ability of engineered adenoviral vectors to infect endothelial cells without similarly enhancing the low basal level of infectivity for a range of other cell types.

The same strategy has also been employed in the targeting of AAV-2 (Liu *et al.*, 2000; Masood *et al.*, 2001; Nicklin and Baker, 2002). Thus, AAV-2 vectors expressing chimeric capsid proteins with either 7-mer or 12-mer peptide sequences selected by phage display inserted at position 587 exhibited selectivity for endothelial cells both *in vitro* and *in vivo* (White *et al.*, 2004). One of the advantages of AAV-2 over adenovirus concerns the ability to generate AAV-2 libraries that directly display random peptide sequences in the capsid protein, allowing vectors with tropism for endothelial cells to be identified and isolated without the need to screen phage display libraries. Initial studies using this approach appear promising (Muller *et al.*, 2003).

Functional targeting

Broadly speaking, functional targeting is an approach in which a biological effect (i.e. the induction of cell death) is targeted to a tumor site as a result of the differential production within the tumor microenvironment of certain initiating signals (soluble mediators, extracellular matrix proteins etc.). Even in those circumstances where the parlicular gene transfer approach employed results in widespread expression of the effector transgene, the corresponding effector function is only triggered at sites where the required secondary signal is produced. For example, we have generated a series of 'molecular bioreductives' that exploit the presence of high levels of the pro-angiogenic cytokine VEGF within many solid tumors (Carpenito *et al.*, 2002). The approach employs a series of chimeric proteins, in which the extracellular ligand binding domain of the VEGF receptors VEGFR-1/Flt-1 or VEGFR-2/Flk-1 (Cross *et al.*, 2003) are fused in frame to the cytoplasmic 'death domain' derived from the pro-apoptotic protein Fas (Carpenito *et al.*, 2002). Rather than triggering the diverse signal transduction events normally initiated upon binding of VEGF, these molecules instead induce cell death. Importantly, since induction of the apoptotic response is critically dependent upon oligomerization of the chimeric receptor, death only occurs at sites where VEGF is produced above a certain critical threshold level. In the absence of VEGF, even cells expressing high levels of the chimeric receptor remain viable and proliferate normally (Carpenito *et al.*, 2002). So far, the targeting potential of this novel approach has been confirmed *in vitro* using established tumor cell lines and primary human endothelial cells (Carpenito *et al.*, 2002). *In vivo* studies are currently underway. It is important to emphasize that this is a broadly applicable strategy, and while initial efforts have focused on VEGF one could similarly exploit any differentially expressed soluble mediator, extracellular matrix protein or other molecule that induces receptor oligomerization.

Transcriptional targeting

Transcriptional targeting refers to the use of approaches that regulate the expression of a therapeutic gene in a particular cell type. Generally, this is achieved by cloning a defined promoter and/or enhancer sequence in an appropriate position upstream of the gene of interest. The elements that control the expression of genes that are differentially expressed in endothelial cells are obvious candidates for use in this way and a number have already been tested either in human endothelial cells *in vitro* or in animal studies. While differences in the precise nature of the sequences used by different groups make it difficult to draw meaningful conclusions regarding the relative activity and/or specificity of particular elements, generally favorable results have been obtained for promoter/enhancer sequences derived from the genes encoding endoglin (Graulich *et al.*, 1999), Flt-1 (Nicklin *et al.*, 2001b; Reynolds *et al.*, 2001), Tie 2 (Korhonen *et al.*, 1995; De Palma, Venneri and Naldini, 2003), ICAM-2 (Cowan *et al.*, 1996; Nicklin *et al.*, 2001b; Velasco *et al.*, 2001; Richardson, Kaspers and Porter, 2004), vascular endothelial (VE-) cadherin (Dancer *et al.*, 2003) and pre-proendothelin-1 (Jager, Zhao and Porter, 1999; Mavria, Jager and Porter, 2000; Varda-Bloom *et al.*, 2001; Cho *et al.*, 2003; Greenberger *et al.*, 2004). While cDNA array analysis and other approaches have identified additional genes that appear to be preferentially expressed in endothelial cells and/or the tumor-associated vasculature, defining the precise elements that control the expression of such genes in order that they can be used in gene therapy can be a long and frustrating process. The enhancer elements that determine high-level expression may be located some considerable distance from the gene itself, and because of the size limitations inherent in current vector design it may be necessary to carefully dissect a promising sequence using deletional analysis and site-direct mutagenesis in order to define the precise regions responsible for regulated gene expression.

An alternative strategy that may ultimately supersede such approaches involves the generation of entirely synthetic promoters. Unfortunately, detailed analysis of sequences located 5′ of genes that exhibit endothelial-cell-restricted expression failed to reveal any characteristic arrangement of transcription factor binding sites or common structural feature to help guide the design of synthetic endothelial-cell-specific promoters (Dai, McAninch and Sutton, 2004). Cloning approaches have been rather more fruitful. Thus, following on from earlier studies by Li *et al.* (1999) and Edelman *et al.* (2000) that focused on skeletal muscle, Dai and colleagues have recently developed a promising system that has allowed the isolation of synthetic promoter sequences active in endothelial cells (Dai, McAninch and Sutton, 2004). Briefly, the approach employs a self-inactivating human immunodeficiency virus type 1 (HIV-1-) based library in which short oligonucleotides corresponding to previously defined transcription factor binding sites are randomly ligated together and cloned adjacent to a minimal ICAM-2 promoter upstream of a green fluorescent protein (GFP) indicator gene. Pseudotyped particles expressing vesicular stomatitis virus G protein are then generated and used to infect an established Rhesus monkey choroidal endothelial cell line. The small subset of cells expressing high levels of GFP were isolated by FACS, expanded and the sorting procedure repeated to further enrich. Ultimately, PCR was used to recover the synthetic promoter elements deemed to have the highest activity and their specificity for endothelial cells was determined. Although at an early stage in development, this approach has already yielded several promising elements (Dai, McAninch and Sutton, 2004).

Post-transcriptional targeting

Although little practical work has actually been done in the area, various post-transcriptional processes including mRNA degradation and alternative pre-mRNA splicing could potentially be exploited in the development of vascular-targeted cancer gene therapy. For example, if a particular mRNA transcript has an especially long half-life in tumor-associated endothelial cells, the sequence motifs normally located at the 3′ end of the message that control the degradative process could be incorporated into vectors in order to ensure that the product of a therapeutic gene persists and is expressed at a high level in transduced cells. Similarly, if a certain alternative splicing event occurs preferentially in tumor-associated endothelial cells it may be possible to build constructs in which the expression of a therapeutic gene requires that this particular event occur. In proof of principle studies, we have generated a series of minigene constructs that incorporate alternatively spliced regions derived from the gene encoding the cell surface adhesion protein CD44 cloned in-frame upstream of a cDNA encoding the enzyme alkaline phosphatase (ALP) (Hayes *et al.*, 2002). Expression of a chimeric protein with ALP activity that can convert the inactive prodrug Etopophos® to the potent topoisomerase II inhibitor etoposide requires complete and accurate removal of any intronic sequences. Importantly, we have demonstrated that this is a carefully controlled process and that appropriate splicing only occurs in cells that normally express the corresponding alternatively spliced CD44 isoform (Hayes *et al.*, 2002, 2004). Thus, complete removal of the intron separating the alternatively spliced exons v9 and v10 only occurs in cells that express CD44R1, a CD44 isoform that contains sequences encoded by exons v8, v9 and v10 (Hayes *et al.*, 2004). In cells that express CD44 isoforms that do not contain these particular exons (e.g. CD44H) portions of the v9 intron are retained within the final transcript, and since these contain multiple in-frame stop codons, translation is terminated at this point and no functional ALP protein is produced (Hayes *et al.*, 2002, 2004). Interestingly, although not designed with vascular targeting in mind, there is evidence that v10-containing CD44 isoforms including CD44R1 are upregulated on endothelial cells following stimulation with the pro-angiogenic cytokine bFGF (Griffioen *et al.*, 1997).

14.5 Concluding remarks

Ongoing studies with small molecules have confirmed the therapeutic potential of targeting the vasculature upon which the survival and growth of a tumor depends, particularly when used in conjunction with other modalities. While equivalent gene-therapy-based approaches are less well developed, the exquisite specificity for tumor sites that can potentially be achieved by incorporating multiple targeting strategies into the vectors used for gene delivery is an important advantage that has served to encourage further work in this area. Certainly, targeting the vasculature overcomes some of the difficulties faced in the context of tumor-cell-directed gene therapy, while the fact that vectors are administered intravenously will clearly facilitate translation to a clinical setting. The results of pre-clinical studies have been encouraging and there is considerable optimism that vascular-targeted gene therapy will prove an effective addition to the treatment of solid tumors.

Acknowledgment

Work from the author's laboratory referred to in this article was supported in part by Grant RO1 CA100004 from the National Institutes of Health.

References

Baker, A.H. *et al.* (2005). Cell-selective viral gene delivery vectors for the vasculature. *Exp Physiol* **90**, 27–31.

Bergelson, J.M. (1999). Receptors mediating adenovirus attachment and internalization. *Biochem Pharmacol* **57**, 975–979.

Bilbao, R. *et al.* (2000). A blood–tumor barrier limits gene transfer to experimental liver cancer: the effect of vasoactive compounds. *Gene Ther* **7**, 1824–1832.

Brooks, P.C. *et al.* (1994). Integrin alpha v beta 3 antagonists promote tumor regression by inducing apoptosis of angiogenic blood vessels. *Cell* **79**, 1157–1164.

Brooks, P.C. *et al.* (1995). Antiintegrin alpha v beta 3 blocks human breast cancer growth and angiogenesis in human skin. *J Clin Invest* **96**, 1815–1822.

Carpenito, C. *et al.* (2002). Exploiting the differential production of angiogenic factors within the tumor microenvironment in the design of a novel vascular-targeted gene therapy-based approach to the treatment of cancer. *Int J Radiat Oncol Biol Phys* **54**, 1473–1478.

Cho, J. *et al.* (2003). Development of an efficient endothelial cell specific vector using promoter and 5′ untranslated sequences from the human preproendothelin-1 gene. *Exp Mol Med* **35**, 269–274.

Cowan, P.J. *et al.* (1996). Targeting gene expression to endothelial cells in transgenic mice using the human intercellular adhesion molecule 2 promoter. *Transplantation* **62**, 155–160.

Cross, M.J. *et al.* (2003). VEGF-receptor signal transduction. *Trends Biochem Sci* **28**, 488–494.

Dai, C., McAninch, R.E. and Sutton, R.E. (2004). Identification of synthetic endothelial cell-specific promoters by use of a high-throughput screen. *J Virol* **78**, 6209–6221.

Dancer, A. *et al.* (2003). Expression of thymidine kinase driven by an endothelial-specific promoter inhibits tumor growth of Lewis lung carcinoma cells in transgenic mice. *Gene Ther* **10**, 1170–1178.

De Palma, M., Venneri, M.A. and Naldini, L. (2003). In vivo targeting of tumor endothelial cells by systemic delivery of lentiviral vectors. *Hum Gene Ther* **14**, 1193–1206.

Denekamp, J. (1990). Vascular attack as a therapeutic strategy for cancer. *Cancer Metastasis Rev* **9**, 267–282.

Denekamp, J. (1993). Review article: angiogenesis, neovascular proliferation and vascular pathophysiology as targets for cancer therapy. *Br J Radiol* **66**, 181–196.

Dougherty, G.J., Davis, P.D. and Dougherty, S.T. (2004). Vascular-targeted cancer gene therapy. *Exp Opin Biol Ther* **4**, 1911–1920.

Edelman, G.M. *et al.* (2000). Synthetic promoter elements obtained by nucleotide sequence variation and selection for activity. *Proc Natl Acad Sci USA* **97**, 3038–3043.

Enenstein, J. and Kramer, R.H. (1994). Confocal microscopic analysis of integrin expression on the microvasculature and its sprouts in the neonatal foreskin. *J Invest Dermatol* **103**, 381–386.

Fabbri, M. *et al.* (1996). A functional monoclonal antibody recognizing the human alpha 1-integrin I-domain. *Tissue Antigens* **48**, 47–51.

Gaggar, A., Shayakhmetov, D.M. and Lieber, A. (2003). CD46 is a cellular receptor for group B adenoviruses. *Nat Med* **9**, 1408–1412.

Gao, G.P. *et al.* (2002). Novel adeno-associated viruses from rhesus monkeys as vectors for human gene therapy. *Proc Natl Acad Sci USA* **99**, 11 854–11 859.

Graulich, W. *et al.* (1999). Cell type specificity of the human endoglin promoter. *Gene* **227**, 55–62.

Greber, U.F. *et al.* (1993). Stepwise dismantling of adenovirus 2 during entry into cells. *Cell* **75**, 477–486.

Greenberger, S. *et al.* (2004). Transcription-controlled gene therapy against tumor angiogenesis. *J Clin Invest* **113**, 1017–1024.

Gregorevic, P. *et al.* (2004). Systemic delivery of genes to striated muscles using adeno-associated viral vectors. *Nat Med* **10**, 828–834.

Griffioen, A.W. *et al.* (1997). CD44 is involved in tumor angiogenesis; an activation antigen on human endothelial cells. *Blood* **90**, 1150–1159.

Hayes, G.M. *et al.* (2002). Alternative splicing as a novel of means of regulating the expression of therapeutic genes. *Cancer Gene Ther* **9**, 133–141.

Hayes, G.M. *et al.* (2004). Molecular mechanisms regulating the tumor-targeting potential of splice-activated gene expression. *Cancer Gene Ther* **11**, 797–807.

Jager, U., Zhao, Y. and Porter, C.D. (1999). Endothelial cell-specific transcriptional targeting from a hybrid long terminal repeat retrovirus vector containing human prepro-endothelin-1 promoter sequences. *J Virol* **73**, 9702–9709.

Jain, R.K. (1990). Vascular and interstitial barriers to delivery of therapeutic agents in tumors. *Cancer Metastasis Rev* **9**, 253–266.

Jinno-Oue, A., Oue, M. and Ruscetti, S.K. (2001). A unique heparin-binding domain in the envelope protein of the neuropathogenic PVC-211 murine leukemia virus may contribute to its brain capillary endothelial cell tropism. *J Virol* **75**, 12439–12445.

Korhonen, J. *et al.* (1995). Endothelial-specific gene expression directed by the tie gene promoter in vivo. *Blood* **86**, 1828–1835.

Kozian, D.H. and Augustin, H.G. (1995). Rapid identification of differentially expressed endothelial cell genes by RNA display. *Biochem Biophys Res Commun* **209**, 1068–1075.

Krasnykh, V. *et al.* (1998). Characterization of an adenovirus vector containing a heterologous peptide epitope in the HI loop of the fiber knob. *J Virol* **72**, 1844–1852.

Li, X. *et al.* (1999). Synthetic muscle promoters: activities exceeding naturally occurring regulatory sequences. *Nat Biotechnol* **17**, 241–245.

Liu, L. *et al.* (2000). Incorporation of tumor vasculature targeting motifs into moloney murine leukemia virus env escort proteins enhances retrovirus binding and transduction of human endothelial cells. *J Virol* **74**, 5320–5328.

Masood, R. *et al.* (2001). Retroviral vectors bearing IgG-binding motifs for antibody-mediated targeting of vascular endothelial growth factor receptors. *Int J Mol Med* **8**, 335–343.

Masuda, M. *et al.* (1996). Effects of subtle changes in the SU protein of ecotropic murine leukemia virus on its brain capillary endothelial cell tropism and interference properties. *Virology* **215**, 142–151.

Masuda, M. *et al.* (1997). Capillary endothelial cell tropism of PVC-211 murine leukemia virus and its application for gene transduction. *J Virol* **71**, 6168–6173.

Mavria, G., Jager, U. and Porter, C.D. (2000). Generation of a high titre retroviral vector for endothelial cell-specific gene expression in vivo. *Gene Ther* **7**, 368–376.

Muller, O.J. *et al.* (2003). Random peptide libraries displayed on adeno-associated virus to select for targeted gene therapy vectors. *Nat Biotechnol* **21**, 1040–1046.

Nabel, E.G., Plautz, G. and Nabel, G.J. (1991). Gene transfer into vascular cells. *J Am College Cardiol* **17**, 189B–194B.

Nicklin, S.A. and Baker, A.H. (2002). Tropism-modified adenoviral and adeno-associated viral vectors for gene therapy. *Curr Gene Ther* **2**, 273–293.

Nicklin, S.A. *et al.* (2001a) Efficient and selective AAV2-mediated gene transfer directed to human vascular endothelial cells. *Mol Ther* **4**, 174–181.

Nicklin, S.A. *et al.* (2001b) Analysis of cell-specific promoters for viral gene therapy targeted at the vascular endothelium. *Hypertension* **38**, 65–70.

Nicklin, S.A. *et al.* (2004). In vitro and in vivo characterisation of endothelial cell selective adenoviral vectors. *J Gene Med* **6**, 300–308.

Pajusola, K. *et al.* (2002). Cell-type-specific characteristics modulate the transduction efficiency of adeno-associated virus type 2 and restrain infection of endothelial cells. *J Virol* **76**, 11 530–11 540.

Prols, F., Loser, B. and Marx, M. (1998). Differential expression of osteopontin, PC4, and CEC5, a novel mRNA species, during in vitro angiogenesis. *Exp Cell Res* **239**, 1–10.

Reynolds, P.N. *et al.* (2001). Combined transductional and transcriptional targeting improves the specificity of transgene expression in vivo. *Nat Biotechnol* **19**, 838–842.

Richardson, T.B., Kaspers, J. and Porter, C.D. (2004). Retroviral hybrid LTR vector strategy: functional analysis of LTR elements and generation of endothelial cell specificity. *Gene Ther* **11**, 775–783.

Richter, M. *et al.* (2000). Adeno-associated virus vector transduction of vascular smooth muscle cells in vivo. *Physiol Genom* **2**, 117–127.

Sarkar, R. *et al.* (2004). Total correction of hemophilia A mice with canine FVIII using an AAV 8 serotype. *Blood* **103**, 1253–1260.

Senger, D.R. *et al.* (1997). Angiogenesis promoted by vascular endothelial growth factor: regulation through alpha1beta1 and alpha2beta1 integrins. *Proc Natl Acad Sci USA* **94**, 13612–13617.

Varda-Bloom, N. *et al.* (2001). Tissue-specific gene therapy directed to tumor angiogenesis. *Gene Ther* **8**, 819–827.

Velasco, B. *et al.* (2001). Vascular gene transfer driven by endoglin and ICAM-2 endothelial-specific promoters. *Gene Ther* **8**, 897–904.

Wang, K. *et al.* (1998). Adenovirus internalization and infection require dynamin. *J Virol* **72**, 3455–3458.

White, S.J. *et al.* (2004). Targeted gene delivery to vascular tissue in vivo by tropism-modified adeno-associated virus vectors. *Circulation* **109**, 513–519.

Wickham, T.J. *et al.* (1993). Integrins alpha v beta 3 and alpha v beta 5 promote adenovirus internalization but not virus attachment. *Cell* **73**, 309–319.

Wickham, T.J. *et al.* (1997). Targeted adenovirus-mediated gene delivery to T cells via CD3. *J Virol* **71**, 7663–7669.

Zhang, H.T. *et al.* (1999). Transcriptional profiling of human microvascular endothelial cells in the proliferative and quiescent state using cDNA arrays. *Angiogenesis* **3**, 211–219.

15

Vasculature-disrupting Strategies Combined with Bacterial Spores Targeting Hypoxic Regions of Solid Tumors

G-One Ahn and J. Martin Brown

Abstract

This chapter describes the combination of vascular disrupting agents with genetically engineered anaerobic bacteria in cancer therapy. Though there is evidence that,
at least in mouse tumours, the combination of vascular disrupting agents with
anaerobic bacteria can have an anticancer effect, we believe that the power of this
approach is to target specific genes into tumours. This is not classical gene therapy,
which is defined as the introduction of a gene, or part of a gene, into normal or cancer
cells. Rather, the anaerobic bacteria are used to produce a protein of choice in
tumours. This can be a powerful adjunct to cancer therapy. In this chapter we will
discuss this hypoxic/necrotic-targeted therapy, using the obligate anaerobe Clostridium *sporogenes* as the prototype agent. Second, we will consider how the efficacy of
this therapy using *Clostridium*, termed Clostridia Directed Enzyme Prodrug Therapy
(CDEPT) can be significantly enhanced by combining with vascular disrupting
agents.

Keywords
anaerobic bacteria, prodrug enzyme therapy, hypoxia, cancer therapy

15.1 Hypoxia and necrosis as a selective target for cancer therapy

The presence of hypoxic/necrotic area is a common feature of human solid
tumor. It occurs as a result of unrestrained tumor growth, causing cells to be

Vascular-targeted Therapies in Oncology Edited by Dietmar W. Siemann
© 2006 John Wiley & Sons, Ltd.

forced away from functional blood vessels beyond the effective diffusion distance of oxygen in respiring tissues, thereby becoming hypoxic and eventually necrotic. Given typical values for intracapillary oxygen tensions and oxygen consumption rates, the oxygen diffusion distance is approximately 150 μm (Thomlinson and Gray, 1955), consistent with necrotic regions being observed at distances greater than about 100–150 μm from tumor capillaries. Hypoxic regions have been extensively quantified and characterized by polarographic oxygen electrodes in various tumors or metastases of the head and neck, cervix, brain, melanomas, sarcomas, anal, prostate and pancreatic cancers (Becker et al., 1998; Brizel et al., 1995; 1999; Vaupel and Hockel, 1995; Rampling et al., 1994; Sundfor et al., 1997; Movsas et al., 1999; Koong et al., 2000).

Hypoxic tumor cells adversely affect cancer management because they are resistant to killing by ionizing radiation, and possibly chemotherapy (Brown and Giaccia, 1998; Brown and Wilson, 2004; Wouters et al., 2002). They may also promote tumor progression by transactivating many genes that are associated with a more malignant phenotype (Graeber et al., 1996; Harris, 2002). However, because hypoxic/necrotic regions are unique to tumors compared with other normal tissues, they can be exploited as a selective target for cancer therapy (Brown and Wilson, 2004).

15.2 Use of Clostridia as hypoxia/necrotic selective cancer therapy

The genus *Clostridium* comprises a large and heterogeneous group of Gram-positive spore-forming bacteria that become vegetative and grow only in the absence (or at very low levels) of oxygen. Malmgren and Flanigan were the first to demonstrate that intravenous injection of spores of *C. tetani* colonized solid tumors by observing that tumor-bearing mice died of tetanus within 48 h of their administration, whereas non-tumor-bearing animals were unaffected (Malmgren and Flanigan, 1955). Mose and Mose (1959, 1964) later reported that a non-pathogenic clostridial strain, *C. butyricum* M-55, localized and germinated in solid Ehrlich tumors, causing extensive lysis without any concomitant effect on normal tissues. Such observations were soon confirmed and extended by a number of investigators using tumors in mice, rats, hamsters, and rabbits (Thiele, Arison and Boxer, 1964; Engelbart and Gericke, 1964), and were followed by clinical studies with cancer patients (Carey et al., 1967; Heppner and Mose, 1978; Heppner et al., 1983). While the anaerobic bacteria did not significantly alter tumor control or eradication, these clinical reports established the safety of this approach as well as the fact that colonization of human tumors occurs following intravenous (i.v.) injection of clostridial spores.

The studies showing the specific colonization of tumors by non-pathogenic clostridial species prompted us to suggest in 1994 that they could be used as a tumor-specific gene delivery system (Lemmon et al., 1994), a strategy we have termed clostridia-directed enzyme prodrug therapy (CDEPT). CDEPT involves injection of spores of non-pathogenic clostridia, genetically engineered to produce an enzyme capable of activating a non-toxic 'prodrug' into a toxic, drug when the spores geminate. Because germination to the vegetative form will only occur in the hypoxic/necrotic regions, the enzyme, and therefore activation of the prodrug to a toxic drug should be produced only in the tumor (Figure 15.1).

In early studies with this approach, we showed that the *E. coli* enzyme cytosine deaminase (CD) could be expressed in the clostridium *C. beijerinckii* and could convert the non-toxic prodrug 5-fluorocytosine (5-FC) to the toxic anticancer drug 5-fluorouracil (5-FU) *in vitro* (Fox *et al.*, 1996). In addition, we showed that injection of spores of recombinant *C. beijerinckii* expressing the *E. coli* enzyme nitroreductase (NTR) into tumor-bearing mice produced NTR protein solely in the tumors (Lemmon *et al.*, 1997). These studies therefore established the proof of principle that a foreign protein of choice can be

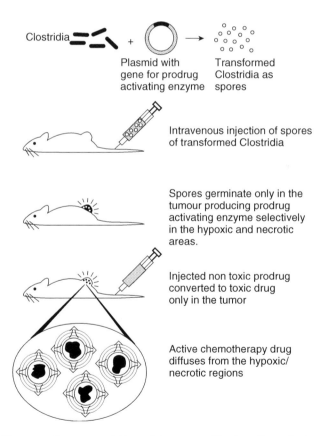

Figure 15.1 Diagrammatic representation of tumor-specific targeting of chemotherapy using obligate anaerobes

expressed exclusively in transplanted tumors in rodents following systemic administration of the recombinant clostridial spores.

However, early *in vivo* studies with genetically engineered *C. beijerinkii* failed to produce antitumor activity when the relevant prodrug was injected systemically (5-FC for CD-expressing tumors and CB1954 for NTR-expressing tumors) due to the insufficient levels of prodrug-activating enzyme resulting from low levels of viable clostridia in the tumors. Indeed, *C. beijerinkii* produced only 10^5–10^6 bacteria per gram of tumor (Lemmon *et al.*, 1997), whereas other clostridial spores such as *C. sporogenes* have a greater colonization efficiency, with levels of 10^8 or more bacteria per gram of tumor in experimental tumor models (Liu *et al.*, 2002). With our recent success in transforming *C. sporogenes* with enzyme-prodrug constructs we have shown that intravenous injection into tumor-bearing mice of spores of *C. sporogenes* transformed with *E. coli*-derived CD produced not only tumor-specific expression of the CD protein (Figure 15.2) but also significant antitumor efficacy when 5-FC was given systemically (Figure 15.3).

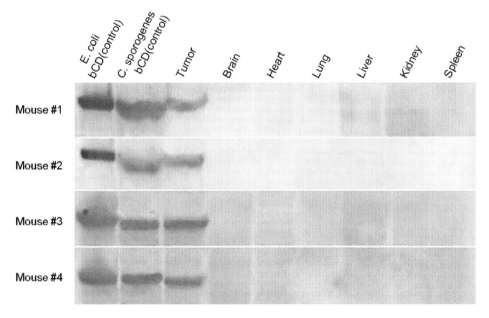

Figure 15.2 Immunoblot for CD in cell extracts from SCCVII tumors and from several normal tissues from the same mice injected i.v. 7 days prior to animal sacrifice with spores of CD-transformed *C. sporogenes*. The tumors were approximately 100 mg at the time of i.v. injection. 100 μg of cell extract from the tumor and normal mouse tissues was loaded on the gel. Shown also are cell extracts from CD-transformed *E. coli* and *C. sporogenes* with 1 and 20 μg cell extract loaded respectively. From Liu *et al.* (2002) with permission

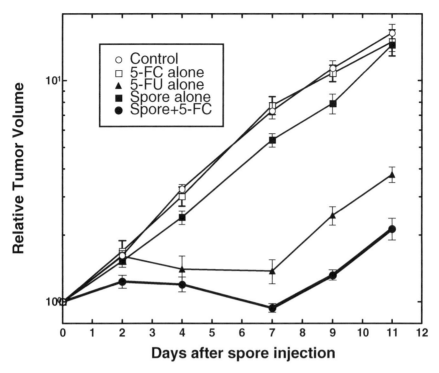

Figure 15.3 Growth delay produced by daily (five times per week) injections of 5-FC (500 mg kg^{-1} day^{-1}) in SCCVII tumors injected on day 0 with 10^8 spores of CD-transformed *C. sporogenes*. Shown also is the growth delay produced by a similar injection schedule of the maximally tolerated dose of 5-FU (15 kg^{-1} day^{-1}) in the same experiment. Data are from five mice per group, with the error bar showing SEM for each group. From Liu *et al.* (2002) with permission

15.3 Advantage of CDEPT over ADEPT and GDEPT

Both ADEPT (antibody-directed) and GDEPT (gene-directed) enzyme prodrug therapy are viable approaches to achieve locally high concentrations of anticancer drugs in tumors and are appropriately receiving significant effort in both preclinical and clinical studies. However, we believe that the clostridial approach to enzyme/prodrug therapy (CDEPT) has a number of intrinsic advantages, as outlined below.

Lack of an immune response

An immune response against the antibody/enzyme conjugates has been a major problem with ADEPT (Melton and Sherwood, 1996). However, clostridial spores elicit an undetectable immune response, and when the spores germinate into vegetative bacteria they are present in necrotic areas of the tumor, which are immune-privileged sites. In fact, it has been found both in clinical (Carey *et al.*, 1967) and preclinical studies (Gericke *et al.*, 1979) that multiple treatments are effective. In studies with intravenous injection of *C. sporogenes* and *C. acetobutylicum* we and others have found no loss of numbers of bacteria in experimental tumors for up to 14–17 days following a single i.v. injection of spores (Liu *et al.*, 2002; Nuyts *et al.*, 2002).

An advantageous intratumor distribution

The necessity of delivering enzyme/antibody conjugates for ADEPT, or vectors for GDEPT, through the bloodstream makes it likely that the highest concentrations of enzyme will be perivascular. However, the resistant cells in the tumor are likely to be the non-proliferating hypoxic cells distant from the vasculature and often close to necrosis. In contrast, the prodrug-activating enzyme from clostridia will be at its highest concentration in areas adjacent to necrosis and far from blood vessels. Not only does this guarantee that the drug activated by the enzyme from clostridia will be at its highest level adjacent to the necrosis and close to the resistant hypoxic cells, it also minimizes the problem of leakage of activated drug back into the blood vessels, a problem that has been reported for ADEPT (Martin *et al.*, 1997).

The same construct will be universally applicable to all cancer patients

As opposed to ADEPT, which requires either tumor-specific or possibly patient-specific enzyme/antibody conjugates, the CDEPT approach, because it depends only on tumor necrosis, will have universal applicability. In a recent publication on the potential of clostridia to target human tumors, Dang and colleagues reported that all 20 liver metastases of colorectal carcinoma $\geq 1\,cm^3$ in size had 25–75 per cent of their volume occupied by necrosis (Dang *et al.*, 2001).

Higher tumor to normal tissue targeting ratios

Major problems with ADEPT and GDEPT are that tumor targeting cannot be 100 per cent effective. In most cases the majority of the injected material will not be localized in the tumor but in the reticular endothelial system. This necessitates efforts to clear such non-bound material. On the other hand, with clostridia it appears that 100 per cent of the novel protein expressed from the recombinant clostridia is within the tumor.

15.4   Combination of CDEPT with vascular-disrupting agents

Rationale of the combination

The need for hypoxic/necrotic areas of tumors for vegetative growth of obligate anaerobes provides a strong rationale for the combination of CDEPT with vascular-disrupting agents such as DMXAA (5,6-dimethylxanthenone-4-acetic acid), combretastatin 4A and ZD 6126. These agents induce rapid and selective disruption of tumor endothelium, severe reduction of tumor blood flow and increased necrosis in the tumor within 16–24 h of the administration. Theoretically, this increase in tumor necrosis should enhance the colonization of the bacteria and expression of the prodrug-converting enzyme. This should in turn lead to a greater efficiency of prodrug conversion into active anticancer drug, leading to an enhanced tumor cell kill. In addition, because the vascular-disrupting agent brings the necrotic region and the well oxygenated zone in the peripheral rim of the tumor closer, this should substantially reduce the depth of viable tumor tissue into which the released active anticancer drug needs to diffuse (Figure 15.4). This diffusing ability (bystander effect) is a very important determinant for the activity of an anticancer drug and is often compromised, particularly for drugs of large molecular weight (Pruijn *et al.*, 2005).

There is a further theoretical advantage to combining a vascular-disrupting agent with CDEPT. Vascular-disrupting agents could open up the possibility that the minimum tumor size for the antitumor efficacy by CDEPT can be substantially reduced by inducing necrosis in small tumors or metastases that do not normally contain necrosis. In support of this, it has recently been reported that ZD6126 induces extensive tumor necrosis (Varghese *et al.*, 2004) and endothelial cell apoptosis (Goto *et al.*, 2002) in liver and lung metastasis models, respectively. Some vascular-disrupting agents producing tubulin depolymerization such as combretastatin A4 have previously been shown to increase colonization (Theys *et al.*, 2001) and antitumor activity (Dang *et al.*, 2001) of non-recombinant clostridia in tumor xenograft models. As shown below, we find that both increased colonization and antitumor activity are achieved

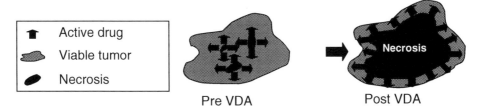

Pre VDA   Post VDA

Figure 15.4   Schematic diagram for combination of CDEPT with vascular-disrupting agents (VDAs). Active drug is the anticancer drug generated from its prodrug form by the enzyme expressed in anaerobes (A color reproduction of this figure can be seen in the color section)

when genetically engineered clostridia are used in combination with vascular-disrupting agents of a variety of modes of action.

CDEPT in combination with DMXAA

DMXAA is a small-molecule vascular-disrupting agent inducing rapid apoptosis of the tumor vascular endothelium (Ching *et al.*, 2002; Baguley and Ching, 2002) followed by multiple tumor and host chemokine production (Baguley and Ching, 2002). A study determining the sequence of administration for the combination of clostridial spores and DMXAA by quantifying colony-forming units of vegetative bacteria per gram of tumor showed that there was approximately four- and 10-fold higher number of bacteria in human HT29 and murine SCCVII tumors, respectively, when DMXAA was administered intraperitoneally 4 h <u>after</u> spore injection (Ahn *et al.*, 2004). In contrast, DMXAA given 24 h before spores resulted in a number of bacteria two to three orders of magnitude <u>lower</u> than that by spores alone (Liu *et al.*, unpublished data), suggesting that the tumor blood flow shutdown by pretreatment with DMXAA interfered the delivery of spores to the tumor. It has been reported that the number of blood vessels (Siemann *et al.*, 2002) and perfusion volume (Siim *et al.*, 2003) in the tumor that fall rapidly by DMXAA (within 5 h) do not reverse at 24 h of the administration, indicating that blood flow in the tumor is severely compromised at this time. With the preferred sequence (spores followed after 4 h by DMXAA) we have shown that the tumor lysis by spores was significantly enhanced with DMXAA treatment, leading to an extensive hemorrhagic necrosis in the tumor (Ahn *et al.*, 2004). The combination of CD-expressing spores with DMXAA in conjunction with the prodrug 5-FC led to a significant antitumor activity (Figure 15.5), and this was superior to non-recombinant spores of the same combination treatment in SCCVII murine tumor models (Ahn *et al.*, unpublished data).

CDEPT in combination with ZD6126

ZD6126 (N-acetylcochinol-O-phosphate) is a phosphate prodrug of the tubulin-binding agent ZD6126 phenol, an inhibitor of microtubule polymerization that selectively disrupts the endothelial cell monolayer lining of tumor vessels, leading to blood vessel congestion and the loss of blood flow in the tumor (Blakey *et al.*, 2002). The observation that these changes occur at a dose well below the maximum tolerated dose enabled us to obtain a dose–response relationship for colonization efficiency of clostridial spores by ZD6126. When followed after 4 h by the recombinant spores, ZD6126 increased the number of vegetative bacteria in HT29 tumor in a dose-dependent manner, reaching approximately 10-fold increase at $150 \, mg \, kg^{-1}$ of ZD6126 intraperitoneal administration (Ahn *et al.*, 2004). This dose-dependent increase in colonization efficiency of spores most likely results from the dose-dependent increase in tumor necrosis by this agent

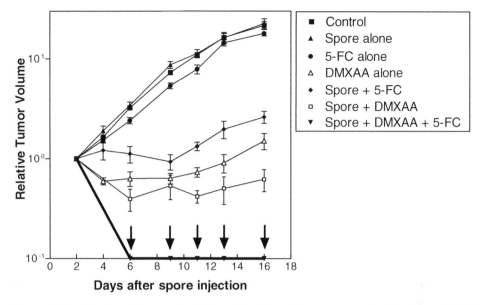

Figure 15.5 Growth delay produced by daily (five times per week) injection of 5-FC ($500\,mg\,kg^{-1}day^{-1}$) in SCCVII tumors injected 2 days after 10^8 spores of CD-transformed *C. spororgenes* with and without DMXAA. DMXAA ($25\,mg\,kg^{-1}$) was given 4 h after the spores on a weekly schedule. Plots are the means for three mice per group, with the error bar showing SEM for each group. From Liu *et al.*, unpublished data

(Robinson *et al.*, 2003). The combination of CD-expressing clostridial spores and ZD6126, in conjunction with the prodrug 5-FC, demonstrated a superior antitumor activity in HT29 human tumor xenograft models compared with the treatment without ZD6126 (Ahn *et al.*, 2004). Intratumoral levels of 5-FU converted from 5-FC in this combination were equivalent to, if not higher than, a single maximally tolerated dose of 5-FU given systemically (Ahn *et al.*, 2004). Importantly, there was no detectable level of 5-FU in the plasma from this combination (Ahn *et al.*, 2004), ruling out the possibility of systemic toxicity induced by 5-FU. This implies that by combining CDEPT with a vascular-disrupting agent, one can repeatedly administer non-toxic prodrug at high doses without systemic toxicity, thereby obtaining intratumoral levels of active anticancer drug greater than could be achieved by administration of the anticancer agent alone.

Applications with other vascular-disrupting agents and future directions

Choosing the vascular-disrupting agent for combination with CDEPT

In addition to the small-molecule vascular-disrupting agents discussed above, other vascular disrupting agents could be considered for combination with

CDEPT. These include analogs of small-molecule vascular-disrupting agents with better systemic toxicity profiles, or ligand-based vascular-disrupting agents such as antibody- or peptide-directed toxins or cytokines, and antiangiogenic agents that shut down tumor blood flow, such as the potent vascular endothelial growth factor (VEGF) antagonist VEGF-Trap (Huang *et al.*, 2003).

An important determinant of the antitumor activity for the combination of CDEPT with a vascular-disrupting agent is the timing and the sequence of the combination. Because most, if not all, vascular-disrupting agents exert their vascular shutdown in the tumor in a highly time-dependent fashion, one should carefully monitor this activity when combining with CDEPT or other treatment modalities. A typical example was demonstrated above with DMXAA and ZD6126. Although both agents induce rapid reduction in tumor blood flow (Siim *et al.*, 2003; Goertz *et al.*, 2002) and the number of endothelial cells in the tumor (Siemann *et al.*, 2002; Siemann and Rojiani, 2002), the blood flow does not reverse even 24 h after the administration for DMXAA (Siim *et al.*, 2003; Siemann *et al.*, 2002) whereas it returns to pre-treatment levels within 24 h following ZD6126 (Goertz *et al.*, 2002; Horsman and Murata, 2003). CDEPT is absolutely dependent upon reaching the necrotic area of the tumor to exert its antitumor activity. Hence, in order to achieve the enhanced antitumor activity by CDEPT with vascular-disrupting agents, the vascular-disrupting agent should not compromise the delivery of spores or accessibility of the prodrug. Prolonged or persistant reduction in tumor blood flow resulting from vascular disruption by the vascular-disrupting agent is likely to interfere the delivery of CDEPT. The timing requirement is different for other treatment modalities such as radiation or anticancer drugs, the cell killing of which are not affected by tumor necrosis. In fact, a significant (1–2 log) tumor cell killing is generally observed when tumor blood flow is reduced by the vascular-disrupting agents ZD6126 or DMXAA in combination with radiation (Siemann and Rojiani, 2002; Murata *et al.*, 2001), or with cisplatin (Siemann *et al.*, 2002; Siemann and Rojiani, 2002; Siim *et al.*, 2003). This is probably due to the different modes of tumor cell kill by these agents, such that vascular-disrupting agents kill necrotic/hypoxic cells while radiation or anticancer drugs kill well oxygenated cells in the tumor.

Optimizing prodrug design

In general, a viable rim of the tumor survives from the treatment of vascular-disrupting agents and this region is often responsible for regrowth of the tumor. This may be also true for CDEPT in combination with vascular-disrupting agents. This means that the best prodrug will be one that produces an anticancer drug with a significant diffusing ability, thereby allowing additional cell killing of the adjacent viable rim of the tumor. 5-FU, the active anticancer drug generated by 5-FC from CD-transformed clostridia, fulfills this requirement, as the anticancer drug has good bystander activity (Kuriyama *et al.*, 1998). However, because 5-FU primarily kills rapidly proliferating tumor cells (Longley, Harkin and Johnston, 2003) and many cells in tumors proliferate only slowly, studies of other prodrug–active anticancer drug systems are warranted. Several physico-chemical features should be considered when designing prodrugs. First the prodrug should be stable in the tumor microenvironment (reviewed by Denny, 2003). This is especially true close to hypoxic/necrotic areas of the tumor, where anaerobic glycolysis produces an excess amount of lactic acid, leading to an acidic environment (Brown and Giaccia, 1998). Hence, prodrugs with basic functional groups are unlikely to be useful because they may undergo chemical change in these conditions. Moreover, the prodrug should not be metabolized by cells or enzymes unless this is the activating mechanism. Second, the prodrug should effectively mask cytotoxicity of the corresponding active anticancer drug. Third, the prodrug should efficiently release the anticancer drug upon activation. Fourth, and most importantly, the prodrug should have a sufficient diffusing ability to penetrate multiple layers of tumor cells. This is critical for CDEPT, because the necrotic area of the tumor where the prodrug needs to reach is likely to be distant from the functional blood vessels in the tumor. The *in vitro* multi-cellular layer (MCL) culture model, diffusion-limited structures in which tumor cells are grown at tissue-like density, has been validated to be a useful technique in quantifying such extravascular diffusion and bystander effects for various prodrugs (Pruijn *et al.*, 2005; Wilson *et al.*, 2002).

Some of the features for the active anticancer drug that is released or con-verted from the prodrug might include that it should have potent cytotoxicity, efficiently killing slowly as well as rapidly proliferating tumor cells. As for the prodrug, the active anticancer drug should also have a good diffusing ability to kill adjacent and surrounding viable tumor cells.

Other enzyme–prodrug combinations for CDEPT

In order to be tumor specific, CDEPT utilizes enzymes of non-human origin. In addition to the *E. coli*-derived cytosine deaminase discussed above, other potential enzymes that can be used for CDEPT include β-glucuronidase and β-galactosidase. These enzymes are particularly attractive because their prodrug forms, which incorporate glucuronide and galactoside sugar moieties, are extremely hydrophilic, offering an improved extravascular transportation (by the paracellular route) and very high cytotoxic differential between the pro-drug and the active drug (up to three orders of magnitude). β-galactoside and β-glucoside analogs of duocarmycin and CC1065, very potent DNA minor groove alkylators, have been reported as potential prodrugs for activation by β-galactosidase and β-glucosidase (Tietze *et al.*, 2001).

Other ways to potentiate antitumor activity by CDEPT in combination with vascular-disrupting agents

Adding another treatment modality such as ionizing radiation or an anticancer drug that would preferentially kill the well oxygenated, peripheral rim of the tumor would be expected to lead to greater antitumor activity by CDEPT in combination with the vascular-disrupting agent. This is particularly the case for the combination of ionizing radiation with CD-expressing clostridial spores and the 5-FC prodrug because 5-FU generated from 5-FC by CD is also an effective radiosensitizer (Kievit *et al.*, 2000). With radiation and CDEPT (CD-expressing clostridial spores and 5-FC) in combination with ZD6126, we have observed an even enhanced antitumor activity over any single or combination of two treatments in human tumor xenograft models (Ahn *et al.*, unpublished data).

15.5   Clinical significance

It was the lack of any adverse effects in preclinical testing of C. *butyricum* that led Mose and Mose to inject themselves with the spores, thereby demonstrating the lack of human pathogenicity. Clinical studies with cancer patients followed using i.v. injection of 10^9–10^{10} spores per individual (Carey *et al.*, 1967; Heppner and Mose, 1978; Heppner *et al.*, 1983). Typically, a low-grade fever occurs 1–3 days following injection, with further increase in temperature on days 5–8, which coincides with lysis in the centre of the tumor. In subsequent clinical studies with 49 patients with malignant gliomas, Heppner and Mose injected clostridial spores into the carotid artery on the side of the tumor (Heppner *et al.*, 1983). All tumors showed lysis, following which the tumors were removed surgically. However, there was no prolongation of the recurrence-free interval. In more recent studies with the non-pathogenic clostridial strain C. *butyricum*, CNRZ 528, Fabricius and colleagues (1993) injected 68 clinical volunteers with 3.5–7.0×10^9 spores per patient in order to determine the half-life of blood clearance of the spores. This was found to be 1–2 days in man. No adverse effects were noted.

   These clinical reports demonstrate that spores of non-pathogenic strains of clostridia can be given safely, that the spores germinate in the necrotic regions of tumors and that in the case of C. *oncolyticum* lysis of the tumors can occur. Also in preclinical studies with mice and rabbits, a similar lack of C. *oncolyticum* pathogenicity has been seen (Thiele, Arison and Boxer, 1964). In our own studies we have seen no adverse effects following i.v. injections in control and tumor-bearing mice with up to 10^9 genetically engineered C. *sporogenes* per mouse.

   An important question is whether there will be an immune response against the clostridial spores, the vegetative bacteria or the secreted protein that might preclude treatment of patients on multiple occasions. However, both the clinical (Carey *et al.*, 1967) and experimental data (Gericke *et al.*, 1979) so far suggest that multiple treatments are effective. In our own studies we have found undiminished expression of CD and no loss of numbers of bacteria in experimental tumors for up to 14 days following a single intravenous injection.

   The combination of CDEPT with vascular-disrupting agents opens an exciting possibility that clinical antitumor efficacy of CDEPT can be substantially enhanced by these agents. Not only by these agents themselves inducing massive vascular shutdown and necrosis leading to some antitumor activity, but by combining with CDEPT one can observe more than additive yet tumor-selective efficacy from this combination. Moreover, if systemic administration of vascular-disrupting agents can produce necrosis in small metastases, which normally do not have necrosis, this would make them susceptible to colonization of obligate anaerobes and hence treatable with CDEPT. In summary, we believe that CDEPT has established its likelihood of being effective in the clinic and that vascular-disrupting agents could be an important adjunct to CDEPT in potentiating its effectiveness over a wide range of tumor sizes.

References

Ahn, G., Liu, S.C., Menke, D., Dorie, M.J. and Brown, J.M. (2004). Enhanced antitumor activity of 5-FC by genetically engineered anaerobic bacteria *C. sporogenes* expressing cytosine deaminase when combined with a vascular targeting agent, ZD6126 or DMXAA. In *2nd International Conference on Vascular Targeting*, Miami, FL.

Baguley, B.C. and Ching, L.M. (2002). DMXAA: an antivascular agent with multiple host responses. *Int J Radiat Oncol Biol Phys* 54, 1503–1511.

Becker, A., Hansgen, G., Bloching, M., Weigel, C., Lautenschlager, C. and Dunst, J. (1998). Oxygenation of squamous cell carcinoma of the head and neck: comparison of primary tumors, neck node metastases, and normal tissue. *Int J Radiat Oncol Biol Phys* 42, 35–41.

Blakey, D.C., Westwood, F.R., Walker, M., Hughes, G.D., Davis, P.D., Ashton, S.E. and Ryan, A.J. (2002). Antitumor activity of the novel vascular targeting agent ZD6126 in a panel of tumor models. *Clin Cancer Res* 8, 1974–1983.

Brizel, D.M., Dodge, R.K., Clough, R.W. and Dewhirst, M.W. (1999). Oxygenation of head and neck cancer: changes during radiotherapy and impact on treatment outcome. *Radiother Oncol* 53, 113–117.

Brizel, D.M., Rosner, G.L., Prosnitz, L.R. and Dewhirst, M.W. (1995). Patterns and variability of tumor oxygenation in human soft tissue sarcomas, cervical carcinomas, and lymph node metastases. *Int J Radiat Oncol Biol Phys* 32, 1121–1125.

Brown, J.M. and Giaccia, A.J. (1998). The unique physiology of solid tumors: opportunities (and problems) for cancer therapy. *Cancer Res* 58, 1408–1416.

Brown, J.M. and Wilson, W.R. (2004). Exploiting tumour hypoxia in cancer treatment. *Nat Rev Cancer* 4, 437–447.

Carey, R.W., Holland, J.F., Whang, H.Y., Neter, E. and Bryant, B. (1967). Clostridial oncolysis in man. *Eur J Cancer* 3, 37–46.

Ching, L.M., Cao, Z., Kieda, C., Zwain, S., Jameson, M.B. and Baguley, B.C. (2002). Induction of endothelial cell apoptosis by the antivascular agent 5,6-dimethylxanthenone-4-acetic acid. *Br J Cancer* 86, 1937–1942.

Dang, L.H., Bettegowda, C., Huso, D.L., Kinzler, K.W. and Vogelstein, B. (2001). Combination bacteriolytic therapy for the treatment of experimental tumors. *Proc Natl Acad Sci USA* 98, 15155–15160.

Denny, W.A. (2003). Prodrugs for gene-directed enzyme–prodrug therapy (suicide gene therapy). *J Biomed Biotechnol* 2003, 48–70.

Engelbart, K. and Gericke, D. (1964). Oncolysis by Clostridia. V. Transplanted tumors of the hamster. *Cancer Res* 24, 239–243.

Fabricius, E.M., Schneeweiss, U., Schau, H.P., Schmidt, W. and Benedix, A. (1993). Quantitative investigations into the elimination of in vitro-obtained spores of the non-pathogenic Clostridium butyricum strain CNRZ 528, and their persistence in organs of different species following intravenous spore administration. *Res Microbiol* **144**, 741–753.

Fox, M.E., Lemmon, M.J., Mauchline, M.L., Davis, T.O., Giaccia, A.J., Minton, N.P. and Brown, J.M. (1996). Anaerobic bacteria as a delivery system for cancer gene therapy: in vitro activation of 5-fluorocytosine by genetically engineered clostridia. *Gene Ther* **3**, 173–178.

Gericke, D., Dietzel, F., Konig, W., Ruster, I. and Schumacher, L. (1979). Further progress with oncolysis due to apathogenic clostridia. *Zentralb Bakteriol [Orig A]* **243**, 102–112.

Goertz, D.E., Yu, J.L., Kerbel, R.S., Burns, P.N. and Foster, F.S. (2002). High-frequency Doppler ultrasound monitors the effects of antivascular therapy on tumor blood flow. *Cancer Res* **62**, 6371–6375.

Goto, H., Yano, S., Zhang, H., Matsumori, Y., Ogawa, H., Blakey, D.C. and Sone, S. (2002). Activity of a new vascular targeting agent, ZD6126, in pulmonary metastases by human lung adenocarcinoma in nude mice. *Cancer Res* **62**, 3711–3715.

Graeber, T.G., Osmanian, C., Jacks, T., Housman, D.E., Koch, C.J., Lowe, S.W. and Giaccia, A.J. (1996). Hypoxia-mediated selection of cells with diminished apoptotic potential in solid tumours. *Nature* **379**, 88–91.

Harris, A.L. (2002). Hypoxia – a key regulatory factor in tumour growth. *Nat Rev Cancer* **2**, 38–47.

Heppner, F. and Mose, J.R. (1978). The liquefaction (oncolysis) of malignant gliomas by a non pathogenic clostridium. *Acta Neurol* **12**, 123–125.

Heppner, F., Mose, J., Ascher, P.W. and Walter, G. (1983). *13th Int Congr Chemother* **226**, 38–45.

Horsman, M.R. and Murata, R. (2003). Vascular targeting effects of ZD6126 in a C3H mouse mammary carcinoma and the enhancement of radiation response. *Int J Radiat Oncol Biol Phys* **57**, 1047–1055.

Huang, J., Frischer, J.S., Serur, A., Kadenhe, A., Yokoi, A., McCrudden, K.W., New, T., O'Toole, K., Zabski, S., Rudge, J.S., Holash, J., Yancopoulos, G.D., Yamashiro, D.J. and Kandel, J.J. (2003). Regression of established tumors and metastases by potent vascular endothelial growth factor blockade. *Proc Natl Acad Sci USA* **100**, 7785–7790.

Kievit, E., Nyati, M.K., Ng, E., Stegman, L.D., Parsels, J., Ross, B.D., Rehemtulla, A. and Lawrence, T.S. (2000). Yeast cytosine deaminase improves radiosensitization and bystander effect by 5-fluorocytosine of human colorectal cancer xenografts. *Cancer Res* **60**, 6649–6655.

Koong, A.C., Mehta, V.K., Le, Q.T., Fisher, G.A., Terris, D.J., Brown, J.M., Bastidas, A.J. and Vierra, M. (2000). Pancreatic tumors show high levels of hypoxia. *Int J Radiat Oncol Biol Phys* **48**, 919–922.

Kuriyama, S., Masui, K., Sakamoto, T., Nakatani, T., Kikukawa, M., Tsujinoue, H., Mitoro, A., Yamazaki, M., Yoshiji, H., Fukui, H., Ikenaka, K., Mullen, C.A. and Itsujii, T. (1998). Bystander effect caused by cytosine deaminase gene and 5-fluorocytosine in vitro is substantially mediated by generated 5-fluorouracil. *Anticancer Res* **18**, 3399–3406.

Lemmon, M.J., Elwell, J.H., Brehm, J.K., Mauchline, M.L., N, M., Minton, N.P., Giaccia, A.J. and Brown, J.M. (1994). Anaerobic bacteria as a gene delivery system to tumors. *Proc Am Assoc Cancer Res* **35**, 374.

Lemmon, M.L., Van Zijl, P., Fox, M.E., Mauchline, M.L., Giaccia, A.J., Minton, N.P. and Brown, J.M. (1997). Anaerobic bacteria as a gene delivery system that is controlled by the tumor microenvironment. *Gene Ther* **4**, 791–796.

Liu, S.C., Minton, N.P., Giaccia, A.J. and Brown, J.M. (2002). Anticancer efficacy of systemically delivered anaerobic bacteria as gene therapy vectors targeting tumor hypoxia/necrosis. *Gene Ther* **9**, 291–296.

Longley, D.B., Harkin, P. and Johnston, P.G. (2003). 5-fluorouracil: mechanisms of action and clinical strategies. *Nat Rev Cancer* **3**, 330–338.

Malmgren, R.A. and Flanigan, C.C. (1955). Localization of the vegetative form of *Clostridium tetani* in mouse tumors following intravenous spore administration. *Cancer Res* **15**, 473–478.

Martin, J., Stribbling, S.M., Poon, G.K., Begent, R.H., Napier, M., Sharma, S.K. and Springer, C.J. (1997). Antibody-directed enzyme prodrug therapy: pharmacokinetics and plasma levels of prodrug and drug in a phase I clinical trial. *Cancer Chemother Pharmacol* **40**, 189–201.

Melton, R.G. and Sherwood, R.F. (1996). Antibody-enzyme conjugates for cancer therapy. *J Natl Cancer Inst* **88**, 153–165.

Mose, J.R. and Mose, G. (1959). Onkolyseversuche mit apathogenen anaeroben Sporenbildern am Ehrlich Tumor des Maus. *Z Krebsforsch* **63**, 63–74.

Mose, J.R. and Mose, G. (1964). Oncolysis by clostridia. I. Activity of *Clostridium butyricum* (M-55) and other nonpathogenic clostridia against the Ehrlich carcinoma. *Cancer Res* **24**, 212–216.

Movsas, B., Chapman, J.D., Horwitz, E.M., Pinover, W.H., Greenberg, R.E., Hanlon, A.L., Iyer, R. and Hanks, G.E. (1999). Hypoxic regions exist in human prostate carcinoma. *Urology* **53**, 11–18.

Murata, R., Siemann, D.W., Overgaard, J. and Horsman, M.R. (2001). Improved tumor response by combining radiation and the vascular-damaging drug 5,6-dimethylxanthenone-4-acetic acid. *Radiat Res* **156**, 503–509.

Nuyts, S., Van Mellaert, L., Theys, J., Landuyt, W., Lambin, P. and Anne, J. (2002). Clostridium spores for tumor-specific drug delivery. *Anticancer Drugs* **13**, 115–125.

Pruijn, F.B., Sturman, J., Liyanage, S., Hicks, K.O., Hay, M.P. and Wilson, W.R. (2005). Extravascular transport of drugs in tumor tissue: effect of lipophilicity on diffusion of tirapazamine analogues in multicellular layer cultures. *J Med Chem* **48**, 1079–1087.

Rampling, R., Cruickshank, G., Lewis, A.D., Fitzsimmons, S.A. and Workman, P. (1994). Direct measurement of pO_2 distribution and bioreductive enzymes in human malignant brain tumors. *Int J Radiat Oncol Biol Phys* **29**, 427–431.

Robinson, S.P., McIntyre, D.J., Checkley, D., Tessier, J.J., Howe, F.A., Griffiths, J.R., Ashton, S.E., Ryan, A.J., Blakey, D.C. and Waterton, J.C. (2003). Tumour dose response to the antivascular agent ZD6126 assessed by magnetic resonance imaging. *Br J Cancer* **88**, 1592–1597.

Siemann, D.W., Mercer, E., Lepler, S. and Rojiani, A.M. (2002). Vascular targeting agents enhance chemotherapeutic agent activities in solid tumor therapy. *Int J Cancer* **99**, 1–6.

Siemann, D.W. and Rojiani, A.M. (2002). Enhancement of radiation therapy by the novel vascular targeting agent ZD6126. *Int J Radiat Oncol Biol Phys* **53**, 164–171.

Siim, B.G., Lee, A.E., Shalal-Zwain, S., Pruijn, F.B., McKeage, M.J. and Wilson, W.R. (2003). Marked potentiation of the antitumour activity of chemotherapeutic drugs by the antivascular agent 5,6-dimethylxanthenone-4-acetic acid (DMXAA). *Cancer Chemother Pharmacol* **51**, 43–52.

Sundfor, K., Lyng, H., Kongsgard, U.L., Trope, C. and Rofstad, E.K. (1997). Polarographic measurement of pO_2 in cervix carcinoma. *Gynecol Oncol* **64**, 230–236.

Theys, J., Landuyt, W., Nuyts, S., Van Mellaert, L., Bosmans, E., Rijnders, A., Van Den Bogaert, W., van Oosterom, A., Anne, J. and Lambin, P. (2001). Improvement of

Clostridium tumour targeting vectors evaluated in rat rhabdomyosarcomas. *FEMS Immunol Med Microbiol* **30**, 37–41.

Thiele, E.H., Arison, R.N. and Boxer, G.E. (1964). Oncolysis by clostridia. III. Effects of clostridia and chemotherapeutic agents on rodent tumors. *Cancer Res* **24**, 234–238.

Thomlinson, R.H. and Gray, L.H. (1955). The histological structure of some human lung cancers and the possible implications for radiotherapy. *Br J Cancer* **9**, 539–549.

Tietze, L.F., Lieb, M., Herzig, T., Haunert, F. and Schuberth, I. (2001). A strategy for tumor-selective chemotherapy by enzymatic liberation of *seco*-duocarmycin SA-derivatives from nontoxic prodrugs. *Bioorg Med Chem* **9**, 1929–1939.

Varghese, H.J., Mackenzie, L.T., Groom, A.C., Ellis, C.G., Ryan, A., MacDonald, I.C. and Chambers, A.F. (2004). In vivo videomicroscopy reveals differential effects of the vascular-targeting agent ZD6126 and the anti-angiogenic agent ZD6474 on vascular function in a liver metastasis model. *Angiogenesis* **7**, 157–164.

Vaupel, P.W. and Hockel, M. (1995). Oxygenation status of human tumors: a reappraisal using computerized pO_2 histography. In *Tumor Oxygenation* (Ed. P.W. Vaupel, D.K. Kelleher and M. Gunderoth) Fischer, Stuttgart, pp. 219–232.

Wilson, W.R., Pullen, S.M., Hogg, A., Helsby, N.A., Hicks, K.O. and Denny, W.A. (2002). Quantitation of bystander effects in nitroreductase suicide gene therapy using three-dimensional cell cultures. *Cancer Res* **62**, 1425–1432.

Wouters, B.G., Weppler, S.A., Koritzinsky, M., Landuyt, W., Nuyts, S., Theys, J., Chiu, R.K. and Lambin, P. (2002). Hypoxia as a target for combined modality treatments. *Eur J Cancer* **38**, 240–257.

16

Imaging the Effects of Vasculature-targeting Agents

Susan M. Galbraith

16.1 Introduction

A variety of methods have been used to image the effects of vascular-targeting agents in pre-clinical and clinical settings. The techniques chosen have been designed to measure tissue microcirculatory parameters such as blood flow rate and hypoxia, which would be expected to change following treatment with such an agent. In the traditional model of oncology drug development for cytotoxic compounds, phase I doses are escalated until dose-limiting toxicity is seen, and the maximum tolerated dose (MTD) is taken forward into single-arm phase II trials with primary endpoints of response rate. For vascular-targeting agents the traditional model has been perceived to be inappropriate, since the rate of acute tumor regressions is lower than with cytotoxic compounds. Therefore, endpoints in addition to response rate are required in phase I/II trials in order to optimize dose and schedule selection and confirm anti-tumor efficacy prior to initiation of phase III trials.

There are several important questions in development of these agents, which imaging techniques might assist in answering.

1. What is the pharmacokinetic exposure–response relationship for changes in the tumor microcirculation?

2. What is the time course of response, and therefore what are the optimal timepoints for imaging?

3. How does the imaging endpoint relate to induction of tumor necrosis?

Vascular-targeted Therapies in Oncology   Edited by Dietmar W. Siemann
© 2006 John Wiley & Sons, Ltd.

4. What duration and extent of change in tumor microcirculation are enough for anti-tumor efficacy?

5. What is the optimal dosing schedule?

6. How should anti-vascular drugs be combined with other anti-cancer agents?

7. How well do pre-clinical models predict for clinical efficacy?

8. Why do some tumors not respond?

9. What is happening in normal tissues?

10. What are the mechanisms of toxicity?

There is an opportunity to answer some of these questions in the pre-clinical setting, preferably using a range of tumor models, but early phase clinical trials also need to be designed appropriately to enable useful conclusions from the imaging data. It is desirable to be able to compare the findings seen in the clinic with the pre-clinical assessments to maximize the understanding gained, and thereby to come to the appropriate decision following the early clinical trial results. This desire to translate methodologies from pre-clinical experiments to early clinical trials drives some pragmatic choices, since the range of imaging techniques available for pre-clinical experiments is generally wider than that readily available across a sufficient number of potential clinical sites. This chapter will review the available imaging methodologies, concentrating on those that can be used in both pre-clinical and clinical settings, and discuss the available data on the use of these techniques in pre-clinical experiments as well as in the clinical trials with vascular-targeting agents. The contribution of the imaging data to the pre-clinical and clinical development of these drugs, and to answering the above questions, will also be discussed.

16.2 Methods for imaging tissue blood flow rate

There are several methods for measuring blood flow rate in a tissue, of which imaging techniques form a sub-set. There are direct methods, for example by insertion of electromagnetic flowmeters into or around a vessel, and a variety of indirect methods, some of which are invasive, and some which require only intravenous injection. There are three general principles underlying the indirect methods:

(a) measurement of the mean transit time of a tracer through a tissue

(b) measurement of the uptake of a tracer into a tissue, or clearance from it

(c) measurement of the fractional distribution of cardiac output.

In addition, there are methods such as laser Doppler flowmetry and color Doppler ultrasound that do not measure tissue blood flow rate itself, but micro-regional red cell flux, and flow velocities within the larger vessels in a tissue respectively.

16.3   Central volume theorem

The first method is based on Stewart's central volume theorem (Stewart, 1894). This states that the tissue blood flow rate F is determined by

$$F = \frac{V}{\text{MTT}} \tag{16.1}$$

where V is the volume of distribution of the agent within the tissue, and MTT is the mean transit time, or the average time it takes for a tracer to pass through the tissue.

There are several reasons why this apparently simple equation may be difficult to solve. First, the volume of distribution of the tracer may be biologically multi-compartmental, with transfer of the tracer between different tissue volumes occurring at different rates. The passage of the tracer through tissue compart-ments must therefore be modeled. Second, even for single-compartment models such as pure intravascular markers, the theorem assumes an instantaneous bolus injection, which is not achievable *in vivo*, and measurement of the MTT requires an adequate temporal sampling rate. The actual measured tissue-concentration time curve, Tissue(t), is the convolution of the arterial input function Art(t) and the residue function RF(t)

$$\text{Tissue}(t) = \text{Art}(t) \otimes \text{RF}(t) \tag{16.2}$$

Therefore, to measure RF(t), and the associated MTT, Art(t) is required. This can be measured directly with arterial blood sampling, or indirectly if a non-invasive method exists with sufficient temporal resolution. For pure intravascu-lar markers the volume of distribution is the blood volume and is determined by

$$V = \frac{\int \text{Tissue}(t)}{\int \text{Art}(t)} \tag{16.3}$$

This principle has been used for calculation of cerebral blood volume (Rosen *et al.*, 1990), and cerebral blood flow rate by MRI, after intravenous injection of gadopentetate dimeglumine (Gd-DTPA) (Ostergaard *et al.*, 1996a, 1996b), which behaves as an intravascular tracer in brain, due to the blood–brain barrier. Perfusion-weighted images can be obtained with T2* weighted sequences using rapid temporal resolution (1–2 s) in order to track the bolus of paramagnetic contrast material as it passes through a capillary bed (Sorensen *et al.*, 1997; Barbier, Lamalle and Decorps, 2001). Within blood vessels, the contrast agent produces magnetic field inhomogeneities that result in a decrease in the signal intensity of surrounding tissues. The degree of signal intensity loss is dependent on the concentration of the contrast agent within the vessel, microvessel size and density (Dennie *et al.*, 1998). This technique is most reliable in brain applications because the blood–brain barrier ensures the contrast medium is largely retained within the intravascular space (Knopp *et al.*, 1999). The advent of higher-molecular-weight MRI contrast agents, which remain in the vascular compartment, would enable this principle to be used in other tissues (Furman-Haran *et al.*, 1998; Su *et al.* 1998), although such agents are not currently available for clinical use. This principle has also been used with ultrasound techniques, using microbubbles injected intravenously as contrast agents (Albrecht *et al.*, 1999).

16.4   Kety model

In 1948 Kety described a model of tissue uptake of a freely diffusible, inert tracer, based upon the Fick principle, that was originally used for the determination of cerebral blood flow rate using nitrous oxide (Kety and Schmidt, 1948), and adapted for determining regional blood flow rate by measuring the local clearance of a radioactive tracer (Kety, 1949). The model was further developed to allow quantitative regional blood flow rate determination using an intravenous bolus of an inert, freely diffusible tracer, iodoantipyrine (Kety, 1960a, 1960b). The Fick principle in turn is based on the theory of mass conservation. That is, for a substance distributed to a tissue in the blood within a time Δt, the quantity brought in, Q_a, is equal to the quantity accumulated in the tissue, Q_t, metabolized, Q_m, or removed from the tissue, Q_e:

$$\frac{Q_a}{\Delta t} = \frac{\Delta Q_t}{\Delta t} + \frac{Q_m}{\Delta t} + \frac{Q_e}{\Delta t} \tag{16.4}$$

A freely diffusible substance injected as a rapid intravenous bolus will accumulate in the tissue until its tissue concentration, C_t, is equivalent to that in the arterial blood, C_a. If the substance is inert, $Q_m = 0$, and as Q_a is the product of blood flow F and C_a then

$$\frac{dQ_t}{dt} = F(C_a - C_v) \tag{16.5}$$

After a sufficient period of time (T), there will be equilibration between the concentration of the substance in the tissue and the venous blood, so

$$C_t = \frac{Q_t(T)}{V} = C_v(T)\lambda \tag{16.6}$$

where λ is the tissue–blood partition coefficient of the substance, and V is the volume of the tissue. Integrating (16.5) and substituting (16.6) yields

$$\frac{F}{V} = \frac{C_v(T)\lambda}{\int_0^T (C_a - C_v)\mathrm{d}t} \tag{16.7}$$

which requires knowledge of the arterial and venous concentrations in order to determine blood flow rate. This has been used to determine cerebral blood flow rate using nitrous oxide (Kety and Schmidt, 1948). If the substance is not freely diffusible then Equation (16.5) needs to be modified to include the extraction fraction E (fractional loss from blood to tissue in a single passage). Also, in other organs, determination of C_v may not be practical:

$$\frac{\mathrm{d}Q_t}{V\mathrm{d}t} = \frac{\mathrm{d}C_t}{\mathrm{d}t} = \frac{EF}{\lambda V}(\lambda C_a - C_t) \tag{16.8}$$

Integrating and solving this equation when C_a is negligible, as for interstitial injection of an inert radioactive tracer,

$$C_t(T) = C_t(0)e^{-\left(\frac{EF}{\lambda V}\right)t} \tag{16.9}$$

This equation has been used to calculate blood flow rate in superficial tumors after local injection of xenon-133, argon-41 and krypton-85 (Mantyla et al., 1988). This method is obviously invasive, only gives information about a region of a tumor and is not suitable for large or deep-seated tumors.

When C_a is variable, but zero at time 0, and where F is blood flow rate per unit mass of tissue rather than total blood flow rate, then

$$C_t(T) = EF\int_0^T C_a\, e^{\frac{-EF}{\lambda}(T-t)}\mathrm{d}t \tag{16.10}$$

This equation, known as the Kety equation, has been used to derive blood flow rate using radiolabeled iodoantipyrine (IAP) as a tracer, for which $E = 1$ (Kety, 1960b; Tozer et al., 1994). It requires knowledge of the arterial input function $\equiv \int_0^T C_a \mathrm{d}t$, which can be obtained by direct arterial sampling and the partition coefficient for the tracer in the tissue of interest. This method is widely established for measurement of blood flow rate in experimental tumors, but has not been used clinically.

The same principle is used in positron emission tomography (PET) studies using the positron-emitting isotope $^{15}\mathrm{O}$ in water, $H_2{}^{15}\mathrm{O}$, to determine tissue blood flow rate (Beaney et al., 1984; Lammertsma and Jones, 1992). This tracer, like IAP, is freely diffusible, but has the disadvantage that its half-life is only 2.5 minutes, thus requiring a cyclotron to generate the isotope on the same site as the experiment.

Dynamic contrast-enhanced magnetic resonance imaging (DCE-MRI) also uses models based on the Kety equation (Tofts *et al.*, 1999), although the tracer used, gadopentetate dimeglumine (Gd-DTPA), is neither freely diffusible, nor a pure intravascular marker. Gd-DTPA, being an extracellular agent, diffuses from the blood into the extracellular extravascular space (EES) at a rate determined by a combination of tissue perfusion, vascular permeability of the capillaries and vascular surface area. The presence of the paramagnetic contrast medium in the EES produces an increase in signal intensity in T1-weighted images due to shortening of the T1 relaxation rate. The Kety equation can be adapted for intravenous bolus injection of Gd-DTPA (Tofts *et al.*, 1999):

$$C_t(T) = K^{trans} \int_0^T C_p(t) e^{-k_{ep}(T-t)} dt \qquad (16.11)$$

where C_p is arterial plasma concentration of Gd-DTPA, K^{trans} is the volume constant for the transfer of Gd-DTPA from the vessel into the extracellular extravascular space (EES) and k_{ep} is the rate constant for the transfer of Gd-DTPA from the EES back into the plasma. From the above two equations,

$$K^{trans} = EF\rho(1-Hct) \qquad (16.12)$$

where ρ is tissue density (g ml^{-1}) and Hct is hematocrit. K^{trans} has several physiologic interpretations, depending on the balance between capillary permeability to Gd-DTPA and blood flow rate in the tissue of interest. In tissues with highly permeable vessels, where flux across the endothelium is flow limited, E is close to unity so K^{trans} is equal to the blood plasma flow rate per unit volume of tissue (ml plasma per ml tissue per minute):

$$K^{trans} = F\rho(1-Hct) \qquad (16.13)$$

Adapting Renkin's equation (Renkin, 1959) for extraction fraction for a freely diffusible tracer to an extracellular tracer,

$$E = 1 - e^{\frac{PS}{F(1-Hct)}} \qquad (16.14)$$

where PS is the permeability (P) vessel surface area (S) product. Therefore, when $PS \ll F$, as in tissues such as brain with low vessel permeability, flux across the endothelium is permeability limited,

$$E = \frac{PS}{F(1-\text{Hct})} \qquad (16.15)$$

and K^{trans} is equal to the permeability surface area product per unit volume of tissue:

$$K^{\text{trans}} = PS\rho \qquad (16.16)$$

In tumors there is heterogeneity of vessel permeability, and K^{trans} is determined by a combination of flow, permeability and vessel surface area. The ratio of K^{trans} to k_{ep} gives the volume of EES per unit volume of tissue, v_{e}, otherwise known as the Gd-DTPA leakage space:

$$v_{\text{e}} = \frac{K^{\text{trans}}}{k_{\text{ep}}} \qquad (16.17)$$

This model assumes an instantaneous bolus and instant mixing of Gd-DTPA within the blood and within the leakage space after transfer from the vessel, and ignores the contribution of intravascular tracer to the tissue concentration.

In order to use Equation (16.11) to derive the parameters K^{trans}, k_{ep} and v_{e}, tissue concentration of Gd-DTPA has to be derived from the MRI signal intensity information. It has been assumed by some groups that for the range of concentrations of Gd-DTPA used in clinical studies there is a linear relationship between 1/T1 and tissue concentration of Gd-DTPA (Belfi *et al.*, 1992). This has been confirmed by measuring tissue concentration and relaxation rate (Strich *et al.*, 1985). However, it is also dependent on the initial T1 of the tissue (Tweedle *et al.*, 1991):

$$\frac{1}{\text{T1}(t)} - \frac{1}{\text{T1}(0)} = \beta C_{\text{a}}(t) \qquad (16.18)$$

and signal intensity on a T1-weighted image is not linearly related to 1/T1, as it also depends on aspects of the RF pulse sequence used and the tissue proton density (Evelhoch, 1999). However, the T1 of the tissue can be calculated by obtaining a proton-density-weighted image prior to contrast injection. Providing the machine scaling factors are not altered during the sequence of T1-weighted images, only one proton density image is required, as signal from this image should not vary with contrast agent concentration. Using a calibration curve generated from measurements on a variety of phantoms with known T1 levels, the ratio of the T1-weighted images to the proton density image can allow T1 values to be calculated (Parker *et al.*, 1997), and the concentration of Gd-DTPA can be obtained.

Tofts *et al.* set out a consensus of opinion about the standard quantities and symbols that should be adopted when using DCE-MRI to obtain fully quantitative parameters that relate to tissue perfusion, vessel permeability and surface area (Tofts *et al.*, 1999). However, some groups still use semi-quantitative parameters, such as the initial gradient of the signal enhancement derived from the signal intensity–time curves, which are simpler to obtain. In the absence of absolute T1 measurements, or the use of a proton density image to derive T1, the relative change in signal intensity (S) divided by the initial signal (S_0) has been used. This is called the enhancement (E):

$$E = \frac{S_t - S_0}{S_0} \qquad (16.19)$$

The gradient (G) is calculated from the rate of change of enhancement:

$$G = \frac{\mathrm{d}E}{\mathrm{d}T} \qquad (16.20)$$

The maximum enhancement and maximum or initial gradient are usually used. Relative changes in such semi-quantitative parameters can be examined, which may be indirectly related to changes in the physiological end-point of interest, such as blood flow rate (Bonnerot *et al.*, 1992; Mayr *et al.*, 1996; Beauregard *et al.*, 1998; Ostergaard *et al.*, 1998; Hawighorst *et al.*, 1999). If there is no correction for initial T1 relaxation time, then variations in this value will affect enhancement to some degree, as illustrated in Figure 16.1, which shows the signal intensity–time curves for regions of interest (ROIs) in fat and muscle from the same patient. At the top is the normalized signal intensity plotted against time for fat, which has a high T1, and muscle, which has a lower T1. The enhancement and gradient in muscle is ~4 times greater than that in fat.

At the bottom the data is corrected for initial T1 level, using the method described above, to calculate Gd-DTPA concentration which is plotted against time. The gradient in fat is now greater than that in muscle, and the enhancement is only slightly greater in muscle than fat. Semi-quantitative parameters that are not corrected for initial T1 could not therefore be used to compare relative levels of blood flow in different tissues or patients, although they could be used to compare changes within the same tissue after an intervention.

For accurate estimates of the kinetic parameters, the Gd-DTPA concentration–time curve in the artery supplying the tissue of interest (arterial input function) should be measured. Reliable methods for measuring arterial input function for routine DCE-MRI studies have been described but are still not widely available (Rijpkema *et al.*, 2001), and most studies reported to date have used an assumed arterial input function. This may lead to systematic errors in the calculated values of kinetic parameters (Buckley, 2002), as well as affecting the reproducibility of serial measurements within the same subject. Where it is

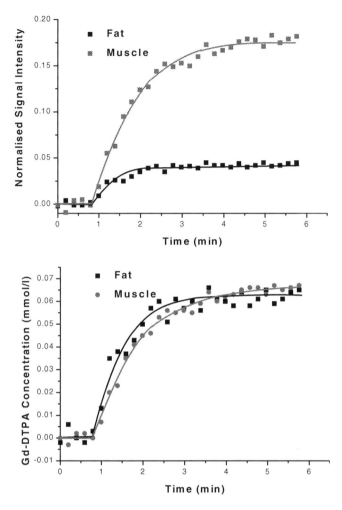

Figure 16.1 Illustration of the influence of initial T1 level on signal enhancement and gradient (A color reproduction of this figure can be seen in the color section)

not possible to obtain an arterial input function, Evelhoch recommends using the uptake integral (the area under the concentration time curve over the first 90 seconds after the onset time, IAUC), and normalizing to a normal tissue such as muscle (Evelhoch, 1999), as this minimizes errors due to variations in the arterial input. This assumes that the agent being investigated does not have a direct effect on the muscle microcirculation, and another potential disadvantage of this proposal is that the signal to noise ratio in muscle is poor due to low resting blood flow and the interstitial fluid content will vary in dependent muscles.

The above discussion demonstrates that the values derived from DCE-MRI analysis will not give a pure measure of blood flow rate, but will also be affected by the permeability of the tissue's vessels and the vascular surface area. Non-invasive measurement of the arterial input function is also problematic, making it difficult to obtain fully quantitative measurements. It has advantages over PET however, as it does not use ionizing radiation, has much better spatial resolution and is more widely applicable due to the greater number of MRI machines in clinical centers.

16.5 Fraction of cardiac output or 'first-pass' methods

Methods employing the uptake of an agent as a fraction of cardiac output include technetium-99m labeled hexamethyl-propyleneamine oxime, $^{99}Tc^mHM$-PAO, which is mainly used as a tracer for cerebral blood flow rate, measured by SPECT (single-photon emission computed tomography). This compound is unstable and converts rapidly from the lipophilic form, which passes the blood–brain barrier, to the hydrophilic form, which is then trapped in the brain, and levels remain stable for 24 h (Andersen, 1989). It has also been used to measure tumor blood flow rate in sites other than brain (Hammersley *et al.*, 1987), when it was shown to correlate well with $^{86}RbCl$ uptake. Rowell *et al.* used this technique to measure blood flow in human lung tumors (Rowell *et al.*, 1993). Its main disadvantage is poor spatial resolution, and cardiac output measurement is required for absolute flow calculation.

Dynamic CT measurements made in the first 30–40 s after intravenous bolus injection of contrast agent (during the 'first pass' of the agent through the vascular bed) also provide quantitative blood flow measurements, based on the principle of delivery in relation to cardiac output (Blomley *et al.*, 1993; Hermans *et al.*, 1999). This technique provides good spatial and temporal resolution, although the ionizing radiation dose received has disadvantages when several serial measurements are required in each patient. In addition, only a single slice through the tumor can be obtained, and there are artifacts produced from sites that move with arterial pulsation or respiration.

16.6 Color Doppler ultrasonography

The principle described by Doppler underlying this method is that the frequency of sound waves reflected from an object moving relative to an observer is shifted. The Doppler frequency shift is used in this ultrasound technique to give a measure of flow velocities in tissue blood vessels. The resolution of ultrasound, and the reduced blood velocity in smaller arterioles and capillaries means that flow in these vessels is not measured by this technique. In addition bulk tissue movements produce artifacts, which can be a problem in some organs (Eriksson *et al.*, 1991). Parameters obtained include vascularity index, peak flow velocity and flow resistance index. Although these parameters have been used to monitor the changes in tumor vascularity after treatment (Kedar *et al.*, 1994; van der Woude *et al.*, 1995), it has not been possible to directly relate them to other measures of angiogenesis such as microvessel density (Peters-Engl *et al.*, 1998). The technique has been improved by the use of power Doppler, which also encodes the power in the Doppler signal, therefore giving a measure of blood volume as well as velocity (Martinoli *et al.*, 1998), as well as improving the sensitivity. A measure of the total integrated power (IP) can be calculated within a tumor volume at each time point as follows:

$$IP = \sum P(i, j, k)$$

where i, j and k are the volumetric pixel indices, and the power P is in linear rather than in logarithmic form (Goertz *et al.*, 2002). The IP is related to the volume of moving blood within the tumors (Foster *et al.*, 2000) and, as such, it reflects the functional vascular volume.

16.7 Imaging hypoxia

It is possible to use intrinsic MR contrast within tissues to image the distortion of magnetic field homogeneity caused by the presence of deoxyhemoglobin, which acts as an intrinsic, oxygen-sensitive paramagnetic marker. BOLD (blood-oxygen-level-dependent) and FLOOD (flow- and oxygen-dependent) sequences are examples (Robinson, Howe and Griffiths, *et al.*, 1995). These sequences are sensitive to both microvascular blood flow as well as oxygen level. However, these techniques are limited by lower contrast to noise compared to those that use extrinsic paramagnetic contrast agents.

Nitroimidazole compounds have been developed for the detection of hypoxic cells. Such agents, which were originally developed as radiation sensitizers, contain an RNO_2 side chain that becomes rapidly reduced in the absence of oxygen (Chapman, Baer and Lee, 1983; Koch, Evans and Lord, 1995) then binds to cellular macromolecules. Nitroimidazole-based hypoxic markers have been used extensively in preclinical evaluations of tumor hypoxia (Evans, Hahn and Mapavelli, 2001; Koch, Evans and Lord, 1995) using immunohistochemistry or flow cytometry techniques. Various nitroimidazole hypoxia markers have also been developed for non-invasive detection by methods including SPECT (Koch and Evans, 2003), ^{18}F PET (Koch and Evans, 2003; Koh *et al.*, 1992; Barthel *et al.*, 2004; Piert *et al.*, 2005; Rajendran *et al.*, 2004). and ^{19}F MRS (Aboagye *et al.*, 1997; Kwock *et al.*, 1992). However, the signals generated by such nuclear medicine techniques are comprised of multiple tracer components including parent, reduced unbound and reduced bound hypoxic cell markers, rather than just the selective binding of the marker to hypoxic tumor cells. The potential problems with interpretation of ^{19}F MRS imaging of one of these nitroimidazole markers, EF5, were illustrated by a study showing that the signal observed *in vivo* 6 h after EF5 injection was most likely the consequence of parent and/or reduced unbounded EF5 and not bound EF5 metabolites in hypoxic KHT tumor cells (Salmon and Siemann, 2004). Thus the difference in signals observed between tumor and normal tissues might be based predominantly on differences in the tracer clearance rates of the tissues, making discrimination between hypoxia and alterations in tumor perfusion or vessel density difficult.

Technetium-99m (99mTc) labeling for imaging tissue hypoxia has also been investigated because of the ready availability of 99mTc in nuclear medicine departments, (Archer *et al.*, 1994). 99mTc-labeled HL-91 (Prognox) is a non-nitroimidazole that is selectively taken up by hypoxic cells in culture (Zhang *et al.*, 1998). It appears to localize in hypoxic regions of murine tumors, as demonstrated by selective binding in poorly perfused regions near necrosis (Tatsumi *et al.*, 1999), and by the correlation between the uptake of 99mTc-labeled HL-91 and the levels of hypoxia as measured with an oxygen electrode (Honess *et al.*, 1998).

16.8   Imaging glucose metabolism

^{18}F-labeled 2-fluoro-2-deoxy-D-glucose ([^{18}F] FDG) is the most common PET radiotracer used for clinical oncology applications. The basis for [^{18}F] FDG imaging lies in its ability to reflect the increased demand for glucose in malignant cells. FDG, after entering the cell, is phosphorylated by hexokinase. Once phosphorylated, it becomes trapped within the cell as it is not a substrate for the subsequent enzymatically driven pathways for glucose and the rate of dephosphorylation is slow. Tumors in general show an increased uptake of FDG compared with normal tissues (Warburg, 1956), and changes in FDG-PET uptake have been shown to be an early indicator of tumor response (Young *et al.* 1999) and to be related to overall survival (Vansteenkiste *et al.*, 1998; MacManus *et al.*, 2001; Pardo *et al.*, 2004). Therefore, whilst FDG-PET does not measure a specific effect of vascular targeting agents, this technique could be utilized as a pharmacodynamic endpoint predictive of clinical benefit.

Table 16.1 summarizes the different imaging techniques discussed above. Several different methods are suitable for clinical use, but differ in their potential for giving fully quantitative results, spatial resolution and repeatability. As many of the models used to describe the uptake of contrast agents into tissues were initially developed for the cerebral circulation, it is important that clinical techniques are also validated for the measurement of blood flow rate in extracranial sites. No systematic comparisons of the different methods in human tumors have been performed. However, Feldmann *et al.* have compared thermal washout techniques, dynamic CT and dynamic MRI in pelvic tumors, with good correlations (Feldmann *et al.*, 1993). DCE-MRI and CT both provide excellent spatial

Table 16.1 Indirect methods of measuring blood flow

Principle	Methods	Invasive	Quantitative	Serial measurements	Used clinically	Whole tumor	Resolution
Bolus tracking (Stewart theorum)	MRI–DCE or T2*	No	Yes	Yes	Yes	Yes	Excellent
	Ultrasound with microbubble contrast	No	Yes	Yes	Yes	Yes	Good
Tracer uptake/ clearance (Kety model)	^{133}Xe, ^{85}Kr, ^{41}Ar clearance	Yes	Yes	Yes (radiation dose)	Yes	No	Region
	Radiolabeled iodoantipyrine	Yes	Yes	No	No	Yes	Good
	^{15}O PET		Yes	Yes (radiation dose)	Yes	Yes	Moderate
	DCE-MRI	Arterial line	Possible	Yes	Yes	Yes	Excellent
	^{133}Xe enhanced CT	No No	Yes	Yes (radiation dose)	Yes	Yes	Good
Cardiac output fraction (first pass)	Microspheres	Cardiac catheter	Yes	Limited	Yes	Yes	Poor
	RbCl	Yes	Yes	No	No	Yes	Whole tissue
	HMPAO	No	Yes	Yes (radiation dose)	Yes	Yes	Poor
	Dynamic CT	No	Yes	Yes (radiation dose)	Yes	Yes	Good
Conservation of energy	Thermal clearance	Yes	Yes	Yes	Yes	Yes	Whole tissue

resolution, and DCE-MRI has the advantage of no ionizing radiation dose. The extracellular MR contrast agents used introduce an additional level of complexity in analysis due to their size, being neither freely diffusible nor purely intravascular, and because the increase in signal intensity they produce is not necessarily linearly related to concentration. The most common techniques used in the assessment of vascular targeting agents are DCE-MRI, ^{15}O-PET and ultrasound.

16.9   Preclinical experience of imaging vascular-disrupting agents

The effects of combretastatin A4 phosphate (CA4P) on the vasculature of tumors in mice and rats have been demonstrated using radioactive tracer uptake methods such as radiolabeled IAP (Dark *et al.*, 1997; Tozer *et al.*, 1999; Prise *et al.*, 2002), histological assessment of functional vascular volume using Hoescht dye (Dark *et al.*, 1997) and non-invasively by DCE-MRI (Beauregard *et al.*, 1998, 2001; Maxwell *et al.*, 2002). Beauregard *et al.*, demonstrated that DCE-MRI parameters decreased significantly in central regions of the tumor after treatment with CA4P (Beauregard *et al.*, 1998). This was attributed to disruption of the vasculature and was consistent with necrosis and hemorrhage seen in histological sections. Localized ^{31}P-MRS also showed that there was decline in cellular energy status in the tumor after treatment with the drug. This group also examined DCE-MRI and spectroscopy effects after CA4P treatment in a range of different tumor types (Beauregard *et al.*, 2001). LoVo and RIF-1 tumors responded well to drug treatment, with significant increases in the P(i)/ nucleoside triphosphate ratio within 3 hours, whereas SaS, SaF and HT29 tumors did not respond to the same extent. This variable response was also seen in DCE-MRI experiments. The differential susceptibility of the tumors to CA4P showed a positive correlation with prior MRI measurements of tumor vascular permeability, which was determined by measuring the inflow of a macromolecular contrast agent, bovine albumin-GdDTPA (Beauregard *et al.*, 2002).

The limitations of DCE-MRI discussed above meant that prior to the use of this technique in clinical trials with CA4P it was important to determine how well DCE-MRI measurements compared with the absolute blood flow rate measurements possible with IAP. Two studies have demonstrated that although the magnitude of changes in K^{trans} and IAUC was smaller than that in tumor blood flow measured by IAP the time course and dose-dependency patterns were very similar (Maxwell *et al.*, 2002; Galbraith *et al.*, 2003). There was a large and statistically significant reduction in mean IAUC at 1 and 6 hours in the tumor of 90 and 95 per cent respectively after injection of CA4P 30 mg kg^{-1}. K^{trans} was also reduced by 73 and 64 per cent at 1 and 6 h respectively in tumor. For comparison, another study in the same tumor model (Prise *et al.*, 2002) showed 87 and 98 per cent reductions in blood flow for the P22 tumor with this dose at the same timepoints using IAP. When the semi-quantitative parameter gradient from the signal intensity–time curve was used, the correlation with IAP measurements remained good ($R = 0.97$ $p = 0.002$) (unpublished data). However, the maximum reduction in gradient was only 30 per cent after $100\,mg\,kg^{-1}$ at 6 and 24 h. This suggests that whilst the semi-quantitative gradient method can be used as a relative measure of blood flow, with a treatment producing a blood flow reduction, the gradient change is likely to underestimate the true size of the treatment effect. IAUC and K^{trans} gave a better estimate of treatment effect than gradient – they accurately reflected true changes in tumor blood flow in this animal model after treatment with CA4P, thus justifying their use in human experiments with this agent. However, similar comparisons across a range of tissues and different tumor types would not necessarily confirm that K^{trans} accurately reflects differences in blood flow in general. As discussed above, blood flow, vessel permeability and surface area all contribute to K^{trans} values, and the relative contribution of each of these will vary in different tissues. There is evidence that tumor blood vessel permeability increases early after CA4P treatment in an isolated tumor model, using radiolabeled albumin and correcting for blood flow changes with ^{86}RbCl (Kanthou et al., 2001). At the same time, both blood flow and vessel surface area decrease. The above data demonstrate that in this tumor model these latter two effects predominate, and the resultant K^{trans} values reflect blood flow changes. The time-course demonstrating maximal response on DCE-MRI at around 6 h helped to drive the choice of imaging timepoints in the clinical phase I study.

One group has looked at the effects of CA4P on ^{18}F-fluorodeoxyglucose (FDG)-PET imaging of liver metastases in B6D2F1 mice. FDG-PET changes correlated with histological assessments, demonstrating a 30 per cent decrease in viable tumor after a single dose of CA4P (Zhao et al., 1999). No comparison of FDG-PET with DCE-MRI changes has been reported however.

Like CA4P, ZD6126 is a tubulin-depolymerizing agent, which produces rapid tumor blood flow shutdown. In GH3 prolactinomas, ZD6126 at $50\,mg\,kg^{-1}$ produced significant changes in DCE-MRI measurements, which were maintained for up to 96 h (McIntyre et al., 2004). The same group also examined the dose response to ZD6126 across the dose range $12.5–50\,mg\,kg^{-1}$, using both DCE-MRI as well as T2*-based BOLD measurements reflecting deoxyhemoglobin levels (Robinson et al., 2003). Tumor IAUC and $R(2)^*$ $(=1/T(2)^*)$ decreased post-treatment with ZD6126 in a dose-dependent manner. Lower doses of ZD6126 reduced the IAUC close to zero within restricted areas of the tumor, typically in the centre, while the highest dose reduced the IAUC to zero over the majority of the tumor. A decrease in both MRI end-points was associated with a dose-dependent increase in central tumor necrosis measured histologically from a baseline level of 40–50 per cent to a maximum of around 80 per cent after treatment with $50\,mg\,kg^{-1}$. This dose reduced the IAUC close to zero across the vast majority of the tumor, with more than 50 per cent fewer highly enhancing pixels on DCE-MRI compared to baseline. Most of the remaining enhancing pixels were in the tumor rim, a pattern consistent with the histological distribution of necrotic and viable tumor. The preservation of a viable rim of tumor is a common finding after treatment with vascular-disrupting agents. Lower doses of ZD6126 (12.5–25 mg kg^{-1}) reduced the IAUC close to zero within more restricted central areas of the tumor.

DCE-MRI studies with ZD6126 have also been performed in subcutaneous C38 colon xenografts (Evelhoch et al., 2004) 24h after doses of 50, 100 and 200 mg kg^{-1}. Median IAUC was decreased by 6–48 per cent at 50 mg kg^{-1}, 58–91 per cent at 100 mg kg^{-1} and 11–93 per cent at 200 mg kg^{-1}. This was again associated with an increase in necrotic fraction from around 40 per cent to greater than 90 per cent for the same dose range.

Goertz et al., used high-frequency Doppler ultrasound to image subcutaneous MeWo melanoma xenografts following treatment with ZD6126 (Goertz et al., 2002). Volumetric imaging detected a significant reduction in integrated power (IP), which represents functional vascular volume 4h after injection of ZD6126 followed by recovery 24h after injection. Measurements of tumor functional vascular volume using Hoechst 33342 staining correlated with the ultrasound results. At 4h there was 80–90 per cent reduction in IP and 70 per cent decrease in Hoechst staining.

Dimethylxanthenone-4-acetic acid (DMXAA) is a vascular disrupting agent that acts via local induction of tumor necrosis factor (TNF). Siim et al. compared the effects of DMXAA and CA4P on RIF-1 tumor-bearing mice using ^{99m}Tc-labeled HL-91 (Prognox) (Siim et al., 2000). The administration of DMXAA or CA4P resulted in a selective and statistically significant increase (3.5-fold and 3.0-fold, respectively) in tumor concentrations of Prognox. A DMXAA-induced inhibition of tumor blood flow was associated with a 2.0-fold or 3.1-fold increase in tumor uptake of Prognox for MDAH-MCa-4 or NZMN10 tumors, respectively. Comparison of anti-tumor activity measured by quantification of clonogenic cells in RIF-1 tumors with Prognox uptake 18h after treatment with DMXAA demonstrated a significant correlation at doses above 50 μmol kg^{-1}. Unfortunately, Prognox is not available for clinical studies.

In summary, imaging techniques have proved useful in the pre-clinical assessment of vascular-disrupting agents. It has been possible to determine dose–response relationships, but few studies have examined the exposure–response relationship or identified a target exposure threshold above which imaging parameter changes might be expected in clinical trials. Histological correlations have demonstrated that changes in DCE-MRI, MRS, FDG-PET and hypoxia imaging are correlated with histological changes, particularly with the induction of necrosis, and reinforced the pattern of increased effects in the central portion of tumors with preservation of a viable rim. Correlation with a measure of absolute blood flow has also helped to justify the use of DCE-MRI in clinical trials with vascular-disrupting drugs. Determination of the time course of response has been helpful when designing clinical trials. Only one study has examined imaging parameters potentially predictive of response to treatment with these agents, suggesting that tumors with high vascular permeability are more likely to respond.

16.10   Clinical experience of imaging vascular-disrupting agents

DMXAA was the first vascular-disrupting agent for which imaging effects were examined in clinical trials (Galbraith *et al.*, 2002b). The semi-quantitative parameters gradient, enhancement and IAUC were used, but there was no determination of initial T1, thus changes in tissue T1 could potentially bias the results. In the phase I trial 9 of 16 patients across a wide dose range had statistically significant reductions in IAUC 24 h after the first dose of DMXAA, and 8 of 11 patients had significant reductions of up to 66 per cent in IAUC 24 h after the last dose. Mean reductions in gradient, enhancement and IAUC were 25, 18 and 31 per cent respectively 24 h after the last dose, which were significantly greater than the 95 per cent limits of change for a group of 11 patients determined by assessment of the reproducibility from two baseline DCE-MRI assessments performed a few days apart (Galbraith *et al.*, 2002a). While there were significant mean reductions in enhancement and IAUC in muscle 24 h after the first dose, no significant changes were seen 24 h after the last dose.

In the phase I trial with CA4P dosed weekly, both DCE-MRI and O^{15}PET were used (Galbraith *et al.*, 2003; Anderson *et al.*, 2003). The results with both techniques measuring effects on tumor blood flow were broadly comparable. No significant change in K^{trans} was seen in those patients treated at doses up to $40 \, mg \, m^{-2}$, but 6 of 16 patients treated at $\geq 52 \, mg \, m^{-2}$ had significant reductions in K^{trans} at either 4 or 24 hours. The mean reduction in K^{trans} at well tolerated doses of $52–68 \, mg \, m^{-2}$ was 37 per cent at 4 h and 29 per cent at 24 h after the first dose. There was evidence for an exposure–response relationship with a significant correlation between the concentration of CA4 area under the curve derived from plasma pharmacokinetic studies with maximum relative reduction in K^{trans} after the first dose of CA4P, although the cohort size used was too small to allow direct comparisons of one dose level with another. Several patients' tumors demonstrated the same pattern of increased effect in the central portion of the tumor, with sparing of a peripheral rim, as has been well described in pre-clinical models. This pattern was not universal, however. Four of eight patients treated at $\geq 88 \, mg \, m^{-2}$ had an increase in the number of completely non-enhancing pixels. This is shown for one patient in Figure 16.2, where there is a marked increase in black (non-enhancing) pixels after treatment, from 20 per cent pre-treatment to 64 per cent at the end of treatment. There were no significant mean changes in muscle or kidney DCE-MRI parameters.

Pre treatment   4 hours post 1st dose   24 hours post 1st dose

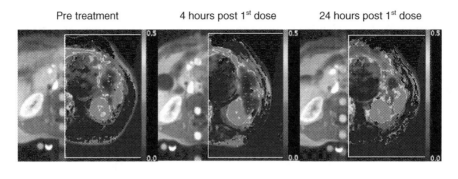

13 days post 3rd dose   13 days post 6th dose

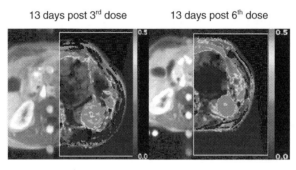

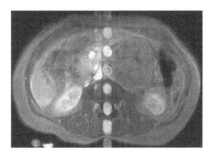

Figure 16.2 Serial K^{trans} parametric maps overlain on transverse T1-weighted images for a patient in the phase I trial of CA4P. Scale = K^{trans} ml ml^{-1} min^{-1}. Bottom, T2-weighted anatomical image. Note the increase in non-enhancing pixels by the end of treatment (A color reproduction of this figure can be seen in the color section)

PET data were obtained for 13 patients in this trial, imaging 30 min and 24 h after infusion of CA4P (Anderson *et al.*, 2003). Significant dose-dependent reductions were seen in tumor perfusion at the 30 min timepoint (mean change −49 per cent at >52 mg m^{-2}; $p = 0.001$). Significant reductions were also seen in tumor blood volume (mean change −15 per cent at >52 mg m^{-2}; $p = 0.007$).

Although by 24 h there was tumor vascular recovery, for doses >52 mg m^{-2} the reduction in perfusion remained significant ($p = 0.013$). Thirty minutes after CA4P administration borderline significant changes were seen in spleen perfusion (mean change −35 per cent; $p = 0.018$), spleen blood volume (mean change −18 per cent; $p = 0.022$), kidney perfusion (mean change −6 per cent; $p = 0.026$) and kidney blood volume (mean change −6 per cent; $p = 0.014$). No significant changes were seen at 24 h in spleen or kidney. The DCE-MRI data in both rats and patients suggested that at 4–6 h after administration of CA4P there was a relatively selective effect on tumor, with no significant reduction in mean kinetic parameters in muscle or kidney. In the PET study a significant mean reduction in cardiac output of nine per cent was seen at 30 min after treatment with CA4P, which coincided with a peak rise in blood pressure and fall in heart rate (Rustin et al., 2003), a pattern of changes also observed in pre-clinical models (Prise et al., 2002). At the time of the 4 h DCE-MRI examination, blood pressure was reduced and heart rate increased. The effects on cardiac output at the examination times in the PET and DCE-MRI studies may therefore be different. Indeed, there was no reduction in stroke volume seen in the PET study, suggesting that the observed changes in heart rate were reflected in the cardiac output changes.

Comparisons of the exposure–response relationship in pre-clinical and clinical studies for CA4P are of interest. The plasma exposure to the active agent, combretastatin-A4, in rats at 10 mg kg^{-1} was 3.76 μmol h l^{-1}. At this exposure a study with IAP observed a substantial blood flow reduction (92 per cent at 6 h) and histological changes including hemorrhage and the development of moderate central necrosis (Prise et al., 2002). This is comparable to the mean exposure achieved at 52–114 mg m^{-2} in patients (2–3.29 μmol h l^{-1}) (Rustin et al., 2003).

A reduction in the semi-quantitative parameter gradient was seen in six of seven patients at 60 mg m^{-2} in another phase I trial of CA4P (Dowlati et al., 2002), 4–6 h after CA4P administration. A third phase I trial used a different schedule of CA4P dosing – daily for 5 days, repeated every three weeks (Stevenson et al., 2003). Patients dosed at 52 mg m^{-2} and above also had DCE-MRI examinations at baseline and 6–8 hours after the fifth daily dose of CA4P. In 8 of 10 patients, there was at least a mild decrease in the K^{trans} value, with a mean decrease of 45 per cent; three patients demonstrated marked loss of vascularity after CA4P. Tumors with the largest baseline K^{trans} demonstrated the greatest drop in K^{trans} after CA4P ($r = -0.89$, $p = 0.001$). There was also a significant negative correlation between the change in K^{trans} and the day 5 exposure to CA4.

Similar effects have been observed with ZD6126 (Evelhoch et al., 2004). At doses of 80 mg m^{-2} and higher in patients, the median IAUC post-ZD6126 treatment was reduced to 36–72 per cent from the baseline value. As with CA4P, there was a significant correlation of change in IAUC with increasing exposure ($p < 0.01$). No drug-induced changes in muscle or spleen IAUC were observed. This study also examined the reproducibility of the technique, reporting within-patient coefficient of variation for IAUC in tumor of 18 per cent. Again, the pattern of increased effects in the central part of tumors was seen.

A preliminary report on a phase I trial with another combretastatin analog, AVE8062, mentioned that some evidence of decreases in DCE-MRI parameters was seen at $15.5 \, \mathrm{mg \, m^{-2}}$, but no details were given (Tolcher *et al.*, 2003).

16.11 Conclusions

The above studies demonstrate that imaging techniques have added to the information gained from early clinical trials with vascular disrupting agents. It has been possible to determine dose– and exposure–response relationships for the imaging effects, demonstrating biological activity even when the rates of tumor regression were very low. In addition, the exposure seen in patients at doses producing significant effects on DCE-MRI and $O^{15}PET$ corresponded with that seen in pre-clinical models at efficacious doses. The pattern seen pre-clinically of particularly marked blood flow reduction in the central portion of tumors and sparing of a viable rim has also been seen in some patients' tumors, and the time course of response in patients has been shown to be similar to that observed in pre-clinical models. Thus, although animal models of cancer are often criticized for not predicting clinical effects, in the case of vascular-disrupting agents the pre-clinical models have predicted many features that have been confirmed with clinical experience.

In general, there has also been evidence for greater effects on tumor microcirculation than on normal tissues, although there were minor changes observed in kidney and spleen perfusion. Detailed examination of cardiac perfusion effects have not been published, but this remains a concern, since there have been reports of patients experiencing cardiac ischemia following treatment with these agents. The pre-clinical observation that tumors with higher initial permeability are more susceptible to vascular-disrupting agents is also supported by the observation that those patients with the highest initial K^{trans} level have the greatest decrease post-treatment.

Questions that remain unanswered include determination of what level of change in imaging parameters is needed for anti-tumor efficacy. This might come from phase II trials, particularly when combinations of vascular-disrupting agents with other anti-cancer therapies are tested. Correlation with tumor shrinkage is not the optimal method for measuring anti-tumor efficacy for such agents, so studies designed to compare the imaging effects with time to tumor progression would be helpful.

Most clinical trials reported to date with DCE-MRI have used an assumed arterial input function. This may lead to systematic errors in the calculated values of kinetic parameters, as well as affecting the reproducibility of serial measurements within the same patient. In particular, the assumption that the arterial input function itself has not changed as a result of the treatment should ideally be tested, at least in pre-clinical models, but preferably in patients. Consideration also needs to be given to imaging tumors in regions such as the lungs and liver, which move significantly during respiration. This motion can invalidate kinetic parameter estimates particularly for pixel-by-pixel analyses. Navigator techniques have been described which register individual images in the sequence to the diaphragm (Taylor *et al.*, 2003). Alternatively, imaging in the non-axial plane reduces the motion and enables image registration prior to analysis (Noseworthy *et al.*, 2001).

Care should be taken about the method used for selecting a region of interest. Even for a high resolution methodology such as MRI, this is a key aspect that can significantly affect reproducibility of measurements. In different studies outlining of the whole tumor, choosing an ROI 'within the area of highest contrast agent uptake' or exclusion of 'necrotic' areas of tumor have been used. Since choosing an ROI within a region of high uptake is more likely to be affected by subjective decisions, this should be avoided. Preferably, one person should be responsible for ROI selection throughout a study, and inter- and intra-observer variability should be known or measured.

Rather than having a small number of patients with varying levels of change in the end-point, it is desirable to determine *a priori* quantitative criteria for the minimum change in the imaging end-point needed to have confidence that a real effect is being measured, of relevance to the drug's mechanism of action. To achieve this it is important both to understand the relationship of change in imaging end-point to antitumor efficacy from pre-clinical or prior clinical studies and to understand the reproducibility of the technique as used in the clinical trial. The multiplicity of imaging methods available, and the continual refinement of techniques, means that wherever possible clinical trials should incorporate two baseline measurements in order to document the reproducibility of the technique used in the trial. The published data on reproducibility illustrates that a cohort size of three patients is insufficient to discriminate clinically important differences in the imaging end-point. It therefore seems more logical to obtain the safety and pharmacokinetic information across cohorts of three as is standard practice in phase I and then to expand two or three cohorts at dose levels that are well tolerated to a size of 10–15 patients, depending on the chosen imaging methodology and effect size of interest. Selecting a single tumor type for this imaging phase will also be likely to improve the consistency of the response seen.

There are other practical implications of the above analysis. In order to accrue 30–45 patients for detailed imaging studies within an acceptable time period, multiple sites will be required. The imaging technology used has therefore to be reasonably widely available with the sites chosen having prior experience in its use. It is not always possible to combine datasets from imaging equipment made by different manufacturers, so this needs to be determined prior to site selection. It is clearly preferable that imaging data from all sites should be combined in one database, so sites need to be able to agree on a common imaging protocol and adhere to it. Quality assurance in as near real time as possible is important.

In conclusion, DCE-MRI has been the predominant imaging technique used to assess vascular-disrupting agents in clinical trials. The results have influenced decisions in early clinical development of these agents. In order to maximize their utility, clinical trial design needs to be adapted to accommodate such endpoints rather than using imaging as an 'optional' add-on to a standard design. Understanding of the relation between DCE-MRI effects and antitumor efficacy is a key challenge for the next clinical trials with these agents.

References

Aboagye, E.O., Maxwell, R.J., Kelson, A.B., Tracy, M., Lewis, A.D., Graham, M.A., Horsman, M.R., Griffiths, J.R. and Workman, P. (1997). Preclinical evaluation of the fluorinated 2-nitroimidazole N-(2-hydroxy-3,3,3-trifluoropropyl)- 2-(2-nitro-1-imidazolyl) acetamide (SR-4554) as a probe for the measurement of tumor hypoxia. *Cancer Res* 57, 3314–3318.

Albrecht, T., Blomley, M.J., Cosgrove, D.O., Taylor-Robinson, S.D., Jayaram, V., Eckersley, R., Urbank, A., Butler-Barnes, J. and Patel, N. (1999). Non-invasive diagnosis of hepatic cirrhosis by transit-time analysis of an ultrasound contrast agent. *Lancet* 353, 1579–1583.

Andersen, A. (1989). 99mTc-D,L-hexamethylene-propyleneamine oxime (99mTc-HMPAO): basic kinetic studies of a tracer of cerebral blood flow. *Cerebrovasc Brain Metab Rev* 1, 288–318.

Anderson, H.L., Yap, J.T., Miller, M.P., Robbins, A., Jones, T. and Price, P.M. (2003). Assessment of pharmacodynamic vascular response in a phase I trial of combretastatin A4 phosphate. *J Clin Oncol* 21, 2823–2830.

Archer, C.M., Edwards, B., Kelly, J.D., King, A.C., Burke, J.F. and Riley, A.L.M. (1994). Technetium labelled agents for imaging tissue hypoxia in vivo. In *Technetium and Rhenium in Chemistry and Nuclear Medicine*, M. Nicolini, G. Bandoli and U. Mazzi (eds). Proceedings 4th International Symposium on Technetium in Chemistry and Nuclear Medicine, Bressanone, Italy, pp. 535–539.

Barbier, E.L., Lamalle, L. and Decorps, M. (2001). Methodology of brain perfusion imaging. *J Magn Reson Imaging* 13, 496–520.

Barthel, H., Wilson, H., Collingridge, D.R., Brown, G., Osman, S., Luthra, S.K., Brady, F., Workman, P., Price, P.M. and Aboagye, E.O. (2004). In vivo evaluation of [18F]fluoroetanidazole as a new marker for imaging tumour hypoxia with positron emission tomography. *Br J Cancer* 90, 2232–2242.

Beaney, R.P., Lammertsma, A.A., Jones, T., McKenzie, C.G. and Halnan, K.E. (1984). Positron emission tomography for in-vivo measurement of regional blood flow, oxygen utilisation, and blood volume in patients with breast carcinoma. *Lancet* 1, 131–134.

Beauregard, D.A., Hill, S.A., Chaplin, D.J. and Brindle, K.M. (2001). The susceptibility of tumors to the antivascular drug combretastatin A4 phosphate correlates with vascular permeability. *Cancer Res* 61, 6811–6815.

Beauregard, D.A., Pedley, R.B., Hill, S.A. and Brindle, K.M. (2002). Differential sensitivity of two adenocarcinoma xenografts to the anti-vascular drugs combretastatin A4 phosphate and 5,6-dimethylxanthenone-4-acetic acid, assessed using MRI and MRS. *NMR Biomed* **15**, 99–105.

Beauregard, D.A., Thelwall, P.E., Chaplin, D.J., Hill, S.A., Adams, G.E. and Brindle, K.M. (1998). Magnetic resonance imaging and spectroscopy of combretastatin A4 prodrug-induced disruption of tumour perfusion and energetic status. *Br J Cancer* **77**, 1761–1767.

Belfi, C.A., Ting, L.L., Hassenbusch, S.J., Tefft, M. and Ngo, F.Q. (1992). Determination of changes in tumor blood perfusion after hydralazine treatment by dynamic paramagnetic-enhanced magnetic resonance imaging. *Int J Radiat Oncol Biol Phys* **22**, 477–482.

Blomley, M.J., Coulden, R., Bufkin, C., Lipton, M.J. and Dawson, P. (1993). Contrast bolus dynamic computed tomography for the measurement of solid organ perfusion. *Invest Radiol* **28** (Suppl. 5), S72–77.

Bonnerot, V., Charpentier, A., Frouin, F., Kalifa, C., Vanel, D. and Di Paola, R. (1992). Factor analysis of dynamic magnetic resonance imaging in predicting the response of osteosarcoma to chemotherapy. *Invest Radiol* **27**, 847–855.

Bruehlmeier, M., Roelcke, U., Schubiger, P.A. and Ametamey, S.M. (2004). Assessment of hypoxia and perfusion in human brain tumors using PET with 18F-fluoromisonidazole and 15O-H_2O. *J Nucl Med* **45**, 1851–1859.

Buckley, D.L. (2002). Uncertainty in the analysis of tracer kinetics using dynamic contrast-enhanced T(1)-weighted MRI. *Magn Reson Med* **47**, 601–606.

Chapman, J.D., Baer, K. and Lee, J. (1983). Characteristics of the metabolism induced binding of misonidazole to hypoxic mammalian cells. *Cancer Res* **43**, 1523–1528.

Dark, G.G., Hill, S.A., Prise, V.E., Tozer, G.M., Pettit, G.R. and Chaplin, D.J. (1997). Combretastatin A-4, an agent that displays potent and selective toxicity toward tumor vasculature. *Cancer Res* **57**, 1829–1834.

Dennie, J., Mandeville, J.B., Boxerman, J.L., Packard, S.D., Rosen, B.R. and Weisskoff, R.M. (1998). NMR imaging of changes in vascular morphology due to tumor angiogenesis. *Magn Reson Med* **40**, 793–799.

Dowlati, A., Robertson, K., Cooney, M., Petros, W.P., Stratford, M., Jesberger, J., Rafie, N., Overmoyer, B., Makkar, V., Stambler, B., Taylor, A., Waas, J., Lewin, J.S., McCrae, K.R. and Remick, S.C. (2002). A phase I pharmacokinetic and translational study of the novel vascular targeting agent combretastatin a-4 phosphate on a single-dose intravenous schedule in patients with advanced cancer. *Cancer Res* **62**, 3408–3416.

Eriksson, R., Persson, H.W., Dymling, S.O. and Lindstrom, K. (1991). Evaluation of Doppler ultrasound for blood perfusion measurements. *Ultrasound Med Biol* **17**, 445–452.

Evans, S.M., Hahn, S.M. and Magarelli, D.P. (2001). Hypoxic heterogeneity in human tumors: EF5 binding, vasculature, necrosis, and proliferation. *Am J Clin Oncol* **24**, 467–472.

Evelhoch, J.L. (1999). Key factors in the acquisition of contrast kinetic data for oncology. *J Magn Reson Imaging* **10**, 254–259.

Evelhoch, J.L., LoRusso, P.M., He, Z., DelProposto, Z., Polin, L., Corbett, T.H., Langmuir, P., Wheeler, C., Stone, A., Leadbetter, J., Ryan, A.J., Blakey, D.C. and Waterton, J.C. (2004). Magnetic resonance imaging measurements of the response of murine and human tumors to the vascular-targeting agent ZD6126. *Clin Cancer Res* **10**, 3650–3657.

Feldmann, H.J., Sievers, K., Füller, J., Molls, M. and Löhr, E. (1993). Evaluation of tumor blood perfusion by dynamic MRI and CT in patients undergoing thermoradiotherapy. *Eur J Radiol* **16**, 224–229.

Foster, F.S., Pavlin, C.J., Harasiewicz, K.A., Christopher, D.A. and Turnbull, D.H. (2000). Advances in ultrasound biomicroscopy. *Ultrasound Med Biol* **26**, 1–27.

Furman-Haran, E., Margalit, R., Grobgeld, D. and Degani, H. (1998). High resolution MRI of MCF7 human breast tumors: complemented use of iron oxide microspheres and Gd-DTPA. *J Magn Reson Imaging* **8**, 634–641.

Galbraith, S.M., Lodge, M.A., Taylor, N.J., Rustin, G.J., Bentzen, S., Stirling, J.J. and Padhani, A.R. (2002a). Reproducibility of dynamic contrast-enhanced MRI in human muscle and tumours: comparison of quantitative and semi quantitative analysis. *NMR Biomed* **15**, 132–142.

Galbraith, S.M., Maxwell, R.J., Lodge, M.A., Tozer, G.M., Wilson, J., Taylor, N.J., Stirling, J.J., Sena, L., Padhani, A.R. and Rustin, G.J. (2003). Combretastatin A4 phosphate has tumor antivascular activity in rat and man as demonstrated by dynamic magnetic resonance imaging. *J Clin Oncol* **21**, 2831–2842.

Galbraith, S.M., Rustin, G.J., Lodge, M.A., Taylor, N.J., Stirling, J.J., Jameson, M., Thompson, P., Hough, D., Gumbrell, L. and Padhani, A.R. (2002b). Effects of 5,6-dimethylxanthenone-4-acetic acid on human tumor microcirculation assessed by dynamic contrast-enhanced magnetic resonance imaging. *J Clin Oncol* **20**, 3826–3840.

Goertz, D.E., Yu, J.L., Kerbel, R.S., Burns, P.N. and Foster, F.S. (2002). High-frequency Doppler ultrasound monitors the effects of antivascular therapy on tumor blood flow. *Cancer Res* **62**, 6371–6375.

Hammersley, P., McCready, V., Babich, J. and Coghlan, G. (1987). 99mTc-HMPAO as a tumour blood flow agent. *Eur J Nucl Med* **13**, 90–94.

Hawighorst, H., Libicher, M., Knopp, M.V., Moehler, T., Kauffmann, G.W. and Gv, K. (1999). Evaluation of angiogenesis and perfusion of bone marrow lesions: role of semi-quantitative and quantitative dynamic MRI. *J Magn Reson Imaging* **10**, 286–294.

Hermans, R., Lambin, P., Van der Goten, A., Van den Bogaert, W., Verbist, B., Weltens, C. and Delaere, P.R. (1999). Tumoural perfusion as measured by dynamic computed tomography in head and neck carcinoma. *Radiother Oncol* **53**, 105–111.

Honess, D.J., Hill, S.A., Collingridge, D.R., Edwards, B., Brauers, G., Powell, N.A. and Chaplin, D.J. (1998). Preclinical evaluation of the novel hypoxic marker 99mTc- HL91 (Prognox) in murine and xenograft systems in vivo. *Int J Radiat Oncol Biol Phys* **42**, 731–735.

Kanthou, C., Prise, V.E., Milson, J. and Tozer, G.M. (2001). The vascular targeting agent combretastatin A4 phosphate alters the andothelial cell actin cytoskeleton and mediates changes in vascular permeability in vitro and in vivo. *Proc Am Assoc Cancer Res*, New Orleans.

Kedar, R., Cosgrove, D., Smith, I., Mansi, J. and Bamber, J. (1994). Breast carcinoma: measurement of tumor response to primary medical therapy with color Doppler flow imaging. *Radiology* **190**, 825–830.

Kety, S. (1949). Measurement of regional circulation by the local clearance of radioactive sodium. *Am Heart J* **38**, 321.

Kety, S. (1960a). Blood–tissue exchange methods. Theory of blood–tissue exchange and its application to measurement of blood flow. *Meth Med Res* **8**, 223–227.

Kety, S. (1960b). Measurement of local blood flow by the exchange of an inert, diffusible substance. *Meth Med Res* **8**, 228–236.

Kety, S. and Schmidt, C. (1948). Nitrous oxide method for quantitative determination of cerebral blood flow in man: theory, procedure and normal values. *J Clin Invest* **27**, 476.

Knopp, E.A., Cha, S., Johnson, G., Mazumdar, A., Golfinos, J.G., Zagzag, D., Miller, D.C., Kelly, P.J. and Kricheff, I.I. (1999). Glial neoplasms: dynamic contrast-enhanced T2*-weighted MR imaging. *Radiology* **211**, 791–798.

Koch, C.J. and Evans, S.M. (2003). Non-invasive PET and SPECT imaging of tissue hypoxia using isotopically labeled 2-nitroimidazoles. *Adv Exp Med Biol* **510**, 285–292.

Koch, C.J., Evans, S.M. and Lord, E.M. (1995). Oxygen dependence of cellular uptake of EF5 [2-(2-nitro-1H-imidazol-1-yl)-N-(2,2,3,3,3-pentafluoropropyl) acetamide]: analysis of drug adducts by fluorescent antibodies vs. bound radioactivity. *Br J Cancer* **72**, 869–874.

Koh, W.J., Rasey, J.S., Evans, M.L., Grierson, J.R., Lewellen, T.K., Graham, M.M., Krohn, K.A. and Griffin, T.W. (1992). Imaging of hypoxia in human tumors with [F-18]fluoromisonidazole. *Int J Radiat Oncol Biol Phys* **22** (1), 199–212.

Kwock, L., Gill, M., McMurry, H.L., Beckman, W., Raleigh, J.A. and Joseph, A.P. (1992). Evaluation of a fluorinated 2-nitroimidazole binding to hypoxic cells in tumor-bearing rats by 19F magnetic resonance spectroscopy and immunohistochemistry. *Radiat Res* **129**, 71–78.

Lammertsma, A.A. and Jones, T. (1992). Low oxygen extraction fraction in tumours measured with the oxygen-15 steady state technique: effect of tissue heterogeneity. *Br J Radiol* **65**, 697–700.

MacManus, M.P., Hicks, R.J., Ball, D.L., Kalff, V., Matthews, J.P., Salminen, E., Khaw, P., Wirth, A., Rischin, D. and McKenzie, A. (2001). F-18 fluorodeoxyglucose positron emission tomography staging in radical radiotherapy candidates with nonsmall cell lung carcinoma: powerful correlation with survival and high impact on treatment. *Cancer* **92**, 886–895.

Martinoli, C., Pretolesi, F., Crespi, G., Bianchi, S., Gandolfo, N., Valle, M. and Derchi, L.E. (1998). Power Doppler sonography: clinical applications. *Eur J Radiol* **27** (Suppl. 2), S133–140.

Mantyla, M., Heikkonen, J. and Perkkio, J. (1988). Regional blood flow in human tumours measured with argon, krypton and xenon. *Br J Radiol* **61**, 379–382.

Maxwell, R.J., Wilson, J., Prise, V.E., Vojnovic, B., Rustin, G.J., Lodge, M.A. and Tozer, G.M. (2002). Evaluation of the anti-vascular effects of combretastatin in rodent tumours by dynamic contrast enhanced MRI. *NMR Biomed* **15**, 89–98.

Mayr, N.A., Yuh, W.T., Magnotta, V.A., Ehrhardt, J.C., Wheeler, J.A., Sorosky, J.I., Davis, C.S., Wen, B.C., Martin, D.D., Pelsang, R.E., Buller, R.E., Oberley, L.W., Mellenberg, D.E. and Hussey, D.H. (1996). Tumor perfusion studies using fast magnetic resonance imaging technique in advanced cervical cancer: a new noninvasive predictive assay. *Int J Radiat Oncol Biol Phys* **36**, 623–633.

McIntyre, D.J., Robinson, S.P., Howe, F.A., Griffiths, J.R., Ryan, A.J., Blakey, D.C., Peers, I.S. and Waterton, J.C. (2004). Single dose of the antivascular agent, ZD6126 (N-acetyl-colchinol-O-phosphate), reduces perfusion for at least 96 hours in the GH3 prolactinoma rat tumor model. *Neoplasia* **6**, 150–157.

Noseworthy, M.D., Sussman, M.S., Haider, M. and Baruchel, S. (2001). Dynamic contrast enhanced liver MRI using a motion tracking algorithm. *Proc Int Soc Magn Reson Med* Glasgow, p. 2240.

Ostergaard, L., Sorensen, A.G., Kwong, K.K., Weisskoff, R.M., Gyldensted, C. and Rosen, B.R. (1996a). High resolution measurement of cerebral blood flow using intravascular tracer bolus passages. Part II: Experimental comparison and preliminary results. *Magn Reson Med* **36**, 726–736.

Ostergaard, L., Weisskoff, R.M., Chesler, D.A., Gyldensted, C. and Rosen, B.R. (1996b). High resolution measurement of cerebral blood flow using intravascular tracer bolus passages. Part I: Mathematical approach and statistical analysis. *Magn Reson Med* **36**, 715–725.

Ostergaard, M., Stoltenberg, M., Lovgreen-Nielsen, P., Volck, B., Sonne-Holm, S. and Lorenzen, I. (1998). Quantification of synovitis by MRI: correlation between dynamic and static gadolinium-enhanced magnetic resonance imaging and microscopic and macroscopic signs of synovial inflammation. *Magn Reson Imaging* **16**, 743–754.

Pardo, F.S., Aronen, H.J., Fitzek, M., Kennedy, D.N., Efird, J., Rosen, B.R. and Fischman, A.J. (2004). Correlation of FDG-PET interpretation with survival in a cohort of glioma patients. *Anticancer Res* **24**, 2359–2365.

Parker, G.J., Suckling, J., Tanner, S.F., Padhani, A.R., Revell, P.B., Husband, J.E. and Leach, M.O. (1997). Probing tumor microvascularity by measurement, analysis and display of contrast agent uptake kinetics. *J Magn Reson Imaging* **7**, 564–574.

Peters-Engl, C., Medl, M., Mirau, M., Wanner, C., Bilgi, S., Sevelda, P. and Obermair, A. (1998). Color-coded and spectral Doppler flow in breast carcinomas – relationship with the tumor microvasculature. *Breast Cancer Res Treat* **47**, 83–89.

Piert, M., Machulla, H.J., Picchio, M., Reischl, G., Ziegler, S., Kumar, P., Wester, H.J., Beck, R., McEwan, A.J., Wiebe, L.I. and Schwaiger, M. (2005). Hypoxia-specific tumor imaging with 18F-fluoroazomycin arabinoside. *J Nucl Med* **46**, 106–113.

Prise, V.E., Honess, D.J., Stratford, M.R., Wilson, J. and Tozer, G.M. (2002). The vascular response of tumor and normal tissues in the rat to the vascular targeting agent, combretastatin A-4-phosphate, at clinically relevant doses. *Int J Oncol* **21**, 717–726.

Rajendran, J.G., Mankoff, D.A., O'Sullivan, F., Peterson, L.M., Schwartz, D.L., Conrad, E.U., Spence, A.M., Muzi, M., Farwell, D.G. and Krohn, K.A. (2004). Hypoxia and glucose metabolism in malignant tumors: evaluation by [18F]fluoromisonidazole and [18F]fluorodeoxyglucose positron emission tomography imaging. *Clin Cancer Res* **10**, 2245–2252.

Renkin, E. (1959). Transport of potassium-42 from blood to tissue in isolated mammalian skeletal muscles. *Am J Physiol* **197**, 1205–1210.

Rijpkema, M., Kaanders, J.H., Joosten, F.B., van der Kogel, A.J. and Heerschap, A. (2001). Method for quantitative mapping of dynamic MRI contrast agent uptake in human tumors. *J Magn Reson Imaging* **14**, 457–463.

Robinson, S.P., Howe, F.A. and Griffiths, J.R. (1995). Noninvasive monitoring of carbogen-induced changes in tumor blood flow and oxygenation by functional magnetic resonance imaging. *Int J Radiat Oncol Biol Phys* **33**, 855–859.

Robinson, S.P., McIntyre, D.J., Checkley, D., Tessier, J.J., Howe, F.A., Griffiths, J.R., Ashton, S.E., Ryan, A.J., Blakey, D.C. and Waterton, J.C. (2003). Tumour dose response to the antivascular agent ZD6126 assessed by magnetic resonance imaging. *Br J Cancer* **88**, 1592–1597.

Rosen, B.R., Belliveau, J.W., Vevea, J.M. and Brady, T.J. (1990). Perfusion imaging with NMR contrast agents. *Magn Reson Med* **14**, 249–265.

Rowell, N., Flower, M., Cronin, B. and McCready, V. (1993). Quantitative single-photon emission tomography for tumour blood flow measurement in bronchial carcinoma. *Eur J Nucl Med* **20**, 591–599.

Rustin, G.J., Galbraith, S.M., Anderson, H., Stratford, M., Folkes, L.K., Sena, L., Gumbrell, L. and Price, P.M. (2003). Phase I clinical trial of weekly combretastatin A4 phosphate: clinical and pharmacokinetic results. *J Clin Oncol* **21**, 2815–2822.

Salmon, H.W. and Siemann, D.W. (2004). Utility of (19)F MRS detection of the hypoxic cell marker EF5 to assess cellular hypoxia in solid tumors. *Radiother Oncol* **73**, 359–366.

Seddon, B.M. and Workman, P. (2003). The role of functional and molecular imaging in cancer drug discovery and development. *Br J Radiol* **76** (Spec No. 2), S128–138.

Siim, B.G., Laux, W.T., Rutland, M.D., Palmer, B.N. and Wilson, W.R. (2000). Scintigraphic imaging of the hypoxia marker (99m)technetium-labeled 2,2'-(1,4-diaminobutane)bis(2-methyl-3-butanone) dioxime (99mTc-labeled HL-91; Prognox): noninvasive detection of tumor response to the antivascular agent 5,6 dimethylxanthenone-4-acetic acid. *Cancer Res* **60**, 4582–4588.

Sorensen, A.G., Tievsky, A.L., Ostergaard, L., Weisskoff, R.M. and Rosen, B.R. (1997). Contrast agents in functional MR imaging. *J Magn Reson Imaging* **7**, 47–55.

Stevenson, J.P., Rosen, M., Sun, W., Gallagher, M., Haller, D.G., Vaughn, D., Giantonio, B., Zimmer, R., Petros, W.P., Stratford, M., Chaplin, D., Young, S.L., Schnall, M. and O'Dwyer, P.J. (2003). Phase I trial of the antivascular agent combretastatin A4 phosphate on a 5-day schedule to patients with cancer: magnetic resonance imaging evidence for altered tumor blood flow. *J Clin Oncol* 21, 4428–4438.

Stewart, J. (1894). Researches on the circulation time in organs and on the influences which affect it. Parts I–III. *J Physiol* 15, 1.

Strich, G., Hagan, P.L., Gerber, K.H. and Slutsky, R.A. (1985). Tissue distribution and magnetic resonance spin lattice relaxation effects of gadolinium-DTPA. *Radiology* 154, 723–726.

Su, M.Y., Mühler, A., Lao, X. and Nalcioglu, O. (1998). Tumor characterization with dynamic contrast-enhanced MRI using MR contrast agents of various molecular weights. *Magn Reson Med* 39, 259–269.

Tatsumi, M., Yutani, K., Kusuoka, H. and Nishimura, T. (1999). Technetium-99m HL91 uptake as a tumour hypoxia marker: relationship to tumour blood flow. *Eur J Nucl Med* 26, 91–94.

Taylor, N.J., Lankester, K.J., Stirling, J.J., *et al.* (2003). Application of navigator techniques to breath-hold DCE-MRI studies of the liver. *Proc Int Soc Magn Reson Med*, Toronto, p. 1306.

Tofts, P., Brix, G., Buckley, D., Evelhoch, J., Henderson, E., Knopp, M., Larsson, H., Lee, T., Mayr, N., Parker, G., Port, R., Taylor, J. and Weisskoff, R. (1999). Estimating kinetic parameters from dynamic contrast-enhanced T(1)-weighted MRI of a diffusable tracer: standardized quantities and symbols. *J Magn Reson Imaging* 10, 223–232.

Tolcher, A.W., Forero, L., Celio, P., Hammond, L.A., Patnaik, A., Hill, M., Verat-Follet, C., Haacke, M., Besenval, M. and Rowinsky, E.K. (2003). Phase I, pharmacokinetic, and DCE-MRI correlative study of AVE8062A, an antivascular combretastatin analogue, administered weekly for 3 weeks every 28-days. *Proc Am Soc Clin Oncol* 22, 208 (abstract 834).

Tozer, G.M., Prise, V.E., Wilson, J., Locke, R.J., Vojnovic, B. and Stratford, M.R. (1999). Combretastatin A-4 phosphate as a tumor vascular-targeting agent: early effects in tumors and normal tissues. *Cancer Res* 59, 1626–1634.

Tozer, G.M., Shaffi, K.M., Prise, V.E. and Cunningham, V.J. (1994). Characterisation of tumour blood flow using a 'tissue-isolated' preparation. *Br J Cancer* 70, 1040–1046.

Tweedle, M., Wedeking, P., Telser, J., Sotak, C., Chang, C., Kumar, K., Wan, X. and Eaton, S. (1991). Dependence of MR signal intensity on Gd tissue concentration over a broad dose range. *Magn Reson Med* 22, 191–194.

van der Woude, H.J., Bloem, J.L., van Oostayen, J.A., Nooy, M.A., Taminiau, A.H., Hermans, J., Reynierse, M. and Hogendoorn, P.C. (1995). Treatment of high-grade bone sarcomas with neoadjuvant chemotherapy: the utility of sequential color Doppler sonography in predicting histopathologic response. *Am J Roentgenol* 165, 125–133.

Vansteenkiste, J.F., Stroobants, S.G., De Leyn, P.R., Dupont, P.J. and Verbeken, E.K. (1998). Potential use of FDG-PET scan after induction chemotherapy in surgically staged IIIa-N2 non-small-cell lung cancer: a prospective pilot study. *Ann Oncol* 9, 1193–1198.

Warburg, O., Posener, K. and Negelein, E. (1924). Uber den stoffwechsel der carcinomzelle. *Biochem Zeitschrift* 152, 309–335.

Young, H., Baum, R., Cremerius, U., Herholz, K., Hoekstra, O., Lammertsma, A.A., Pruim, J. and Price, P. (1999). *Measurement of Clinical and Subclinical Tumour Response Using [18F]-Fluorodeoxyglucose and Positron Emission Tomography: Review and 1999 EORTC Recommendations*. European Organization for Research and Treatment of Cancer (EORTC) PET Study Group.

Zhang, X., Melo, T., Ballinger, J.R. and Rauth, A.M. (1998). Studies of 99mTc-BnAO (HL-91): a non nitroaromatic compound for hypoxic cell detection. *Int J Radiat Oncol Biol Phys* **42**, 737–740.

Zhao, S., Moore, J.V., Waller, M.L., McGown, A.T., Hadfield, J.A., Pettit, G.R. and Hastings, D.L. (1999). Positron emission tomography of murine liver metastases and the effects of treatment by combretastatin A-4. *Eur J Nucl Med* **26**, 231–238.

17

Clinical Progress in Tumor Vasculature-disrupting Therapies

Andrew M. Gaya and **Gordon J. S. Rustin**

Abstract

There are two types of VDA. Biological, or ligand-directed VDAs use antibodies, peptides or growth factors to target toxins or pro-coagulants to the tumour endothelium. To date, small molecule VDAs work either as tubulin binding agents or through induction of local cytokine production. VDAs can potentially kill tumour cells resistant to conventional chemotherapy and radiotherapy, and work best on cells in the poorly perfused hypoxic core of tumours, leaving a viable rim of well-perfused tumour tissue at the periphery, which rapidly regrows. Consequently, responses of tumours to VDAs given as single agents have been poor, however combination therapy with cytotoxic chemotherapy, external beam radiotherapy, and radioimmunotherapy, which target the peripheral tumour cells, have produced some excellent responses in animal tumours. VDAs are generally well tolerated with different side effect profiles to current oncological therapies. Dynamic MRI is most frequently used to obtain a pharmacodynamic endpoint to determine whether the VDA is acting on its intended target.

Keywords

combretastatin A4 phosphate, phase 1 trial

17.1 Introduction

The genetic heterogeneity of advanced tumors leads to resistance against conventional anticancer therapies through the acquisition of drug resistant phenotypes. Novel approaches using 'targeted therapies' to cancer cells and the tumor

---

Vascular-targeted Therapies in Oncology   Edited by Dietmar W. Siemann
© 2006 John Wiley & Sons, Ltd.

microenvironment are therefore becoming important additions to the oncologists' arsenal.

One such strategy focuses on agents that selectively block or destroy the established blood vessels of tumors, leading to rapid shutdown of the tumor's blood supply, thereby killing tumor cells by depriving them of oxygen and nutrients. Vascular-disrupting agents (VDAs) exploit the known differences between the vascular endothelium and basement membranes of tumors and normal tissues (Chapters 1 and 2).

Two classes of VDA are being developed: the biological or ligand-directed VDAs, which use antibodies or peptides to target toxins or pro-coagulants to the tumor endothelium (Chapters 10–14), and the small-molecule VDAs (Chapters 1, 4–9, which exploit the differences between normal and tumor endothelium to induce vascular shutdown of tumor blood vessels. Both types of VDA produce a characteristic pattern of central necrosis, leaving a peripheral rim of viable tumor cells (Huang *et al.*, 1997; Ching *et al.*, 1999; Blakey *et al.*, 2002b; Tozer *et al.*, 2002; Thorpe *et al.*, 2003; Siemann Chuplin and Horseman, 2004).

17.2 Potential clinical advantages of vascular-disrupting agents

There are a number of potential advantages of VDAs over other classes of anticancer drug. There can be a significant bystander effect as one single blood vessel may provide oxygen and nutrients for thousands of tumor cells. Blockage or destruction of this solitary vessel may then result in thousands of downstream cell deaths. The endothelial cell itself does not need to be killed by the VDA – a change of structure or local initiation of the coagulation cascade may be all that is needed. As the endothelium comprises normal untransformed cells, it is unlikely to become drug resistant by genetic alteration (Boehm *et al.*, 1997). However, it has already been shown that some tumors can form luminal blood vessels lined with tumor cells and devoid of endothelium entirely (Maniotis *et al.*, 1999; Folberg *et al.*, 2000; McDonald *et al.*, 2000; Griggs *et al.*, 2001b). Another advantage of VDAs is that there are surrogate markers for their activity – for example local tumor blood flow, which can be measured by non-invasive techniques such as gadolinium dynamic contrast enhanced magnetic resonance imaging (Gd-DCE-MRI), positron emission tomography using ^{15}O-PET, dynamic perfusion CT and three-dimensional micro-bubble ultrasound (Chapter 16).

17.3 Biological (ligand-directed) VDAs

This class of VDA uses a targeting molecule such as an antibody or growth factor that selectively tracks to tumor endothelium.

The result may be thrombosis within tumor vasculature caused by direct injury or apoptosis, initiation of an immune attack on the tumor vasculature, or a change of conformation of the tumor endothelium, which leads to occlusion of the tumor vessels. Phase I clinical trials of these agents in humans are imminent. Further detailed information on these agents can be found in Chapters 10–14.

17.4 Small-molecule VDAs

Flavonoids

Flavone acetic acid (FAA) was originally synthesized as a non-steroidal anti-inflammatory agent, but was found to have widespread anticancer effects in preclinical studies (Smith *et al.*, 1987), inducing hemorrhagic necrosis within animal tumors (Corbett *et al.*, 1986). Unfortunately, it was inactive in human clinical trials (Kerr and Kaye, 1989). DMXAA (5,6-dimethylxanthenone-4-acetic acid) was developed as a more potent and active analogue (Rewcastle *et al.*, 1991), and has shown marked antivascular effects in a wide range of preclinical tumor models (Chapter 9).

Two DMXAA phase I trials in patients with advanced cancer were conducted in parallel by Cancer Research UK in New Zealand and the UK (Jameson *et al.*, 2003; Rustin *et al.*, 2003). In the UK study 46 patients received 247 20-minute weekly infusions of DMXAA over 15 dose levels ranging from 6 to 4900 mg m^{-2}. In New Zealand, 63 patients received DMXAA every 3 weeks, also as a 20-minute infusion. Reversible dose limiting toxicities at 4900 mg m^{-2} were neurological – tremor, anxiety, visual disturbance, urinary incontinence and expressive dysphasia. There was also an episode of left ventricular failure in one patient. The drug was otherwise well tolerated; the most frequent side-effects were visual disturbance, tumor pain, nausea, vomiting, headache, change in blood pressure and malaise. There was no significant hematological toxicity. Maximum tolerated dose was 3700 mg m^{-2}.

One brief partial response was seen in a patient with metastatic melanoma at 1300 mg m^{-2} in the UK. In New Zealand, a patient with metastatic cervical carcinoma also achieved a brief partial response at 1100 mg m^{-2}. Pharmacokinetics were non-linear due to saturation of protein binding at higher doses (Jameson *et al.*, 2000). Terminal elimination half-life was 8.1 ± 4.3 h. At doses of DMXAA ranging from 500 to 4900 mg m^{-2}, evidence of reduction in tumor blood flow was seen with DCE-MRI (Galbraith *et al.*, 2002). There was also a dose-dependent increase in the plasma concentration of 5-hydoxy indole acetic acid (5HIAA), which is the measurable metabolite of 5HT, at DMXAA dose levels of 650 mg m^{-2} and above, which correlated with the MRI findings. There were no consistent dose-dependent increases in plasma nitrate or TNFα; however, the finding of elevated TNF in tumor biopsies suggests that DMXAA actions are predominantly local (M. Jameson, personal communication, 2003).

It is too early to know whether there is sufficient local TNF induction after tolerable doses of DMXAA to induce tumor regression in humans when given alone. The way forward is to try combination therapy with DMXAA and cytotoxic agents, other vascular targeting agents or immunomodulatory agents (Cliffe *et al.*, 1994; Pruijn *et al.*, 1997; Lash *et al.*, 1998; Wilson *et al.*, 1998). In particular, Pedley *et al.* (1996, 1999) have demonstrated cure of human colorectal tumor xenografts in mice treated with a combination of DMXAA and radioimmunotherapy at a dose of DMXAA that produced no growth delay as a single agent. Antisoma, which now holds the license for DMXAA, is planning combination phase II trials once the dose with both acceptable toxicity and reliable reduction in dynamic MRI parameters has been ascertained.

Some toxicity observed with DMXAA resembles the 'serotonin syndrome', attributed to high levels of serotonin in the CNS. There is some evidence that DMXAA increases CNS serotonin release (Jameson *et al.*, 2003).

The visual toxicities of DMXAA such as blurring, color disturbance and photophobia are thought to be due to inhibition of phosphodiesterase type 6 (PDE6), which exists exclusively in the retina. DMXAA has been shown to inhibit this enzyme *in vitro* at therapeutic concentrations (Jameson *et al.*, 2003). In the UK study, all patients receiving $\geq 1750\,\mathrm{mg\,m^{-2}}$ experienced some disturbance of color vision (usually mild) following infusion.

Tubulin-binding agents

These agents work by acting near the colchicine binding site of the β subunit of endothelial cell tubulin, resulting in depolymerization of microtubules and disorganization of actin and tubulin. Endothelial cells are particularly reliant on the cellular cytoskeleton to maintain their shape. A rapid change in endothelial cell shape (Galbraith *et al.*, 2001) causes micro-vessel blockage and loss of flow; it also disrupts the endothelial cell layer, exposing the basement membrane and increasing tumor vascular permeability. This leads to high interstitial pressures, vessel congestion and further loss of flow. Exposure of the basement membrane may also lead to induction of the coagulation cascade and local thrombus formation. Newly formed endothelial cells in tumor vessels are more sensitive to anti tubulin drugs because mature cells have a highly developed actin cytoskeleton, which maintains cell shape despite depolymerization of the tubulin cytoskeleton (Chaplin and Dougherty, 1999).

Based on strong preclinical evidence of selective tumor blood vessel activity and significant antitumor activity in a broad range of human xenografts and rodent models (Chaplin and Petit, 1999; Siemann, Chaplin and Horsman, 2004; Blakey *et al.*, 2002a, 2002b; Davis *et al.*, 2002; Hori and Saito, 2003), lead tubulin-targeting VDAs (CA4P, ZD6126 and AVE8062A) have entered clinical trial evaluation.

Combretastatin A4

Three phase I trials of CA4P in humans investigated three different dose schedules (Dowlati *et al.*, 2002): Case Western Reserve University, Cleveland, OH (CWRU), the University of Pennsylvania, Philadelphia, PA (UPENN) and London (UK) at The Mount Vernon and Hammersmith Hospitals. A small, unpublished study was also carried out by Bristol Myers Squibb (Table 17.1). The UK trial (Anderson *et al.*, 2003; Galbraith *et al.*, 2003; Rustin *et al.*, 2003) used a 10 min weekly infusion of CA4P for three weeks every 28 days, starting at 5 mg m^{-2}, with intra-patient dose escalation and accelerated titration (Simon *et al.*, 1997). Doses were doubled until grade 2 toxicity was seen, after which subsequent

Table 17.1 Phase I trials of CA4P

	UK CRC PH1/066 (Rustin *et al.*, 2003)	UPENN CA4P-102 (Stevenson *et al.*, 2003)	CWRU CA4P-101 (Dowlati *et al.*, 2002)	BMS CA178-002
Schedule	Weekly × 3 every 28 days	Daily × 5 every 21 days	Single dose every 21 days	Initially a single dose every 21 days then changed to weekly × 3 every 28 days
Infusion time	10 min	10 min	10 min 60 min in 7 pts at 54 mg m^{-2}	10 min
Number pts	34	37	25	18
CA4P dose range	5–114 mg m^{-2}	6–75 mg m^{-2}	18–90 mg m^{-2}	30–70 mg m^{-2}
DCE-MRI	Yes	Yes	Yes	No
PET	Yes	No	No	Yes
MTD	68 mg m^{-2}	75 mg m^{-2}	60 mg m^{-2}	70 mg m^{-2}
DLT	Ataxia Motor neuropathy Syncope Diplopia Tumor pain Dyspnea	Tumor pain Sensorimotor neuropathy Syncope Dyspnea	Cardiac ischemia Dyspnea	Tumor pain Cardiac ischemia
RP2D	52–68 mg m^{-2}	52 mg m^{-2}	"60 mg m^{-2}	–
No. doses of CA4P given	167	700	104	–
Terminal half-life CA4P (h)	0.489	0.36	0.47	–
Terminal half-life CA4 (h)	2.23	3.3	4.26	–

dose escalation was by a factor of 1.3. Thirty-four patients with advanced solid tumors received 167 infusions. The MTD was 68 mg m^{-2} and the recommended phase II dose was 52–68 mg m^{-2}. The University of Pennsylvania trial (Stevenson *et al.*, 2003), the most dose intense of the phase I trials, used a 10 min infusion daily for five days every three weeks. Thirty-seven patients with advanced solid tumors received 133 cycles at doses ranging from 6 to 75 mg m^{-2}. All patients were assessable for toxicity. The MTD was 65 mg m^{-2} and recommended phase II dose was 52 mg m^{-2}. The CWRU trial (Dowlati *et al.*, 2002) used a single-dose schedule of CA4P every 21 days using doses up to 90 mg m^{-2} in a variety of advanced solid tumors. Both 10 min and 60 min infusion schedules were investigated. Twenty-five patients received 107 cycles of treatment (dose ranges 18–90 mg m^{-2}). The MTD was 60 mg m^{-2}. Bristol Myers Squibb also conducted a small, unpublished phase I study, initially with single doses of CA4P, 30–70 mg m^{-2}, every 21 days, in 18 patients.

CA4P pharmacokinetics (PK)

Pharmacokinetics of CA4P was assessed from plasma and urine for all patients in the three phase I trials. Plasma was analysed for CA4, CA4P and the metabolite CA4 glucuronide (CA4G) using a high-performance liquid chromatography and fluorescence detection method. Urine was analysed for CA4G. PK data was estimated using non-compartmental methods. PK data from all three trials was in agreement that plasma AUC and plasma C_{max} of CA4P and CA4 have dose-proportional linear kinetics. There was rapid dephosphorylation of CA4P to CA4 and rapid glucuronidation of CA4. There was no evidence of accumulation of CA4P over time with repeated doses. Linear kinetics was also seen in the terminal half-life and systemic clearance of CA4P across all dose levels in all studies. 58–67 per cent of the dose was excreted as CA4G in the first 24 h of urine collection. The mean plasma half-life ($t_{1/2}$) across the three trials for CA4P, CA4 and CA4G was 0.4, 3.8 and 4.5 h respectively. Volume of distribution ranged from 3.8 to 7.5 l, and clearance ranged from 24.5 to 28.2 l h^{-1}. C_{max} (µM) of CA4P ranged from 4.9 at 6 mg m^{-2} to 48.7 at 114 mg m^{-2}. Corresponding AUC values (µM h^{-1}) for CA4P were 1.31 and 11.6 respectively. CA4 C_{max} ranged from 0.31 at 6 mg m^{-2} to 4.2 at 114 mg m^{-2} with corresponding AUC values of 0.24 and 2.49 respectively.

CA4P safety profile/toxicity (non-dose-limiting)

Across all three studies, adverse events were generally mild and manageable, and very different from the usual cytotoxic effects of alopecia, myelosuppression, nausea and mucositis. No significant hematological toxicity was seen in any of the studies. Cardiotoxicity was reported in one study (discussed below).

In the UK study the only drug-related toxicity seen up to $40\,mg\,m^{-2}$ was grade 1 tumor pain in 35 per cent of infusions. It is not clear whether this pain relates to tumor ischemia or to acute swelling of the tumor caused by alteration in endothelial cell permeability after CA4P. The most common site of pain was in the abdomen, which was the most frequent site of tumors. It is not possible to exclude mesenteric angina as a possible cause of pain in some patients. Median time to onset of tumor pain was 40 min from the start of the CA4P infusion (range 2 min–10 h, duration 1–180 min). Other side-effects noted were mainly cardiovascular–tachycardia (53 per cent), hypertension (35 per cent), hypotension (30 per cent), bradycardia (24 per cent), fatigue (23 per cent), nausea (21 per cent), visual disturbance (nine per cent) and dyspnoea (six per cent).

Mean increase in blood pressure at doses $\geq 52\,mg\,m^{-2}$ was 8–10 per cent over the first hour followed by a mean decrease in blood pressure of six to seven per cent, most obvious at 4 h. Microtubule depolymerization is known to affect vasomotor tone and total peripheral resistance – the changes in heart rate and BP probably reflect this.

Toxicity in the UPENN and CWRU studies was very similar to the UK experience. Tumour pain did not appear to correlate with either clinical response or DCE-MRI parameters, and appeared more common following the 60 min infusion schedule.

Gastrointestinal side-effects were considered to be the DLT in animals. Whilst GI side-effects were common in the human phase I trials (diarrhea, nausea, vomiting, abdominal pain), they were usually mild (grade 1 or 2). A wide range of neurological effects was seen in the phase I studies, mainly at the higher doses. Effects such as perineal and perirectal paresthesia, peripheral neuropathy, visual blurring, diplopia, ataxia and leg weakness were seen; they were transient, mild and fully reversible at lower doses, becoming more severe at higher doses (see DLTs below).

CA4P dose-limiting toxicity (DLT)

In the UK study, four DLTs were reported. The first was a grade 3 vasovagal episode that occurred on the patient's second dose ($88\,mg\,m^{-2}$). This began 4½ hours following CA4P and lasted three minutes. The patient recovered fully with supportive treatment. It is possible that an early swelling of this patient's neck mass might have contributed to the vasovagal episode by pressing on the carotid body. There were two cases of transient and reversible grade 2 ataxia at $114\,mg\,m^{-2}$. Upon reducing the dose back to $88\,mg\,m^{-2}$ there was an episode of reversible grade 4 ataxia, grade 3 double vision and grade 3 leg weakness in one of the patients who experienced ataxia at the higher dose level. The final DLT in this study was an episode of grade 4 small-bowel ischemia at $52\,mg\,m^{-2}$, which led to the patient's death. Autopsy revealed the small-bowel ischemia was confined to the area of a previously treated radical radiation field, which contained evidence of late radiation change and small-vessel damage. The patient's tumor also involved the mesentery of the affected bowel segment. Concern that normal tissue vasculature might be compromised by previous radical radiotherapy has led to patients who have received radical radiotherapy being excluded from future CA4P trials.

In the CWRU study, four DLTs were also reported. The first was an episode of grade 3 dyspnea at $90\,mg\,m^{-2}$ in a patient with advanced ovarian cancer with pleural involvement. The second was grade 2 stridor and grade 3 apnea at $60\,mg\,m^{-2}$ in a patient with advanced thyroid cancer. The third and fourth DLTs were cardiac, and are discussed below.

In the UPENN study, there were also four DLTs. Two episodes of grade 3 tumor pain at $75\,mg\,m^{-2}$ were reported. At the same dose, one patient with advanced NSCLC experienced transient and reversible grade 3 hypoxia and grade 4 dyspnea. This patient had poor lung function at baseline and had been requiring home oxygen therapy. Finally, also at $75\,mg\,m^{-2}$, there was a syncopal episode secondary to dehydration induced grade 2 hypotension and grade 3 hypoxia.

CA4P cardiotoxicity

Significant cardiotoxicity was only reported in the CWRU phase I trial (the least dose intense CA4P regimen). This was probably related to chance or patient selection. The other studies reported no cardiotoxicity. Cardiovascular effects such as transient hypertension, hypotension, tachycardia or bradycardia were seen in all three studies.

In the CWRU trial, two cases of cardiotoxicity were reported at $60\,mg\,m^{-2}$ and one at $90\,mg\,m^{-2}$. The first ($60\,mg\,m^{-2}$) was a diabetic patient with known ischemic heart disease, although this was not initially disclosed. The patient's screening ECG also revealed a QTc interval in excess of $450\,ms$. Shortly after CA4P he experienced shoulder and neck pain, followed by bradycardia and hypoxia. He was treated with opiate analgesia and oxygen. Approximately $90\,min$ later he developed stridor, lethargy, sinus tachycardia, ventricular arrhythmia and dizziness, and after $3\,h$, apnea. Naloxone (Narcan®) was given successfully to reverse the effects of this opiate toxicity. The following day the patient's QTc interval peaked at $533\,ms$, most likely due to hypomagnesemia, hyperglycemia and myocardial ischemia (T-wave changes on ECG). There was no evidence of ischemia on cardiology review, and cardiac enzymes remained in normal limits. Autopsy several weeks later revealed metastatic carcinoma within the heart in addition to the known ischemic disease.

The second cardiac event occurred in a male with a 30 year history of hypertension, on triple antihypertensive therapy. The patient was hypomagnesemic and bradycardic at baseline, so the β-blocker was stopped. The following morning the patient's BP rose as high as 210/88. Following CA4P the BP rose to 229/95. Approximately 90 min following the CA4P, the ECG revealed ST segment depression, and an hour later there was evidence of septal myocardial infarction (MI) associated with raised serum Troponin. It was subsequently shown that the patient's ejection fraction had declined prior to the study from 60 per cent (eight months before) to 42 per cent (post-CA4P) and ischemic heart disease was also diagnosed. Abrupt cessation of β-blockers has been previously documented to cause MI (Astra Zeneca Pharmaceuticals, (Macclesfield).

The third cardiac event occurred at 90 mg m^{-2}, 1 h following the second infusion of CA4P. The patient had ischemic ECG changes and underwent immediate cardiac angiography, which revealed minimal occlusion of the distal left anterior descending coronary artery. There was no rise in cardiac enzymes, and the ECG normalized within a few hours. His only cardiac risk factor was smoking. The patient's heart rate and BP pre- and post-dose are not known, but may have been elevated.

CA4P ECG repolarization (QTc) effects

In vitro ion channel studies have demonstrated that CA4P and CA4 are weak inhibitors of the HERG potassium channel, and CA4P is also a weak inhibitor of the L-type calcium channel. CA4 decreased the action potential duration (APD) and CA4G increased the APD by less than 20 per cent in rabbit Purkinje fibres at a concentration of 30 μM. The human PK data indicates that plasma concentrations of CA4P, CA4 and CA4G are well below these levels and should not have any significant clinical safety effects (Young and Chaplin, 2004). In all three phase I studies, ECGs were performed hourly for 6 h and at 24 h following CA4P. ECGs were analysed centrally, and both Bazett's (QTcB) and Fridericia's (QTcF) formulae were used (Bazett, 1920; Fridericia, 1920).

There was inconsistency of QTc results between the three studies. In the CWRU study, significant QTcB prolongation was found at 2–8 h post-CA4P 60 mg m^{-2} 10 min infusion (maximum 41.3 ms prolongation), 4–5 h post-CA4P 60 mg m^{-2} 60 min infusion (maximum 32.7 ms prolongation) and 4–8 h post-CA4P 90 mg m^{-2} (maximum 42.7 ms prolongation). Using QTcF, significant changes were found only at hours 2 and 7 for 60 mg m^{-2} (maximum 28.8 ms prolongation), and hour 4 for 90 mg m^{-2} (maximum 34.7 ms prolongation). No patients had a QTc >500 ms, and no patients' QTc increased more than 25 per cent over baseline.

In the UK study, two patients had a mean QTc prolongation of ≥30 ms, but less than 60 ms. This study used doses as high as 114 mg m^{-2} CA4P. The UPENN study, the most dose intensive phase I trial, showed mean increases in QTcB of >20 ms at day 1 hours 3–4 at 56 mg m^{-2}, and day 1 hour 4 at 75 mg m^{-2}.

In conclusion, there may be a dose-dependent prolongation of QTc interval at doses ≥56 mg m^{-2}, but the data should be interpreted with caution due to the variable time points of the data collection, large standard deviations, small sample sizes and lack of control groups.

CA4P antitumor activity

In the UK study, one patient with metastatic adrenocortical carcinoma had an unmaintained partial response of their liver metastases to therapy. The tumor shrank by 51 per cent; however, this effect was not sustained for long enough to be classified a partial response. In the UPENN study, one patient with lung metastases from a fibrosarcoma had a partial response at $56\,mg\,m^{-2}$, and 14 patients showed stable disease over 3–29 cycles of CA4P. One patient with metastatic medullary thyroid carcinoma received 29 cycles of CA4P with stable disease and no cumulative toxicity. In the CWRU study, one pathological and radiological complete response was observed in a patient with metastatic anaplastic thyroid cancer ($60\,mg\,m^{-2}$) who received eight cycles of therapy, with the patient disease free 48 months later. Two further patients, one with metastatic colorectal cancer (24 cycles over 19 months at $60\,mg\,m^{-2}$) and another with advanced medullary thyroid cancer (15 cycles over 12 months at $50\,mg\,m^{-2}$) both had prolonged responses to therapy of >12 months. One patient with metastatic kidney cancer had stable disease for 6 months on $18\,mg\,m^{-2}$.

CA4P recommendations

Since these studies were completed, due to the toxicities already described, it has been generally recommended that patients with a history of ischemic heart disease, myocardial infarction, uncontrolled hypertension, arrhythmias, clotting disorders, or patients who have previously received radical doses of radiation therapy should not receive CA4P.

Rat data shows that CA4P-induced hypertension can be effectively controlled with prophylactic antihypertensive therapy, and that these agents do not alter the effects of CA4P on tumor blood flow (Prise *et al.*, 2002). In the current phase I/II CA4P studies, patients experiencing a rise in blood pressure above 160/100 following the first dose of CA4P are subsequently treated with prophylactic doses of the mixed arteriovasodilator hydralazine (given orally 1–2 h before CA4P infusion). It is hoped that these measures will improve the safety profile of this otherwise well tolerated drug. To date, no further significant cardiotoxicity has been reported.

17.5   Potential surrogate markers of CA4P activity

DCE-MRI and PET have important roles in assessing the effects of VDAs on the tumor vasculature (see Chapter 16). Indeed, significant reductions in tumor blood flow were seen in many patients undergoing CA4P treatment when evaluated by PET and DCE-MRI (Anderson *et al.*, 2003; Galbraith *et al.*, 2003). Results of these studies are reviewed in detail by Galbraith in Chapter 16. The MRI data should nonetheless be interpreted with caution due to the small numbers of patients, the wide variety of tumor types and the fact that the imaging techniques were being altered and fine tuned during the course of the studies. Current ongoing CA4P studies are also using these techniques and will increase the volume of data available on the use of DCE-MRI in assessing tumor perfusion.

Interestingly, in the UK study (reference) increases in peripheral blood neutophil counts of on average 80 per cent were seen 4 h following CA4P at doses $\geq 55 \, mg \, m^{-2}$, corresponding to a rise in the patients' core temperature – this would be consistent with an inflammatory/cytokine response to endothelial attack by CA4P. This phenomenon will be researched further to see whether a complete blood count at 4 h post-CA4P might be a surrogate marker of activity.

As CA4P primarily targets dividing endothelial cells, CA4-induced damage or apoptosis of these cells may be associated with release of endothelial-cell-specific markers into the circulation (Bevilacqua and Nelson, 1993). Elevated levels of serum ICAM, VCAM and E-selectin are indicative of endothelial cell dysfunction and small-vessel pathology in patients with essential hypertension and diabetes mellitus (Ferri *et al.*, 1998), and elevated levels of serum VCAM have been seen in patients receiving certain angiogenesis inhibitors (DeVore *et al.*, 1997). In the CWRU study 12 patients had measurements of serum ICAM, VCAM and E-selectin performed just before infusion of CA4P and at 1 h and 24 h post-infusion. Paired comparisons of serum ICAM showed significantly higher levels for pre-treatment versus 1 h or 24 h post-infusion. No significant change was seen in serum VCAM or E-selectin. These results imply that serial measurement of endothelial-cell-specific markers may provide insight into the effects of antiangiogenic drugs and vascular-disrupting agents on the endothelial cell.

ZD6126

In phase I clinical trials (LoRusso *et al.*, 2001; DelProposto *et al.*, 2002; Gadgeel, Wozniak and Wheeler, 2002; Radema *et al.*, 2002; SC, 2002; Thorpe *et al.*, 2003), illustrated in Table 17.2, stable disease lasting four or more cycles was seen in three patients, and one patient had a minor response lasting 19 cycles. Radema *et al.* reported vascular damage in four out of five patients 4–6 h post infusion of ZD6126, indicated by a doubling of circulating endothelial cells, which were viewed as a surrogate marker for vascular damage (Radema *et al.*, 2002). Adverse events noted so far include hypokalemia, anorexia, constipation, dyspnea, fatigue, headache, nausea, pain and vomiting. One patient had asymptomatic, reversible, grade 2 ischemic changes on ECG and grade 3 elevation of Troponin I, with subsequent demonstration of coronary

Table 17.2   Phase I trials of ZD6126

	LoRusso et al. (2001)	Gadgeel, Wozniak and Wheeler (2002)	Radema et al. (2002)	DelProposto et al. (2002)
Schedule	Single dose, q21d	Single dose, q21d	Weekly infusion	Single dose, q21d
Infusion time	10 min	10 min	10 min	–
Number pts	19	27	12	6
ZD6126 dose range	5–40 mg m^{-2}	5–112 mg m^{-2}	5–7 mg m^{-2}	56–112 mg m^{-2}
Elimination $t_{1/2}$	2–3 h	2–3 h	2–3 h	–
DLT	Anemia Cardiac ischemia	Anorexia Constipation Dyspnea Fatigue Headache Pain Nausea	Hypokalemia Reduced LVEF Increased ICP with brain mets	–

artery disease (Gadgeel, Wozniak and Wheeler, 2002). Two other patients have developed transient, reversible declines in left ventricular ejection fraction. Two patients with undiagnosed brain metastases developed symptoms of raised intracranial pressure (somnolence, nausea, vomiting, dizziness) shortly after treatment (Radema et al., 2002).

DCE-MRI analysis was undertaken in six patients following a single dose of ZD6126 every three weeks (three patients at 56 mg m^{-2}, two patients at 80 mg m^{-2} and one patient at 112 mg m^{-2}) (DelProposto et al., 2002). The overall tumor IAUGC$_{60}$ decreased to 13–84 per cent of the baseline value 6 h after ZD6126 administration in all but one subject (56 mg m^{-2}). As expected, the effects were most noticeable in the tumor core. The IAUGC increased to baseline within 24 h in three of the five patients with an initial decrease, but remained below baseline for two patients even after 18–21 days (DelProposto et al., 2002).

Pharmacokinetic analysis showed that C_{max} for plasma ZD6126 was observed 5 min into a 10 min infusion, and levels were undetectable after an hour. An AUC of 1533 ± 556.6 ng h^{-1} ml^{-1} and a $t_{1/2}$ of 2.913 ± 1.11 hours was determined (Scurr et al., 2004). ZD6126 was rapidly hydrolysed to the active metabolite ZD6126 phenol. The majority of the dose was excreted in the feces, showing the importance of biliary excretion.

Because of concerns about the effect of ZD6126 on blood pressure and potential cardiotoxicity, clinical trials of this agent have been temporarily halted. ZD6126 is likely to be tested as a single agent for the treatment of advanced kidney cancer, and a phase II trial of ZD6126 in combination with Oxaliplatin and 5-fluorouracil is under consideration for advanced colorectal cancer.

AVE8062A (AC7700)

AVE8062A (Aventis Pharmaceuticals) is a synthetic water soluble Combretastatin analogue, which is currently undergoing single agent phase I trials in humans (Tolcher *et al.*, 2003). Nine reported patients with advanced cancer have received 48 infusions of AVE8062 (4.5–30 mg m^{-2}) weekly for 3 weeks every 28 days over 30 min (Tolcher *et al.*, 2003). Asymptomatic hypotension without any other cardiac toxicity was dose limiting at 30 mg m^{-2}. Preliminary evidence of decreased vascular flow by DCE-MRI was observed at 15.5 mg m^{-2}. AVE8062A was rapidly eliminated with a $t_{1/2}$ of 15 min and a clearance of 50 L h^{-1} m^{-2}, leading to an active metabolite, RPR258063, with a $t_{1/2}$ of 7 h. The C_{max} values for AVE8062A and RPR258063 were 2.1 and 0.3 µM ml^{-1} at 22 mg m^{-2}. Published data on AVE8062A is, however, very limited.

Other VDAs

A number of other VDAs including OXi4503 (Oxigene) and MN-029 (MediciNova) have begun or will soon enter phase I trial evaluations in humans.

17.6   Combination therapy with VDAs

A well recognized feature of tumors treated with VDAs is the survival of a rim of neoplastic cells at the tumor periphery (Chaplin and Petit, 1999; Siemann, Chaplin and Horsman, 2004). Cells in this viable rim of tumor tissue are likely to be in a state of rapid proliferation and excellent nutrition. These factors may make the surviving tumor cells susceptible to killing by conventional therapies. Indeed, it is now well established that improved tumor responses can be achieved in animals when VDAs are applied in combined modality treatment strategies. The basis and outcomes of studies utilizing VDAs in conjunction with anticancer treatments such chemotherapy, radiotherapy, hyperthermia, radioimmunotherapy or antiangiogenic agents are reviewed in Chapters 1, 7 and 8. The success of the preclinical investigations utilizing VDAs in combination with conventional therapies has resulted in the initiation of several clinical investigations.

Preclinical studies combining CA4P with radioimmunotherapy (Pedley *et al.*, 2001) had shown not only significantly enhanced tumor responses but also an enhancement of the radioimmunotherapy by entrapment of additional radioantibody after CA4P-induced vessel collapse (Lankester and 2004). These findings have led to a Cancer Research UK phase I study of ^{131}I-labeled anti-CEA antibody (1600–1800 MBq m^{-2}) in combination with weekly CA4P (45–63 mg m^{-2}) in humans with advanced colorectal carcinoma, which is ongoing.

A phase I study is also ongoing in humans using 3 weekly CA4P in combination with carboplatin or paclitaxel in advanced cancer, which will progress to a randomized phase II trial of the triplet combination in relapsed ovarian cancer. Preliminary data from a similar study suggest that great care is needed when combining these agents, as CA4P could alter the AUC of a drug such as carboplatin that is renally excreted (Bilenker *et al.*, 2003). CA4P is therefore being administered 18–20 h prior to chemotherapy in the ongoing study. More than 20 patients have been treated to date, with no grade 3 or 4 drug-related toxicity so far seen (Rustin, personal communication).

A phase I trial of CA4P in combination with radiotherapy in patients with advanced lung, prostate or head and neck cancer is also currently recruiting patients in the UK. To date, 12 patients with NSCLC and 10 patients with prostate cancer have received $50\,\text{mg}\,\text{m}^{-2}$ CA4P either as a single dose, or as a weekly infusion, in combination with their radiotherapy treatment, with no grade 3 or 4 drug-related toxicity. The CA4P dose is due to be escalated to $63\,\text{mg}\,\text{m}^{-2}$ (Quan Ng, personal communication).

Other active studies include a phase II trial of single-agent CA4P in advanced anaplastic carcinoma of the thyroid, a phase I/II trial of CA4P in combination with doxorubicin and cisplatin in newly diagnosed anaplastic thyroid carcinoma, a phase I trial of CA4P + cisplatin in advanced or recurrent cervical cancer, and a phase I/II study of CA4P in patients with age-related macular degeneration. ZD6126 is likely to be tested as a single agent for the treatment of advanced kidney cancer, and a phase II trial of ZD6126 in combination with Oxaliplatin and 5-fluorouracil is under consideration for advanced colorectal cancer.

DMXAA when combined with antibody-dependent enzyme prodrug therapy (ADEPT) or radioimmunotherapy in colorectal xenografts also gave significantly enhanced therapy, with no increase in systemic toxicity (Pedley *et al.*, 1996, 1999). The combination of DMXAA with Paclitaxel has been very successful, with some cures seen in animal models (Siim, 2004). Clinical trials of combination therapy with DMXAA are starting soon.

Finally, athough no clinical studies have as yet been initiated, preclinical studies have demonstrated that combining VDAs with antiangiogenic approaches is also likely to achieve a complementary tumor effect (Chapter 1). Cells surviving VDA treatment at the tumor periphery aggressively promote neovascularization to achieve rapid regrowth, thus providing a favourable setting for antiangiogenic therapy (Siemann, 2002; Wedge *et al.*, 2002). The encouraging preclinical data seen with the combination of ZD6126 and the VGFR2 tyrosine kinase inhibitor ZD6474 (Siemann and Shi, 2004; Varghese *et al.*, 2004) suggests that future combinations of such agents may be feasible.

17.7   VDAs in non-malignant diseases

Normal human vasculature is generally in a quiescent state except for processes such as menstruation, growth or wound healing. Since the antivascular effects of CA4P are division specific, CA4P can cause extensive damage to endothelial cells in rapidly proliferating, non-neoplastic tissue undergoing neovascularization, for example goitres (Griggs *et al.*, 2001a). The use of VDAs is currently being explored in diseases such as diabetic retinopathy, psoriasis, rheumatoid arthritis and age-related macular degeneration (ARMD). The abnormal vascular endothelium in these conditions has similarities to tumor endothelium, particularly its immaturity. CA4P has shown benefits in murine models of diabetic retinopathy (Griggs *et al.*, 2002). Phase I/II trials of CA4P in ARMD and myopic macular degeneration are ongoing. See Chapter 18 for further details of non-malignant applications of VDAs.

17.8 Conclusions

Tumours need a vascular supply for progression, survival and dissemination. Targeting the tumor vasculature offers the attractive possibility of inducing responses in all tumor types, and improving the effectiveness of conventional clinically active antitumor therapies.

Many antiangiogenic compounds have already been tested in cancer patients, and the vascular-disrupting agents have shown some potential in early phase clinical trials. In addition, new agents are on the way. Testing these agents for clinical activity is a major challenge.

VDAs can eliminate the central, poorly perfused, hypoxic regions of the tumor; however, combination therapy with cytotoxics, radiation, antiangiogenics or radioimmunotherapy is needed to kill those cells surviving at the the periphery of the tumor. The combinations are complimentary and enhance cell kill. Any benefits of VDAs as possible cancer therapies are likely to be seen when combination studies are completed.

Despite much research, the exact mechanisms that render tumor vasculature more susceptible to VDAs are still uncertain. In addition, the optimum timing and frequency of VDA administration in a clinical setting have yet to be determined. The current data, however, looks interesting for the further development of these agents in the coming years.

References

Anderson, H.L., Yap, J.T. *et al.* (2003). Assessment of pharmacodynamic vascular response in a phase I trial of combretastatin A4 phosphate. *J Clin Oncol* 21 (15), 2823–2830.

Astra Zeneca Pharmaceuticals. *Toprol-XL Product Information.* Macclesfield, U.

Bazett, H.C. (1920). 'An analysis of the time relations of electrocardiograms.' *Heart* 7, 353–367.

Bevilacqua, M.P. and Nelson, R.M. (1993). 'Selectins.' *J Clin Invest* 91 (2), 379–387.

Bilenker, J.H., Stevenson, J.P., Rosen, M.A., Gallagher, M., Flaherty, K.T., Algazy, K., Sun, W., Schnall, M. and O'Dwyer, P.J. (2003). 'Phase Ib trial of combretastatin A4 phosphate (CA4P) in combination with carboplatin in patients with advanced cancer.' *Proc Am Soc Clin Oncol* 22, abstract 889.

Blakey, D.C., Ashton, S.E. *et al.* (2002a). 'ZD6126: a novel small molecule vascular targeting agent.' *Int J Radiat Oncol Biol Phys* **54** (5), 1497–1502.

Blakey, D.C., Westwood, F.R. *et al.* (2002b). 'Antitumor activity of the novel vascular targeting agent ZD6126 in a panel of tumor models.' *Clin Cancer Res* **8** (6), 1974–1983.

Boehm, T., Folkman, J. *et al.* (1997). 'Antiangiogenic therapy of experimental cancer does not induce acquired drug resistance.' *Nature* **390** (6658), 404–407.

Chaplin, D.J. and Dougherty, G.J. (1999). 'Tumour vasculature as a target for cancer therapy.' *Br J Cancer* **80** (Suppl. 1), 57–64.

Chaplin, D.J., Pettit, G.R. *et al.* (1999). 'Anti-vascular approaches to solid tumour therapy: evaluation of combretastatin A4 phosphate.' *Anticancer Res* **19** (1A), 189–195.

Ching, L.M., Goldsmith, D. *et al.* (1999). 'Induction of intratumoral tumor necrosis factor (TNF) synthesis and hemorrhagic necrosis by 5,6-dimethylxanthenone-4-acetic acid (DMXAA) in TNF knockout mice.' *Cancer Res* **59** (14), 3304–3307.

Cliffe, S., Taylor, M.L. *et al.* (1994). 'Combining bioreductive drugs (SR 4233 or SN 23862) with the vasoactive agents flavone acetic acid or 5,6-dimethylxanthenone acetic acid.' *Int J Radiat Oncol Biol Phys* **29** (2), 373–377.

Corbett, T.H., Bissery, M.C. *et al.* (1986). 'Activity of flavone acetic acid (NSC-347512) against solid tumors of mice.' *Invest New Drugs* **4** (3), 207–220.

Davis, P.D., Dougherty, G.J. *et al.* (2002). 'ZD6126: a novel vascular-targeting agent that causes selective destruction of tumor vasculature.' *Cancer Res* **62** (24), 7247–7253.

DelProposto, Z., LoRusso, P.M., Latif, Z. *et al.* (2002). 'MRI evaluation of the effects of the vascular targeting agent ZD6126 on tumor vasculature.' *Proc Am Soc Clin Oncol* **21** (111a), abstract 440.

DeVore, R.F., Hellerqvist, C.G. *et al.* (1997). 'Phase I study of the antineovascularization drug CM101.' *Clin Cancer Res* **3** (3), 365–372.

Dowlati, A., Robertson, K. *et al.* (2002). 'A phase I pharmacokinetic and translational study of the novel vascular targeting agent combretastatin a-4 phosphate on a single-dose intravenous schedule in patients with advanced cancer.' *Cancer Res* **62** (12), 3408–3416.

Ferri, C., Desideri, G. *et al.* (1998). 'Early activation of vascular endothelium in nonobese, nondiabetic essential hypertensive patients with multiple metabolic abnormalities.' *Diabetes* **47** (4), 660–667.

Folberg, R., Hendrix, M.J. *et al.* (2000). 'Vasculogenic mimicry and tumor angiogenesis.' *Am J Pathol* **156** (2), 361–381.

Fridericia, L.S. (1920). 'Die Systolendauer Im Electrokardiogramm Bei Normalen Menchan Und Bei Herzdranken.' *Acta Med Scand* **53**, 469–486.

Gadgeel, S.M., LoRusso, P.M., Wozniak, A.J. and Wheeler, C. (2002). 'A dose escalation study of the novel vascular targeting agent ZD6126 in patients with solid tumors.' *Proc Am Soc Clin Oncol* **21** (110a), abstract 438.

Galbraith, S.M., Chaplin, D.J. *et al.* (2001). 'Effects of combretastatin A4 phosphate on endothelial cell morphology in vitro and relationship to tumor vascular targeting activity in vivo.' *Anticancer Res* **21** (1A), 93–102.

Galbraith, S.M., Maxwell, R.J. *et al.* (2003). 'Combretastatin A4 phosphate has tumor antivascular activity in rat and man as demonstrated by dynamic magnetic resonance imaging.' *J Clin Oncol* **21** (15), 2831–2842.

Galbraith, S.M., Rustin, G.J. *et al.* (2002). 'Effects of 5,6-dimethylxanthenone-4-acetic acid on human tumor microcirculation assessed by dynamic contrast-enhanced magnetic resonance imaging.' *J Clin Oncol* **20** (18), 3826–3840.

Griggs, J., Hesketh, R. *et al.* (2001a). 'Combretastatin-A4 disrupts neovascular development in non-neoplastic tissue.' *Br J Cancer* **84** (6), 832–835.

Griggs, J., Metcalfe, J.C. *et al.* (2001b). 'Targeting tumor vasculature: the development of combretastatin A4.' *Lancet Oncol* **2** (2), 82–87.

Griggs, J., Skepper, J.N. *et al.* (2002). 'Inhibition of proliferative retinopathy by the anti-vascular agent combretastatin-A4.' *Am J Pathol* **160** (3), 1097–1103.

Hori, K. and Saito, S. (2003). 'Microvascular mechanisms by which the combretastatin A-4 derivative AC7700 (AVE8062) induces tumor blood flow stasis.' *Br J Cancer* **89** (7), 1334–1344.

Huang, X., Molema, G. *et al.* (1997). 'Tumor infarction in mice by antibody-directed targeting of tissue factor to tumor vasculature.' *Science* **275** (5299), 547–550.

Jameson, M., Thompson, P., Baguley, B., Evans, B., Harvey, V., Porter, D., McCrystal, M. and Kestell, P. (2000). 'Phase I pharmacokinetic and pharmacodynamic study of 5,6-dimethylxanthenone-4-acetic acid (DMXAA), a novel anti vascular agent.' *Proc ASCO* abstract 705.

Jameson, M.B., Thompson, P.I. *et al.* (2003). 'Clinical aspects of a phase I trial of 5,6-dimethylxanthenone-4-acetic acid (DMXAA), a novel antivascular agent.' *Br J Cancer* **88** (12), 1844–1850.

Kerr, D.J. and Kaye, S.B. (1989). 'Flavone acetic acid – preclinical and clinical activity.' *Eur J Cancer Clin Oncol* **25** (9), 1271–1272.

Lankester, K.P.B. (2004). 'Acute anti vascular effects of combretastatin A4 phosphate (CA4P) on the SW1222 tumour as measured by dynamic contrast enhanced MRI (DCE-MRI).' BCRM (NCRI) Abstract 2004.

Lash, C.J., Li, A.E. *et al.* (1998). 'Enhancement of the anti-tumor effects of the antivascular agent 5,6-dimethylxanthenone-4-acetic acid (DMXAA) by combination with 5-hydroxytryptamine and bioreductive drugs.' *Br J Cancer* **78** (4), 439–445.

LoRusso, S., Gadgeel, S., Wozniak, A. *et al.* (2001). 'A phase I dose escalation trial of ZD6126, a novel vascular targeting agent, in patients with cancer refractory to other treatments.' *Proc AACR-NCI-EORTC* abstract 36.

Maniotis, A.J., Folberg, R. *et al.* (1999). 'Vascular channel formation by human melanoma cells in vivo and in vitro: vasculogenic mimicry.' *Am J Pathol* **155** (3), 739–752.

McDonald, D.M., Munn, L. *et al.* (2000). 'Vasculogenic mimicry: how convincing, how novel, and how significant?' *Am J Pathol* **156** (2), 383–388.

Pedley, R.B., Boden, J.A. *et al.* (1996). 'Ablation of colorectal xenografts with combined radioimmunotherapy and tumor blood flow-modifying agents.' *Cancer Res* **56** (14), 3293–3300.

Pedley, R.B., Hill, S.A. *et al.* (2001). 'Eradication of colorectal xenografts by combined radioimmunotherapy and combretastatin a-4 3-O-phosphate.' *Cancer Res* **61** (12), 4716–4722.

Pedley, R.B., Sharma, S.K. *et al.* (1999). 'Enhancement of antibody-directed enzyme prodrug therapy in colorectal xenografts by an antivascular agent.' *Cancer Res* **59** (16), 3998–4003.

Prise, V.E., Honess, D.J., Stratford, M.R., Wilson, J. and Tozer, G.M. (2002). 'The vascular response of tumor and normal tissues in the rat to the vascular targeting agent, combretastatin A-4-phosphate, at clinically relevant doses.' *Int J Oncol* **21** (4), 717–726.

Pruijn, F.B., van Daalen, M. *et al.* (1997). 'Mechanisms of enhancement of the antitumor activity of melphalan by the tumor-blood-flow inhibitor 5,6-dimethylxanthenone-4-acetic acid.' *Cancer Chemother Pharmacol* **39** (6), 541–546.

Radema, S.A., Beerepoot, L.V., Witteveen, P.O. *et al.* (2002). 'Clinical evaluation of the novel vascular targeting agent ZD6126: assessment of toxicity and surrogate markers of vascular damage.' *Proc Am Soc Clin Oncol* **21** (110a), abstract 439.

Remick, S.C. (2002). 'Vascular Targeting: Clinical Experience.' *Horizons in Cancer Therapeutics: from Bench to Bedside* **3** (2), 16–23.

Rewcastle, G.W., Atwell, G.J. *et al.* (1991). 'Potential antitumor agents. 61. Structure–activity relationships for in vivo colon 38 activity among disubstituted 9-oxo-9H-xanthene-4-acetic acids.' *J Med Chem* **34** (1), 217–222.

Rustin, G.J., Bradley, C. *et al.* (2003). '5,6-dimethylxanthenone-4-acetic acid (DMXAA), a novel antivascular agent: phase I clinical and pharmacokinetic study.' *Br J Cancer* **88** (8), 1160–1167.

Rustin, G.J., Galbraith, S.M. *et al.* (2003). 'Phase I clinical trial of weekly combretastatin A4 phosphate: clinical and pharmacokinetic results.' *J Clin Oncol* **21** (15), 2815–2822.

SC, R. (2002). 'Vascular targeting: clinical experience.' *Horizons in Cancer Therapeutics: from Bench to Bedside* **3** (2), 16–23.

Scurr, M.J., Brock, I., O'Donnell, C., Tan, A., Partridge, S., D'Souza, E.A., R.A. and Roberts, D.W. (2004). 'Assessment of metabolism, excretion & pharmacokinetics of a single dose of 14C-ZD6126 in patients with solid malignant tumours.' *Proc ASCO* **22** (14S), 3083.

Siemann, D.W. (2002). 'Vascular targeting agents.' *Horizons in Cancer Therapeutics: from Bench to Bedside* **3** (2), 4–15.

Siemann, D.W., Chaplin, D.J. and Horsman, M.R. (2004). 'Vascular targeting therapies for cancer treatment.' *Cancer* **100**, 2491–2499.

Siemann, D.W. and Shi, W. (2004). 'Efficacy of combined antiangiogenic and vascular disrupting agents in treatment of solid tumours.' *Int J Radiat Oncol Biol Phys* **60** (4), 1233–1240.

Siim, B. (2004). 'The DMXAA experience.' *Proc 2nd International Conference on Vascular Targeting, Miami, FL*, abstract 5.

Simon, R., Freidlin, B. *et al.* (1997). 'Accelerated titration designs for phase I clinical trials in oncology.' *J Natl Cancer Inst* **89** (15), 1138–1147.

Smith, G.P., Calveley, S.B. *et al.* (1987). 'Flavone acetic acid (NSC 347512) induces haemorrhagic necrosis of mouse colon 26 and 38 tumors.' *Eur J Cancer Clin Oncol* **23** (8), 1209–1211.

Stevenson, J.P., Rosen, M. *et al.* (2003). 'Phase I trial of the antivascular agent combretastatin A4 phosphate on a 5-day schedule to patients with cancer: magnetic resonance imaging evidence for altered tumor blood flow.' *J Clin Oncol* **21** (23), 4428–4438.

Thorpe, P.E., Chaplin, D.J. *et al.* (2003). 'The first international conference on vascular targeting: meeting overview.' *Cancer Res* **63** (5), 1144–1147.

Tolcher, A.W., Forero, L., Celio, P., Hammond, L.A., Patnaik, A., Hill, M., Verat-Follet, C., Haacke, M., Besenval, M. and Rowinsky, E.K. (2003). 'Phase I, pharmacokinetic, and DCE-MRI correlative study of AVE8062A, an antivascular combretastatin analogue, administered weekly for 3 weeks every 28 days.' *Proc Am Soc Clin Oncol* **22**, abstract 834.

Tozer, G.M., Kanthou, C. *et al.* (2002). 'The biology of the combretastatins as tumor vascular targeting agents.' *Int J Exp Pathol* **83** (1), 21–38.

Varghese, H.J., Mackenzie, L.T., Groom, A.C., Ellis, C.G., Ryan, A., MacDonald, I.C. and Chambers, A.F. (2004). 'In vivo videomicroscopy reveals differential effects of the vascular targeting agent ZD6126 and the anti-angiogenic agent ZD6474 on vascular function in a liver metastasis model.' *Angiogenesis* **7** (2), 157–164.

Wedge, S.R., Kendrew, J., Ogilvie, D.J. *et al.* (2002). 'Combination of the VEGF receptor tyrosine kinase inhibitor ZD6474 and vascular targeting agent ZD6126 produces an enhanced anti-tumor response.' *Proc Am Assoc Cancer Res* **43**, 1081.

Wilson, W.R., Li, A.E. *et al.* (1998). 'Enhancement of tumor radiation response by the antivascular agent 5,6-dimethylxanthenone-4-acetic acid.' *Int J Radiat Oncol Biol Phys* **42** (4), 905–908.

Young, S.L. and Chaplin, D.J. (2004). 'Combretastatin A4 phosphate: background and current clinical status.' *Exp Opin Invest Drugs* **13** (9), 1171–1182.

18

Use of Vasculature-disrupting Agents in Non-Oncology Indications

Joseph C. Randall and Scott L. Young

Abstract

Altered regulation of angiogenesis has been implicated in the pathogenesis of a variety diseases that have a vascular component, including but certainly not limited to arthritis, hemangiomas, and psoriasis as well as a number of ophthalmic conditions including diabetic retinopathy, retinopathy of prematurity, age-related macular degeneration (AMD) and choroidal neovascularization secondary to pathologic myopia. Therefore, a pro-angiogenic phenotype can be considered as a final common pathway in neovascular disease and can lead to the development of aberrant vascular phenotypes in the eye and other tissues. The approval of anti-VEGF treatment strategies in oncology and more recently in ophthalmology implies that anti-neovascular therapy is now recognized as having application outside of the oncology setting. The clinical advantage of the vascular disrupting agents may be their ability to intervene with established and proliferating neovasculature as opposed to a more preventative or prophylactic therapy with the anti-angiogenic based therapies. This chapter presents a rationale for the use of vascular disrupting agents in the treatment of neovascular eye diseases and other indications that are characterized by aberrant vascular phenotypes.

Keywords

Aberrant vascular phenotype, neovascular eye diseases, arthritis, hemangiomas, psoriasis, pathologic myopia, choroidal neovasculature (CNV), age-related macular degeneration (AMD), retinopathy of prematurity (ROP), diabetic retinopathy

18.1 Background

While the inhibition and disruption of neovascular growth by either antiangiogenic agents or vascular-disrupting agents (VDAs) in oncologic malignancies

---

Vascular-targeted Therapies in Oncology   Edited by Dietmar W. Siemann
© 2006 John Wiley & Sons, Ltd.

is now a well established area of research and clinical development, other malignancies may too benefit from this type of therapeutic strategy. In healthy adults, very little neovascular growth occurs, with the exception of uterine endometrium thickening associated with the female menstrual cycle. For the most part, neovascular growth in adults is a response to an abnormal condition, whether it is direct physical injury inducing tissue repair and regrowth or a pathologic condition involving the aberrant growth of tissue, bone etc., which thus can elicit neovascular development. Altered regulation of angiogenesis has been implicated in the pathogenesis of a variety of diseases that have a vascular component, including but certainly not limited to arthritis, hemangioma and psoriasis as well as a number of ophthalmic conditions including diabetic retinopathy, retinopathy of prematurity, age-related macular degeneration (AMD) and choroidal neovascularization (CNV) secondary to pathologic myopia (Folkman, 1993; Otani et al., 1999; Carmeliet and Jain, 2000; Sivakumar, Harry and Paleolog, 2004; Wahl, Moser and Pizzo, 2004). In fact, surgically removed CNV membranes from the eye have stained positive for angiopoietin-1, angiopoietin-2, Tie-2 receptor and vascular endothelial growth factors (VEGFs), regardless of the underlying etiology (myopia, AMD or idiopathic) (Otani et al., 1999). Thus, a pro-angiogenic phenotype may be considered a common mechanism by which these and other neovascular ocular pathologies develop. Similarly, aberrant vascular phenotypes have been observed and characterized in other non-cancer indications, including arthritis (Firestein, 1999), hemangiomas (Bruchner and Frieden, 2003) and psoriasis (Ragaz and Ackerman, 1979; Braverman and Sibley, 1985). This chapter aims to describe the underlying vascular component of the pathology of a few of these diseases and how vascular-disrupting agents with their anti-mitotic, anti-proliferative and anti-vascular effects (Tozer et al., 1999; Kanthou et al., 2004) may be a useful approach as a component in their treatment and management.

Therapeutically, vascular-disrupting agents may have several major advantages over anti-angiogenesis-based therapies. First, VDAs are designed to rapidly increase vascular resistance to blood flow by altering the shape of nascent endothelial cells that line actively proliferating blood vessels (Tozer et al., 2001). Since most VDAs are reversibility bound and rapidly metabolized and excreted, systemic effects on other targets or tissues are significantly minimized. The ability of VDAs to acutely disrupt aberrant choroidal neovasculature and to spare the development of normal retinal vasculature (Ozaki et al., 2000) is unique and sets this class of drugs apart from anti-angiogenesis-based therapies (Campochiaro and Hackett, 2003). Anti-angiogenesis-based therapies may require prolonged treatment to slow the growth of neovasculature and this could cause delayed or chronic toxicity that is not observed in short-term studies (Kerbel, 2000).

The second major advantage of VDAs is that the actin cytoskeleton of mature endothelial cells confers resistance to vascular-disrupting effects in normal tissues. Supra-pharmacological doses of the most clinically advanced VDA,

combretastatin A-4 phosphate (CA4P), increase vascular resistance approximately seven-fold in the spleen of rats and up to 300-fold in P22 tumors. Blood
flow in the heart, kidney and small intestine of rats were in the normal range,
because increased vascular resistance in non-target tissues was generally offset
by an increase in tissue perfusion pressure (Tozer *et al.*, 1999).

The third major advantage of VDAs is that they have been shown in a variety
of oncology models to have synergistic activity when given in combination with
radiation and chemotherapy-based therapies. There appears to be a complementary tumor destruction, whereby the VDA causes massive central necrosis while
the other therapy kills tumor cells at the periphery. The clinical development of
VDAs in the field of oncology is presented elsewhere in this book and in recently
published review articles (Chaplin and Hill, 2002; Siemann, Chaplin and
Horsman, 2004; Young and Chaplin, 2004).

The use of vascular disrupting agents to affect ocular neovasculature stems
from published reports that CA4P slows progression and induces regression of
ocular neovasculature in a mouse model of laser-induced CNV (Nambu *et al.*,
2003) and that CA4P inhibits retinal neovasculature in a mouse model of retinopathy of prematurity (Griggs *et al.*, 2002). Daily intraperitoneal (IP) injections
of CA4P in neonatal mice with oxygen-induced ischemic retinopathy (starting
prior to the onset of neovascularization) exhibited a marked suppression of
retinal neovascularization in this model (Griggs *et al.*, 2002). In transgenic mice
that overexpress VEGF in the retina, daily IP injections of CA4P resulted in a
marked reduction in the number of neovascular lesions and total area of neovascularization per retina (Nambu *et al.*, 2003). In adult mice with laser-induced
rupture of Bruch's membrane, treatment with CA4P resulted in significantly
smaller areas of CNV. In addition, CA4P treatment of mice with established
CNV decreased the size of CNV lesions (Nambu *et al.*, 2003). These reports
indicate that this VDA may cause not only significant inhibition of neovascular
growth in the eye but, perhaps more clinically relevant, it appeared to cause
regression of the aberrant neovasculature, regardless of the underlying
pathology.

18.2   Age-related macular degeneration (AMD)

Age-related macular degeneration is a leading cause of severe vision loss in
persons 55 and older in Western countries (Bressler, 2002; Zarbin, 2004). The
exact etiology of this disease is unknown, but the prevalence is expected to rise
as the as the population ages. The pathogenesis of AMD is characterized by the
accumulation of drusden deposits, geographic atrophy, choroidal neovascularization (CNV), disciform scarring and damage (i.e. tearing) or loss of the retinal-
pigmented epithelium (RPE). The most common form of AMD is called 'dry'
or atrophic AMD and is characterized by the slow progressive atrophy of the
RPE, loss of photoreceptors in the macula and eventual loss of central vision

(Shahidi *et al.*, 2002). There is no effective treatment for geographic atrophy or loss of RPE in late stage 'dry' AMD (Sunness, 1999).

'Wet' AMD (wAMD) is a less common and more progressive form of AMD that can result in sudden vision loss, principally due to CNV (Sunness, 1999). In wAMD, multiple blood vessels originating from the choroidal vascular bed behind the retina grow though Bruch's membrane and into the retinal-pigmented epithelial space, which can result in subretinal hemorrhage (Campochiaro *et al.*, 1999). The pathogenesis of wAMD is quite complicated and involves inflammation, hypoxia of the eye, up-regulation of growth factors and development of a pro-angiogenic phenotype (Schlingemann, 2003) as indicated by positive staining for angiopoietin-1, angiopoietin-2 and Tie-2 receptor and VEGF (Otani *et al.*, 1999). In fact, Macugen® or Pegaptanib is the first approved anti-vascular endothelial growth factor (anti-VEGF) for treatment of neovascular AMD (Gragoudas *et al.*, 2004).

The two most common treatment options for wAMD include laser photocoagulation of non-foveal CNV and photodynamic therapy (PDT) of subfoveal CNV using the agent Visudyne® (Verteporfin for injection) (Bressler, 2002; TAP Reports Nos. 1 and 2). Visudyne® is a photoreactive dye injected intravenously that is then activated in the neovascular lesion with a cold diode laser (wavelength of 689 nm). The use of PDT for occult AMD without classic CNV is associated with an increased risk of large submacular hemorrhages (Do, Bressler and Bressler, 2004). Surgical removal of subfoveal CNV (Grossniklaus and Green, 1998) and macular translocation surgery (Pawlek *et al.*, 2004) are more invasive and are less commonly used. These ablation-based therapies target existing CNV and do not address the underlying metabolic changes in the RPE, and recurrence of CNV is common (Campochiaro *et al.*, 1999). There is also a distinct risk of surgical injury to the surrounding/underlying RPE cells, which can result in retinal scarring and localized loss of function (Grossniklaus and Green, 1998).

The VDA combretastatin A-4 phosphate has been shown to disrupt ocular neovasculature and to promote regression of retinal neovasculature in transgenic mice that overexpress vascular endothelial growth factor (VEGF) and rhodopsin (rho). Rho/VEGF mice were administered daily intraperitoneal injections of vehicle or CA4P in vehicle (2.2 or 4.0 mg kg^{-1} day^{-1}) between postnatal day 7 and 21 (P7–P21). On postnatal day 21, the mice were anesthetized and infused with fluorescein-labeled dextran and retinal flat mounts were prepared. Fluorescein angiography was used to quantitate retinal neovascularization (CNV) in hemizygous transgenic mice. On P21, numerous neovascular lesions were observed and there was no difference in the areas of retinal lesions in controls or animals given 2.2 mg kg^{-1} day^{-1} of CA4P. However, mice treated with 4.0 mg kg^{-1} day^{-1} of CA4P showed a significant reduction in the number of lesions per retina and a decrease in the total area of neovascular lesions per retina (77 per cent smaller than vehicle-treated mice; Nambu *et al.*, 2003).

A laser-induced mouse model of CNV was used to evaluate the pharmacological effects of CA4P on the development of ocular neovasculature (Nambu *et al.*, 2003). Daily intraperitoneal injections of vehicle or 10, 20, 50, 75 or 100 mg kg^{-1} day^{-1} of CA4P were given for two weeks after laser-induced rupture of Bruch's membrane. At the time of sacrifice, C57BL/6J mice were anesthetized and infused with fluorescein-labeled dextran and choroidal flat mounts were prepared. Fluorescein angiography was used to quantitate CNV. There was no significant difference in total CNV area in mice treated with 10, 20 or 50 mg kg^{-1} day^{-1} of CA4P when compared with vehicle treated mice. However, mice treated with 75 and 100 mg kg^{-1} day^{-1} CA4P had significantly smaller CNV areas (<50 per cent decrease) than vehicle-treated mice. The same laser burn model was used to determine whether CA4P had an effect on established CNV. A laser-induced rupture of Bruch's membrane was performed on day 1. On day 7, mice were administered daily intraperitoneal injections of vehicle and 100 mg kg^{-1} of CA4P for 1 week. On day 14, histopathology and fluorescein angiography were used to quantitate CNV surrounding the burns. A dose of 100 mg kg^{-1} of CA4P did not significantly reduce the size of neovascular lesions when compared with baseline; it did however reduce the total area of neovascularization per retina, indicating a partial involution of CNV (Nambu *et al.*, 2003).

The ability of VDAs to acutely disrupt aberrant choroidal or retinal neovasculature and to spare the development of normal retinal vasculature is unique and sets this class of drugs apart from anti-angiogenesis-based therapies (Campochiaro and Hackett, 2003).

CA4P is the first VDA to enter the clinic for treatment of wAMD. While the specific dose and schedule for maximum patient benefit has yet to be determined, this trial represents the broadening use and application of these VDAs to potentially treat neovascular abnormalities outside the oncology setting. Moreover, a preliminary body of research is now being develop to determine the feasibility of these compounds to be delivered non-systemically to the eye, either by some form of peri-ocular injection or as a direct topical application. This data may eventually make its way back to the oncology setting and prove useful to treat melanomas for example or other tumor types where local delivery is achievable and desirable.

18.3 Myopic macular degeneration

Pathologic (degenerative) myopia is a progressive eye disease that is characterized by axial elongation of the eye, visual disturbances and high levels of myopia. Common visual disturbances include metamorphosias, where objects appear distorted in shape, and blurring of central vision that cannot be corrected with prescription lenses or refractive surgery. High levels of myopia (pathologic myopia) can cause tears in Bruch's membrane, which leads to subretinal bleeding and CNV (Blacharski, 1988). This progressive condition is called myopic macular degeneration (MMD) and leads to atrophy of the retinal-pigmented epithelium (RPE) and choroid (also called chorioretinal degeneration). In fact, retinal CNV is one of the most common vision-threatening complications of pathologic myopia. In one study, 10.2 per cent of the eyes developed myopic CNV over a three-year period (Ohno-Matsui *et al.*, 2003). The investigators also found that CNV developed at a much higher rate in the eyes of patients with lacquer cracks (29.4 per cent), patchy chorioretinal atrophy (20.0 per cent) and pre-existing CNV (34.8 per cent). In contrast, the rate of CNV over the follow-up period was 6.2 per cent in patients without pre-existing CNV and only 3.7 per cent in patients with diffuse chorioretinal atrophy. Therefore, lacquer cracks, patchy chorioretinal atrophy and existing CNV are considered predisposing factors for later development of myopic CNV or MMD (Ohno-Matsui *et al.*, 2003).

CNV lesions in patients with pathologic myopia tend to be more self-limiting than in patients with wAMD (Tabandeh *et al.*, 1999). Using the technique of optical coherence tomography (OCT), Baba *et al.* (2002) identified three stages in myopic CNV (active, scar and atrophic). On OCT scans, bleeding and a highly reflective concave deflection on top of the RPE characterize the active stage of myopic CNV (Baba *et al.*, 2002). In this study, grayish-white scars developed about 3–6 months after CNV onset. The hemorrhage due to CNV was self-absorbed and dense areas of pigmentation (Fuch's spots) were sometimes noted. A number of studies have found that chorioretinal atrophy is the major cause of poor visual outcome in advanced stages of myopic CNV (Kojima *et al.*, 2004; Yoshida *et al.*, 2003). Based on the mechanism of action, vascular disrupting agents should be administered during the active phase or the early scar stage of myopic CNV in order to disrupt the neovascular network in the eye. A single compassionate use patient at Johns Hopkins University had regression of myopic CNV and improved visual acuity after intravenous CA4P (Heyman, 2003).

The four existing treatment options for myopic CNV include thermal laser treatment (laser photocoagulation), PDT with Visudyne®, surgical removal of CNV and macular translocation surgery. An excellent review of current treatment options for myopic CNV has been published (Tano, 2002). Each of these treatment paradigms has its limitations and liabilities. For example, laser photocoagulation is not commonly used to treat patients with subfoveal myopic CNV, due to laser scarring of the fovea that can cause a sudden and permanent loss of visual acuity (Cohen *et al.*, 1996; Akinori and Thomas, 2000). There is no statistically significant improvement in visual acuity five-years after laser treatment of myopic CNV. In addition, lacquer cracks in Bruch's membrane and a high rate of CNV recurrence (31–72 per cent) have been reported after laser treatment of myopic CNV (Tano, 2002).

Again, PDT with Visudyne® is a recently approved laser treatment for subfoveal CNV in patients with pathologic myopia. According to interim 1 year clinical trial results in patients with pathologic myopia, there was a significant decrease in the size of the CNV and stabilization or improvement of vision compared with placebo controls (VIP Report No. 1). However, at the 24 month follow-up there was no statistically significant difference in visual acuity, with 51 per cent of placebo control eyes and 36 per cent of Verteporfin-treated eyes losing at least eight letters of visual acuity on a standard (EDTRS) eye-chart (VIP Report No. 3). However, PDT-treated eyes had a mean increase of 0.2 lines of vision compared to a mean loss of 1.6 lines of vision in placebo-control eyes at the 24 month follow-up (VIP Report No. 3). In summary, PDT improved vision at the 1 year follow-up and stabilized vision through the 2 year follow-up.

Photodynamic therapy has the advantage of not causing as much foveal scarring and sudden vision loss as reported with thermal laser photocoagulation (Tano, 2002). In fact, a major health care insurer (AETNA) has classified PDT therapy as medically necessary for the treatment of subfoveal CNV caused by age-related macular degeneration (AMD), ocular histoplasmosis and pathologic myopia (AETNA, Policy Bulletin No. 0594). The wide acceptance of PDT by regulatory authorities (Canada, Europe, Japan, United States and others) and medical reimbursement in the United States make this the *de facto* standard of care for subfoveal CNV in pathologic myopia. However, technical training and cost issues may limit the widespread clinical use of PDT to stabilize vision in early stages of myopic CNV.

There are several surgical treatment options for myopic CNV. The first procedure is surgical removal of CNV (Ruiz-Moreno and De La Vega, 2001; Tano, 2002). According to two reports, visual acuity improved in 39–41 per cent of eyes, was unchanged in 26–32 per cent of eyes and worsened in 27–35 per cent of eyes following surgical removal of CNV (Ruiz-Moreno and De La Vega, 2001; Tano, 2002). Another study showed no significant improvement in best-corrected visual acuity after surgical removal of CNV in pathological myopia (Ruiz-Moreno and De La Vega, 2001). Macular translocation is another surgical treatment for subfoveal CNV that involves moving the macula to a healthier part of the retinal pigment epithelium. There are at least two macular translocation procedures. The first is a limited macular translocation procedure and the other involves a 360° retinotomy (Tano, 2002). Postoperative retinal detachments have been reported in 24–29 per cent of eyes following macular translocation surgery (Tano, 2002). Many patients (32.5–70 per cent) also develop cystoid macular edema after macular translocation surgery (Terasaki *et al.*, 2003).

While PDT and the other therapeutic options may have utility in treating CNV in pathological myopia, not all patients respond and not all patients achieve a durable response. The use of VDAs either as an alternative to PDT or other therapies or as a rescue therapy for PDT failures is an option certainly worthy of clinical consideration.

18.4   Retinopathy of prematurity

Retinopathy of prematurity (ROP) is a major cause of vision loss and blindness in low-birth-weight premature infants (Mechoulam and Pierce, 2003). During normal retinal development, blood vessels grow from the optic disk to the ora serrata by week 36 of gestation and extend to the temporal ora serrata by 39–41 weeks of gestation (Recchia and Capone, 2004). At birth, premature infants have areas of relative hypoxia in the retina, which leads to uncontrolled growth or proliferation of the retinal vasculature. In one large clinical study, up to 20 per cent of premature infants developed retinopathy of prematurity if they weighed less than 1.5 kg at birth and stayed in the hospital for more than 28 days (Chiang *et al.*, 2004). This eye disease has many pathological characteristics in common with diabetic retinopathy (Mechoulam and Pierce, 2003). Exposing newborn rat pups to alternating high and low oxygen levels upregulates VEGF and other growth factors in the retina, which results in a pro-angiogenic phenotype and leads to proliferation of the retinal neovasculature (Zhang *et al.*, 2003). Anti-angiogenic compounds are reported to be active in a mouse model of ROP. For example, selective kinase inhibitors that block VEGF signaling also disrupt normal retinal vascular development in the eyes by slowing the growth of capillaries from the optic nerve (Ozaki *et al.*, 2000). Therefore, administration of anti-angiogenic compounds to premature infants could disrupt the normal growth of vascular networks in retina.

In contrast, administration of the vascular-disrupting agent CA4P blocks retinal neovascularization in a mouse model of ROP, but does not alter normal vascular development in the eye (Griggs *et al.*, 2002). Seven-day-old mice were placed in a chamber and exposed to 75 per cent oxygen atmosphere for five consecutive days and were then returned to normal atmospheric conditions. Untreated mice exposed to hyperbaric oxygen served as positive controls and untreated mice exposed to normal atmospheric conditions served as controls. Starting on postnatal day 12 (P12), hyperoxic mice (five per group) were given daily intraperitoneal injections of 0.78, 1.56, 3.125, 6.25 or 12 mg kg^{-1} CA4P. On P17, the mice were euthanized and eyes enucleated for histopathology. To quantify retinopathy, nuclei penetrating the inner limiting membrane were counted in representative ocular sections (Griggs *et al.*, 2002).

Histological analysis of retinas from the untreated hyperoxic mice revealed a substantial amount of neovascular growth. The aberrant vessels penetrated the vitreous in a manner that closely resembled retinopathy of prematurity. Retinas of normal mice had no cellular protrusions beyond the inner limiting membrane. Administration of 6.25 and 12 mg kg^{-1} CA4P exhibited toxicity in hyperoxic neonatal mice. Doses of 3.125 mg kg^{-1} CA4P or lower caused a dose-dependent inhibition of neovascularization with no apparent side, effects. Quantitative analysis revealed a dose-related decrease in the number of nuclei penetrating the inner limiting retinal membrane of mice treated with CA4P, when compared with the untreated hyperoxic controls. There were 34 per cent fewer lesions at

$0.78 \, \text{mg} \, \text{kg}^{-1} \, \text{day}^{-1}$ and 84 per cent fewer lesions at $3.125 \, \text{mg} \, \text{kg}^{-1} \, \text{day}^{-1}$ when CA4P was administered once daily by intraperitoneal injection. The volume of endothelial cells beneath the limiting retinal membrane, as determined using stereology, was similar in negative control and hyperoxic mice treated with $3.125 \, \text{mg} \, \text{kg}^{-1} \, \text{day}^{-1}$ of CA4P. In addition, retinal flat mounts were examined in treated and control mice that were perfused with fluorescently labeled dextrans. Positive control animals had reduced central perfusion and neovascular tufts in the retina. Treatment with CA4P increased retinal perfusion in hyperbaric oxygen-treated mice and completely blocked neovascular tuft formation at $3.125 \, \text{mg} \, \text{kg}^{-1} \, \text{day}^{-1}$. The investigators found no evidence of CA4P-induced microthrombus formation in the retina and they suggested that CA4 has direct anti-angiogenic properties. A more likely explanation is that the active metabolite of CA4P, combretastatin A-4, induces metaphase arrest and has direct cytotoxic activity (Kanthou *et al.*, 2004) against proliferating endothelial cells in the retina.

This published report suggests that CA4P may be active against retinopathy of prematurity in infants, without damaging the normal development of retinal vasculature (Griggs *et al.*, 2002). This finding by Griggs *et al.* suggests that the mechanism by which VDAs exert their effect is influenced by additional factors yet to be elucidated. It suggests that normal neovascular and aberrant neovascular growth are indeed influenced by similar yet distinguishable local parameters that allow the VDA to have a preferential effect.

Again, the use of VDAs in this setting, while yet untested clinically may be an attractive therapy to explore. Local or periocular administration of vascular disrupting agents would be preferred in order to ameliorate systemic effects of these agents on other organ systems (Tozer *et al.*, 1999), particularly in the pediatric setting.

18.5 Proliferative diabetic retinopathy

Diabetes affects nearly 50 million people in the United States (up to six per cent of the population) and is the leading cause of blindness in this population. Most diabetics develop retinopathy within 15 years of diagnosis and this disease tends to progresses from the background stage to the pre-proliferative and finally to the proliferative stage (Khan and Chakrabarti, 2003). The proliferative stage of diabetic retinopathy is characterized by retinal neovascularization, hemorrhages and blindness if left untreated. The most common treatments for diabetic retinopathy are laser photocoagulation and intraocular surgery (Grant *et al.*, 2004). Proliferative retinopathy is more common in type I (up to 50 per cent in 15 years) than type II diabetic patients (up to 10 per cent in 15 years) (Frank, 2004). The etiology of the disease is unknown, but poor control of blood glucose (i.e. hyperglycemia) is believed to induce hypoxia in the eye, which activates growth factors involved in angiogenesis (Khan and Chakrabarti,

2003; Grant *et al.*, 2004). Based on the proliferative retinopathy studies with CA4P (Griggs *et al.*, 2002), VDAs should induce acute vascular shutdown and could lead to regression of retinal neovasculature in diabetic retinopathy patients.

18.6 Pediatric hemangiomas

Hemangiomas are benign vascular tumors that are seen in one to three per cent of neonates and up to 10 per cent of infants by 1 year of age (Morelli, 1996; Dinehart, Kincannon and Geronemus, 2001). Hemangiomas are classified by the number, depth, size and location on the body (Dinehart, Kincannon and Geronemus, 2001). Most hemangiomas are superficial cutaneous lesions in the cervico-facial area that form bright red nodules or plaques (Dinehart, Kincannon and Geronemus, 2001). In addition, visceral or deep hemangiomas can develop in the liver, brain, lungs, intestines or tongue (Dinehart, Kincannon and Geronemus, 2001). There is a gradual reduction in size for 2–6 years after onset with nearly complete involution by 12 years of age (Frischer, 2004). Superficial dermal hemangiomas are not usually problematic unless they become ulcerated and infected (Dinehart, Kincannon and Geronemus, 2001). The pathogenesis of hemangiomas is not fully understood, but reportedly involves an unusual vascular phenotype (Bruchner and Frieden, 2003) and altered regulation of the vascular endothelial growth factors and angiopoietins (Frischer *et al.*, 2004). Common treatment paradigms include surgical removal, laser treatment, cryosurgery and systemic treatment with glucocorticoids or the angiogenesis inhibitor interferon-alpha-2b (Dinehart, Kincannon and Geronemus, 2001). These two pharmaceutical treatments have unacceptable toxicity, such as neurological side-effects, neutropenia and fever with interferon-alpha (Powell, 1999; Dinehart, Kincannon and Geronemus, 2001) and gastrointestinal effects, insomnia and behavior changes in infants given systemic glucocorticoids (George *et al.*, 2004).

Drugs that target proliferation of the vascular endothelium represent an attractive target for pharmaceutical intervention in this disease. For example, intra-lesional injection of bleomycin is reported to cause regression of hemangiomas and congenital vascular malformations, ostensibly through inhibition of angiogenesis (Muir, 2004). CA4P and other VDAs should theoretically cause acute vascular shutdown in hemangiomas, just as it does in tumors (Siemann, Chaplin and Horsman, 2004). However, CA4P may also target hemangiomas through a second mechanism of action, such as direct inhibition of endothelial cell proliferation. CA4P has been shown to cause metaphase arrest and non-caspase-mediated cell death in cultured endothelial cells (Kanthou *et al.*, 2004). The mechanism of CA4P-induced endothelial cell death is believed to involve prolonged metaphase arrest (Kanthou *et al.*, 2004) and therefore VDAs may attenuate the proliferative phase of hemangiomas.

There is precedence in the literature for the use of vascular-disrupting agents in patients with rare and aggressive vascular tumors (hemangiomas), such as Kasabach–Merritt syndrome (KMS) (Wananukul, Nuchprayoon and Seksaru, 2003). In one clinical report, ten infants were treated with oral corticosteroids and dipyridamole and steroid-resistant cases were followed up with interferon-alpha-2b. One interferon-alpha-2b-resistant patient responded to weekly treatment with vincristine and another had vascular tumor regression following treatment with vinblastine (Wananukul, Nuchprayoon and Seksaru, 2003). Based on the limited clinical use of vascular-disrupting agents in KMS, and the anti-proliferative effects of CA4P on endothelial cells, topical, local injection or systemic administration of VDAs could be effective in the treatment of pediatric hemangiomas.

18.7 Arthritis

Rheumatoid arthritis (RA) is a chronic inflammatory condition that causes significant clinical morbidity and mortality (Wolfe *et al.*, 1994). RA is characterized by inflammatory synovitis of the peripheral joints, pannus formation and destruction of cartilage, bone and joints (Shankar and Handa, 2004). Proliferation of synovial fibroblasts, increased synovial vascularity and infiltration of inflammatory cells are also observed in RA. The subsequent release of pro-inflammatory cytokines, such as tumor necrosis factor alpha (TNF-∞), IL-1 and IL-6 stimulates synovial fibroblasts, osteoclasts and chrondrocytes to produce tissue-damaging metalloproteinases (Shankar and Handa, 2004). Treatment of RA has evolved from aspirin and methotrexate to mechanism-based inactivation of IL-1 (Anakinra) or TNF-alpha (Etanercept, Infliximab, Adalimumab). A detailed discussion of cytokine modulators used in the treatment of RA is presented elsewhere (Shankar and Handa, 2004).

There is growing evidence that angiogenesis plays a critical role in the pathogenesis of rheumatory arthritis (Colville-Nash and Scott, 1992; Firestein, 1999; Uchida *et al.*, 2000; Taylor, 2002; DeBusk *et al.*, 2003). The angiogenesis inhibitor AGM-1470 prevents collagen-induced arthritis in rats as determined by clinical, radiographic and histological measures. In fact, neovascularization and pannus formation were absent from the ankle joints of rats treated with collagen on day 1 and AGM-1470 beginning on day 2 (Peacock *et al.*, 1992). Synovial fibroblasts constitutively expressed angiogenic factors, such as angiopoietin 1 (Ang-1, agonist of Tie2 receptor tyrosine kinase) and angiopoietin 2 (Ang-2, Antagonist of Tie2). Tie-2 is an endothelial-specific tyrosine kinase that is involved in embryonic vascular development (DeBusk *et al.*, 2003). Tie-1 and Tie-2 receptors are reportedly up-regulated in synovial tissue of RA patients that underwent joint replacement surgery (Uchida *et al.*, 2000). Up-regulation of Ang-1 is reported to increase Tie-2 signaling in the synovium of RA patients and tumor necrosis factor alpha has been shown to induce Tie-2 and Ang-1 expression in cultured synoviocytes (DeBusk *et al.*, 2003). Therefore, inflammation is believed to alter the regulation of angiogenic factors and ostensibly induces pathological RA angiogenesis (Firestein, 1999) through modulation of Tie-2 signaling (Uchida *et al.*, 2000; DeBusk *et al.*, 2003; Fearon *et al.*, 2003). Endothelial cells in the rheumatoid synovium stain positive for vascular endothelial growth factor and synovial and plasma levels of VEGF are correlated with clinical progression and severity of RA (Taylor, 2002; Clavel *et al.*, 2003).

Up-regulation of angiogenesis in the inflammatory synoviocytes gives the RA synovium an unusual vascular phenotype that has been compared with the microenvironment of tumor cells. For example, synoviocytes have increased metabolic activity and have somatic mutations in regulatory genes such as H-ras and p53 (Firestein, 1999). The synovial fluid is hypoxic and acidotic in RA patients and the microvasculature of the knee is much deeper and less densely arranged in the rheumatory synovium compared with the normal knee joint. In addition, the blood volume is much lower in the rheumatory synovium (1.2 per cent) when compared with controls (2.9 per cent), which suggests there is impaired oxygen transfer in RA (Stevens *et al.*, 1991). Vascular corrosion casts have shown a marked increase in blood volume and extensively interconnected neovascular arrays that project into the inflammatory synovium of rats with CIA.

The potential use of vascular-disrupting agents, such as combretastatin A-4 phosphate, to disrupt the neovasculature of the inflammatory synovium is based upon the increased metabolic activity of synoviocytes, hypoxia and as a result the growth of aberrant neovascularization. There is one report that a targeted pro-apoptotic peptide (RGD-4C-$_D$(KLAKLAK)$_2$ induces apoptosis in endothelial cells of mice with collagen-induced arthritis (CIA). Intravenous administration of this targeted pro-apoptotic peptide caused regression of arthritis in mice with established CIA (Gerlag, 2001). It is also interesting to note that Taxol is reported to block CIA in mice and rats, presumably due to its effect on the cytoskeleton of synoviocytes (Brahn, Tang and Banquerigo, 1994; Arsenault *et al.*, 1998).

18.8 Psoriasis

Psoriasis is a chronic inflammatory condition that is characterized by 'dilated and tortuous blood vessels' and edema in the papillary dermis, epidermal hyperplasia, perivascular infiltrates of lymphocytes and histiocytes in the epidermis and the formation of pin-sized macules, papules and then dermal plaques (Ragaz and Ackerman, 1979). It is interesting to note that prominent and dilated capillaries in the papillary dermis loops (Braverman and Sibley, 1985) is one of the earliest pathological changes in psoriasis and this lesion is the last one to resolve

(Ragaz and Ackerman, 1979). Therefore, an aberrant vascular phenotype is one of the hallmark features of psoriasis. While topical steroids and oral methotrexate can partially reverse psoriatic changes in the epidermis, neither treatment reversed the abnormal dermal microvasculature as indicated by prominent capillary loops in the papillary dermis (Braverman and Sibley, 1985). In the opinion of the investigators, relapses are possible after discontinuation of treatment with steroids (Braverman and Sibley, 1985).

The presence of an abnormal vascular phenotype is bolstered by several mechanistic studies that indicate angiogenesis is involved in the pathogenesis of psoriasis (Kuroda *et al.*, 2001; Xia *et al.*, 2003; Detmar, 2004). In fact, mRNA for VEGF and basic fibroblast growth factor (bFGF), angiopoietin-1, angiopoietin-2, and tyrosine receptor kinase-2 (Tie-2) are greatly up-regulated in psoriatic (involved) skin compared to uninvolved or healthy skin from biopsies of patients with chronic plaque-type psoriasis (Kuroda *et al.*, 2001). In addition, detectable plasma levels of VEGF and genetic VEGF polymorphisms have been reported in patients that develop severe psoriasis between 20 and 40 years of age (Young *et al.*, 2004). There is also supportive evidence from transgenic mice that overexpress VEGF in the skin (K14-VEGF mice, Xia *et al.*, 2003). These mice develop psoriatic-like phenotype with skin lesions, inflammatory infiltrates, along with vascular and epidermal changes that resemble human psoriasis (Xia *et al.*, 2003). There was partial reversal of the histopathology and immunologic changes in six-month-old K14-VEGF transgenic mice that were given subcutaneous injections of a VEGF trap once every 3 days for 12 days (Xia *et al.*, 2003). There are several other published reports that anti-angiogenesis drugs could be effective in the treatment of psoriasis (Braverman and Sibley, 1982; Dupont *et al.*, 1998; Xia *et al.*, 2003).

Vascular-disrupting agents could ostensibly induce regression of the abnormal vascular phenotype (Ragaz and Ackerman, 1979; Braverman and Sibley, 1982) and be used in the treatment of psoriasis. In addition to the abnormal vascular phenotype, vascular proliferation is reportedly required for epidermal hyperplasia (Braverman and Sibley, 1982). Intradermal injection of vinca alkaloids (vincristine and vinblastine) have been shown to induce metaphase in the human psoriatic epidermis (Ralfs *et al.*, 1981). The optimal dose was one microgram of vincristine given intradermally at the periphery of the psoriatic plaque. It is interesting to note that these vascular-disrupting agents induced metaphase arrest for a minimum of 4 hours and this was followed by the death of psoriatic cells in G2 arrest (Ralfs *et al.*, 1981). Therefore, the anti-mitotic and direct cytotoxic properties of CA4P against endothelial cells (Kanthou *et al.*, 2004) could confer activity against proliferating cells in the epidermis and ameliorate or block epidermal hyperplasia. In fact, there are several published reports that topical or systemic administration of vinca alkaloids or colchicine may be effective in the treatment of psoriasis (Kaidbey, Petrozzi and Kligman, 1975; Wahba and Cohen, 1980).

18.9   Conclusions

Because of the pervasive nature of abnormally elicited neovascular development in a variety of pathologic conditions, only a few of which were discussed here, vascular disrupting agents may represent a new therapeutic strategy or component to existing treatments. Thus theoretically, where there is pathologically induced abnormal neovasculature, there may be a use for VDAs. While systemic delivery of VDAs is in large part preferable in the oncology setting to potentially arrest and destroy undetected neoplastic deposits, many of the disease conditions that we can contemplate possessing an underlying neovascular component may benefit more from localized dug administration. The benefit may be derived both from an efficacy standpoint by gaining better dosage and exposure control, as well as limiting or eliminating adverse systemic effects. Thus one can envision the use and utility of VDAs expanding further into these and other clinical indications as drug delivery technology, techniques and methodologies continue to be developed and refined.

References

AETNA. (2003). Visudyne (Verteporfin) photodynamic therapy. *Clinical Policy Bulletin* 0594 (http://www.aetna.com/cpb/data/CPBA0594.html).

Aiello, L.P., Pierce, E.A., Foley, E.D., Takagi, H., Chen, H., Riddle, L., Ferrara, N., King, G.L. and Smith, L.E.H. (1995). Suppression of retinal neovascularization in vivo by inhibition of vascular endothelial growth factor (VEGF) using soluble VEGF-receptor chimeric proteins. *Proc Natl Acad Sci* 92, 10457–10461.

Akinori, U. and Thomas, M.A. (2000). Subretinal surgery for choroidal neovascularization in patients with high myopia. *Arch Ophthalmol* 118 (3), 344–350.

Arsenault, A.L., Lhotak, S., Hunter, W.L., Banquerigo, M.L.C. and Brahn, E. (1998). Taxol involution of collagen-induced arthritis: ultrastructural correlation with the inhibition of synovitis and neovascularization. *Clin Immunol Immunopathol* 86 (3), 280–289.

Baba, T., Ohno-Matsui, K., Yoshida, T., Yasuzumi, K., Futagami, S., Tokoro, T. and Mochizuki, M. (2002). Optical Coherence Tomography of Choroidal Neovascularization in High Myopia. *Acta Ophthalmol Scand* 80, 82–87.

Blacharski, P.A. (1988). Pathological Progressive Myopia. In: *Retinal Dystrophies and Degenerations*. Raven, New York.

Brahn, E., Tang, C. and Banquerigo, M.L. (1994). Regression of Collagen-Induced Arthritis with Taxol, A Microtubule Stabilizer. *Athritis Rheumatism* 37 (6), 839–845.

Brancato, R., Pece, A., Avanza, P. and Radizzani, E. (1990). Photocoagulation Scar Expansion after Laser Therapy in Degenerative Myopia. *Retina* 10 (4), 239–243.

Braverman, I.M. and Sibley, J. (1982). Role of the Microcirculation in the Treatment and Pathogenesis of Psoriasis. *J Invest Dermatol* 78 (1), 12–17.

Braverman, I.M. and Sibley, J. (1985). The Response of Psoriatic Epidermis and Microvessels to Treatment with Topical Steroids and Oral Methotrexate. *J Invest Dermatol* 85 (6), 584–586.

Bruchner, A.L. and Frieden, I.J. (2003). Hemangiomas of Infancy. *J Am Acad Dermatol* 48 (4), 477–493.

Campochiaro, P.A. and Hackett, S.F. (2003). Ocular Neovascularization: A Valuable Model System. *Oncogene* **22**, 6537–6548.

Campochiaro, P.A., Soloway, P., Ryan, S.J. and Miller, J.W. (1999). The Pathogenesis of Choroidal Neovascularization in Patients with Age-Related Macular Degeneration. *Molec Vis* **5**, 34.

Carmeliet, P. and Jain, R.K. (2000). Angiogenesis in Cancer and Other Diseases. *Nature* **407**, 249–257.

Chaplin, D.J. and Hill, S.A. (2002). The Development of Combretastatin A4 Phosphate as a Vascular Disrupting Agent. *Int J Radiat Oncol Biol Phys* **54** (5), 1491–1496.

Chiang, M.F., Aarons, R.R., Flynn, J.T. and Starren, J.B. (2004). Incidence of Retinopathy of Prematurity from 1996 to 2000: Analysis of a Comprehensive New York State Patient Database. *Ophthalmology* **111** (7), 1317–1325.

Ciulla, T.A., Criswell, M.H., Danis, R.P., Williams, J.I., McLane, M.P. and Holroyd, K.J. (2003). Squalamine Lactate Reduces Choroidal Neovascularization in a Laser-Injury Model in the Rat. *Retina* **23** (6), 808–814.

Cohen, S.Y., Larouche, A., Leuguen, Y., Soubrane, G. and Coscas, G.J. (1996). Etiology of Choroidal Neovascularization in Young Patients. *Ophthalmology* **103** (8), 1241–1244.

DeBusk, L.M., Chen, Y., Nishishita, T., Chen, J., Thomas, J.W. and Lin, P.C. (2003). Tie2 Receptor Tyrosine Kinase, a Major Mediator of Tumor Necrosis Factor ∝-Induced Angiogenesis in Rheumatoid Arthritis. *Arthritis Rheumatism* **48** (9), 2461–2471.

Detmar, M. (2004). Evidence for Vascular Endothelial Growth Factor (VEGF) as a Modifier Gene in Psoriasis. *J Invest Dermatol* **122** (1), xiv–xv.

Dinehart, S.M., Kincannon, J. and Geronemus, R. (2001). Hemangiomas: Evaluation and Treatment. *Dermatol Surg* **27** (5), 475–485.

Do, D.V., Bressler, N.M. and Bressler, S.B. (2004). Large Submacular Hemorrhages After Verteporfin Therapy. *Am J Opthalmol* **137**, 558–560.

Fearon, U., Griosios, K., Fraser, A., Reece, R., Emery, P., Jones, P.F. and Veale, D.J. (2003). Angiopoietins, Growth Factors and Vascular Morphology in Early Arthritis. *J Rheumatol* **30** (2), 260–268.

Firestein, G.S. (1999). Starving the Synovium: Angiogenesis and Inflammation in Rheumatoid Arthitis. *J Clin Investig* **103** (1), 3–4.

Folkman, J. (1993). Diagnostic and Therapeutic Applications of Angiogenesis Research. *C.R. Acad Sci Paris* **316**, 914–918.

Frank, R.N. (2004). Medical Progress: Diabetic Retinopathy. *N Engl J Med* **350** (1), 48–58.

George, M.E., Sharma, V., Jacobson, J., Simon, S. and Nopper, A.J. (2004). Adverse Effects of Systemic Glucocorticosteroid Therapy in Infants with Hemangiomas. *Arch Dermatol* **140** (8), 963–969.

Gragoudas, E.S., Adamis, A.P., Cunningham, E.T. Jr., Feinsod, M. and Guyer, D.R. (2004). Pegaptanib for neovascular age-related macular degeneration. *N Engl J Med* **351** (27), 2805–2816.

Grant, M.B., Afzal, A., Spoerri, P., Pan, H., Shaw, L.C. and Mames, R.N. (2004). The role of growth factors in the pathogenesis of diabetic retinopathy. *Expert Opin Investig Drugs* **13** (10), 1275–1293.

Griggs, J., Skepper, J. N., Smith, G.A., Brindle, K.M., Metcalfe, J.C. and Hesketh, R. (2002). Inhibition of Proliferative Retinopathy by the Anti-Vascular Agent Combretastatin A-4. *Am J Path* **160** (3), 1097–1103.

Grossniklaus, H.E. and Green, W.R. (1998). Histopathologic and Ultrastructural Findings of Surgically Excised Choroidal Neovascularization. Submacular Surgery Trials Research Group. *Arch Ophthalmol* **116** (6), 745–749.

Heyman, D. (2003). Eye Ailment Cure Sighted. *Calgary Herald*, 31ˢᵗ Dec, Section B6.

Kaidbey, K.H., Petrozzi, J.W. and Kligman, A.M. (1975). Topical Colchicine Therapy for Recalcitrant Psoriasis. *Arch Dermatol* **111** (1), 33–36.

Kanthou, C., Greco, O., Stratford, A., Cook, I., Knight, R., Benzakour, O. and Tozer, G. (2004). The Tubulin-Binding Agent Combretastatin A-4-Phosphate Arrests Endothelial Cells in Mitosis and Induces Mitotic Cell Death. *Am J Pathol* **165**, 1401–1411.

Kerbel, R.S. (2000). Tumor Angiogenesis: Past, Present and the Near Future. *Carcinogenesis* **21** (3), 505–515.

Khan, Z.A. and Chakrabarti, S. (2003). Growth Factors in Proliferative Diabetic Retinopathy. *Experimental Diab Res* **4**, 287–301.

Kojima, A., Ohno-Matsui, K., Teramukai, S., Yoshida, T., Ishihara, Y., Kobayashi, K., Shimada, N., Yasuzumi, K., Futagami, S., Tokorom T. and Mochizuki, M. (2003). Factors associated with the development of chorioretinal atrophy around choroidal neovascularization in pathologic myopia. *Graefes Arch Clin Exp Ophthalmol*, 23 Nov [Epub ahead of print].

Kojima, A., Ohno-Matsui, K., Teramukai, S., Yoshida, T., Ishihara, Y., Kobayashi, K., Shimada, N., Yasuzumi, K., Futagami, S., Tokoro, T. and Mochizuki, M. (2004). Factors Associated with the Development of Corioretinal Arophy Around Choroidal Novascularization in Pathologic Myopia. *Graefes Arch Clin Exp Ophthalmol* **242** (2), 114–119.

Kuroda, K., Sapadin, A., Shoji, T., Fleischmajer, R. and Lebwohl, M. (2001). Altered Expression of Angiopoietins and Tie2 Endothelium Receptor in Psoriasis. *J Invest Dermatol* **116**, 713–720.

Morelli, J.G. (1996). Hemangiomas and Vascular Malformations. *Pediatric Annals* **25**, 91–96.

Muir, T., Kirsten, M., Fourie, P., Dippenaar, N. and Ionescu, G. (2004). Intralesional Bleomycin Injection (IBI) Treatment for Hemangiomas and Congenital Vascular Malformations. *Pediatr Surg Int* **19** (12), 766–773.

Nambu, H., Nambu, R., Melia, M. and Campochiaro, P.A. (2003). Combretastatin A-4 Phosphate Supresses Development and Induces Regression of Choroidal Neovascularization. *Invest Ophthalmol Vis Sci* **44** (8), 3650–3655.

Ohno-Matsui, K., Yoshida, T., Futagami, S., Yasuzumi, K., Shimada, N., Kojima, A., Tokoro, T. and Mochizuki, M. (2003). Patchy Atrophy and Lacquer Cracks Predispose to the Develelopment of Choroidal Neovascularization in Pathologic Myopia. *Br J Ophthalmol* **87**, 570–573.

Otani, A., Takagi, H., Oh, H., Koyama, S., Matsumura, M. and Honda, Y. (1999). Expressions of Angiopoietins and Tie2 in Human Choroidal Neovascular Membranes. *Invest Ophthalmol Vis Sci* **40** (9), 1912–1920.

Ozaki, H., Seo, M-N, Ozaki, K., Yamada, H., Yamada, E., Okamoto, N., Hofmann, F., Wood, J.M. and Campochiaro, P.A. (2000). Blockade of Vascular Endothelial Cell Growth Factor Receptor Signaling is Sufficient to Completely Prevent Retinal Neovascularization. *Am J Pathol* **156**, 697–707.

Powell, J. (1999). Update on Hemangiomas and Vascular Malformations. *Curr Opin Pediatr* **11** (5), 457–463.

Ragaz, A. and Ackerman, A.B. (1979). Evolution, Maturation, and Regression of Lesions of Psoriasis. New Observations and Correlation of Clinical and Histological Findings. *Am J Dermatopathol* **1** (3), 199–214.

Ralfs, I., Dawber, R., Ryan, T., Duffill, M. and Wright, N.A. (1981). The Kinetics of Metaphase Arrest in Human Psoriatic Epidermis: An Examination of Optimal Experimental Conditions for Determining the Birth Rate. *Br J Dermatol* **104** (3), 231–241.

Recchia, F.M. and Capone, A. Jr. Continuing Medical Education: Contemporary Understanding and Management of Retinopathy of Prematurity. *Retina* 24 (2), 283–292.

Ruiz-Moreno, J.M. and De La Vega, C. (2001). Surgical Removal of Subfoveal Choroidal Neovascularization in Highly Myopic Patients. *Br J Ophthalmol* 85, 1041–1043.

Scott, B.B., Zarantin, P.F., Colombo, A., Hansbury, M.J., Winkler, J.D. and Jackson, J.R. (2000). Constitutive Expression of Angiopoietin-1 and -2 and Modulation of their Expression by Inflammatory Cytokines in Rheumatoid Arthritis Synovial Fibroblasts. *J Rheumatol* 29 (2), 230–239.

Shahidi, M., Blair, N.P., Giesler, J. and Pulido, J.S. (2002). Retinal Topography and Thickness Mapping in Atrophic Age-Related Macular Degeneration. *Br J Ophthalmol* 86, 623–626.

Shankar, S. and Handa, R. (2004). Biological Agents in Rheumatoid Arthitis. *J Postgrad Med* 50 (4), 293–299.

Siemann, D.W., Chaplin, D.J. and Horsman, M.R. (2004). Vascular-Disrupting Therapies for Treatment of Malignant Disease. *Cancer* 100, 2491–2499.

Sivakumar, B., Harry, L.E. and Paleolog, E.M. (2004). Modulating Angiogenesis: More vs Less. *JAMA* 292 (8), 972–977.

Soubrane, G. and Bressler, N.M. (2001). Treatment of Subfoveal Choroidal Neovascularisation in Age-Related Macular Degeneration: Focus on Clinical Application of Verteporfin Photodynamic Therapy. *Br J Ophthalmol* 85, 483–495.

Tabandeh, H., Flynn, H.W., Scott, I.U., Lewis, M.L., Rosenfeld, P.J., Rodriguez, F., Rodriguez, A., Singerman, L.J. and Schiffman, J. (1999). Visual Acuity Outcomes of Patients 50 Years of Age and Older with High Myopia and Untreated Choroidal Neovascularization. *Ophthalmology* 106, 2063–2067.

Tano, Y. (2002). Pathological Myopia: Where are we now? *Am J Ophthalmol* 134 (5), 645–660.

TAP Study Group. (1999). Photodynamic Therapy of Subfoveal Choroidal Neovascularization in Age-related Macular Degeneration with Verteporfin: One-Year Results of 2 Randomized Clinical Trials – TAP Report No. 1. *Arch Ophthalmol* 117, 1329–1345.

TAP Study Group. (2001). Photodynamic Therapy of Subfoveal Choroidal Neovascularization in Age-related Macular Degeneration with Verteporfin: Two-Year Results of 2 Randomized Clinical Trials – TAP Report No. 2. *Arch Ophthalmol* 119, 198–207.

Taylor, P.C. (2002). VEGF and Imaging of Vessels in Rheumatoid Arthitis. *Arthritis Res* 4 (Suppl. 3), S99–S107.

Terasaki, H., Ishikawa, K., Suzuki, T., Nakamura, M., Miyake, K. and Miyake, Y. (2003). Morphological and Angiographic Assessment of the Macular after Macular Translocation Surgery with 360° Retinotomy. *Ophthalmology* 110, 2403–2408.

Tozer, G.M., Prise, V.E., Wilson, J., Cemazar, M., Shan, S., Dewhirst, M.W., Barber, P.R., Vojnovic, B. and Chaplin, D.J. (2001). Mechanisms Associated with Tumor Vascular Shut-Down Induced by Combretastatin A-4 Phosphate: Intravital Microscopy and Measurement of Vascular Permeability. *Cancer Res* 61, 6413–6422.

Tozer, G.M., Prise, V.E., Wilson, J., Locke, R.J., Vojnovic, B., Stratford, M.R.L., Dennis, M.F. and Chaplin, D.J. (1999). Combretastatin A-4 Phosphate as a Tumor Vascular-Disrupting Agent: Early Effects in Tumors and Normal Tissues. *Cancer Res* 59, 1626–1634.

Uchida, T., Nakashima, M., Hirota, Y., Miyazaki, Y., Tsukazaki, T. and Shindo, H. (2000). Immunohistochemical Localisation of Protein Tyrosine Kinase Receptors Tie-1 and Tie-2 in Synovial Tissue of Rheumatoid Arthritis: Correlation with Angiogenesis and Synovial Proliferation. *Ann Rheum Dis* 59, 607–614.

VIP Study Group. (2001). Photodynamic Therapy of Subfoveal Choroidal Neovascularization in Pathologic Myopia with Verteporfin: 1-year Results of a Randomized Clinical Trial – VIP Report No. 1. *Ophthalmology* **108**, 841–852.

VIP Study Group. (2003). Verteporfin Therapy of Subfoveal Choroidal Neovascularization in Pathologic Myopia: 2-year Results of a Randomized Clinical Trial – VIP Report No. 3. *Ophthalmology* **110** (4), 667–673.

Wahba, A. and Cohen, H. (1980). Therapeutic Trials with Oral Colchicine in Psoriasis. *Acta Derm Venereol* **60** (6), 515–520.

Wahl, M.L., Moser, T.L. and Pizzo, S.V. (2004). Angiostatin and Anti-Angiogenic Therapy in Human Disease. *Recent Prog Horm Res* **59**, 73–104.

Wananukul, S., Nuchprayoon, I. and Seksaru, P. (2003). Treatment of Kasabach–Merritt Syndrome: a Step-Wise Regimen of Prednisolone, Dipyridamole and Interferon. *Int J Dermatol* **42** (9), 741–748.

Wolfe, F., Mitchell, D.M., Sibley, J.T., Fries, J.F., Bloch, D.A., Williams, C.A., Spitz, P.W., Haga, M., Kleinheksel, S.M. and Cathey, M.A. (1994). The mortality of rheumatoid arthritis. *Arthritis Rheum* **37** (4), 481–494.

Xia, Y-P, Li, B., Hylton, D., Detmar, M., Yancopoulos, G.D. and Rudge, J.S. (2003). Transgenic Delivery of VEGF to Mouse Skin Leads to an Inflammatory Condition Resembling Human Psoriasis. *Blood* **102** (1), 161–168.

Yoshida, T., Ohno-Matsui, K., Ohtakem Y., Takashima, T., Futagami, S., Baba, T., Yasuzumi, K., Tokoro, T. and Mochizuki, M. (2002). Long-term Visual Prognosis of Choroidal Neovascularization in High Myopia: A Comparison Between Age Groups. *Ophthalmology* **109**, 712–719.

Yoshida, T., Ohno-Matsui, K., Yasuzumi, K., Kojima, A., Shimada, N., Futagami, S., Tokoro, T. and Mochizuki, M. (2003). Myopic Choroidal Neovascularization: A 10-year follow-up. *Ophthalmology* **110** (7), 1297–1305.

Young, S.L. and Chaplin, D.J. (2004). Combretastatin A4 Phosphate: Background and Current Clinical Status. *Exp Opin Investig Drugs* **13** (9), 1171–1182.

Young, H.S., Summers, A.M., Bhushan, M., Brenchley, P.E. and Griffiths, C.E. (2004). Single Nucleotide Polymorphisms of Vascular Endothelial Growth Factor in Psoriasis of Early Onset. *J Invest Dermatol* **122** (1), 209–215.

Zhang, W., Ito, Y., Berlin, E., Roberts, R. and Berkowitz, B.A. (2003). Role of Hypoxia During Normal Retinal Vessel Development and in Experimental Retinopathy of Prematurity. *Invest Ophthalmol Vis Sci* **44**, 3119–3123.

Index

Vascular-targeted Therapies in Oncology   Edited by Dietmar W. Siemann
© 2006 John Wiley & Sons, Ltd.

Index compiled by Geoffrey Jones